THIRD EDITION

The Doctor of Nursing Practice Project

A Framework for Success

Katherine Moran, DNP, RN, CDE, FAADE
Kirkhof College of Nursing
Grand Valley State University
Doctor of Nursing Practice Consultants
Grand Rapids, Michigan

Rosanne Burson, DNP, ACNS-BC, CNE, CDE, FAADE
McAuley School of Nursing
University of Detroit Mercy
Doctor of Nursing Practice Consultants
Detroit, Michigan

Dianne Conrad, DNP, RN, FNP-BC, CDE, FNAP
Kirkhof College of Nursing
Grand Valley State University
Doctor of Nursing Practice Consultants
Grand Rapids, Michigan
Cadillac Family Physicians, PC
Cadillac, Michigan

JONES & BARTLETT
LEARNING

World Headquarters
Jones & Bartlett Learning
5 Wall Street
Burlington, MA 01803
978-443-5000
info@jblearning.com
www.jblearning.com

Jones & Bartlett Learning books and products are available through most bookstores and online booksellers. To contact Jones & Bartlett Learning directly, call 800-832-0034, fax 978-443-8000, or visit our website, www.jblearning.com.

Substantial discounts on bulk quantities of Jones & Bartlett Learning publications are available to corporations, professional associations, and other qualified organizations. For details and specific discount information, contact the special sales department at Jones & Bartlett Learning via the above contact information or send an email to specialsales@jblearning.com.

16434-3

Production Credits

VP, Product Management: Amanda Martin
Director of Product Management: Matthew Kane
Product Manager: Tina Chen
Product Assistant: Anna-Maria Forger
Director of Project Management: Jenny L. Corriveau
Director, Relationship Management: Carolyn Rogers Pershouse
Project Manager: Kristen Rogers
Project Specialist: Kelly Sylvester
Project Specialist, Navigate: Kelly Sylvester
Senior Marketing Manager: Jennifer Scherzay
Product Fulfillment Manager: Wendy Kilborn
Composition: S4Carlisle Publishing Services
Cover Design: Michael O'Donnell
Director, Content Services and Licensing: Joanna Gallant
Rights & Media Manager: Shannon Sheehan
Relationship Manager: Merideth Tumasz
Media Development Editor: Troy Liston
Rights & Media Specialist: John Rusk
Cover Image (Title Page): © Rabbit Photo/Shutterstock
Printing and Binding: McNaughton & Gunn
Cover Printing: McNaughton & Gunn

Library of Congress Cataloging-in-Publication Data
Names: Moran, Katherine J., 1959- editor. | Burson, Rosanne, 1957- editor. |
  Conrad, Dianne, 1956- editor.
Title: The doctor of nursing practice project : a framework for success /
  edited by Katherine J. Moran, Rosanne Burson, Dianne Conrad.
Other titles: Preceded by (work): Doctor of nursing scholarly project.
Description: Third edition. | Burlington, MA : Jones & Bartlett Learning,
  [2020] | Preceded by: The doctor of nursing practice scholarly project /
  edited by Katherine Moran, Rosanne Burson, Dianne Conrad. 2017. | Includes
  bibliographical references and index.
Identifiers: LCCN 2018053652 | ISBN 9781284156959 (paperback)
Subjects: | MESH: Advanced Practice Nursing--education | Education, Nursing,
  Graduate | Nursing Research--education | Program Development | United States
Classification: LCC RT75 | NLM WY 18.5 | DDC 610.73071/1--dc23
LC record available at https://lccn.loc.gov/2018053652

6048

Printed in the United States of America
22 21 20 19   10 9 8 7 6 5 4 3 2 1

Brief Contents

SECTION III   Doctor of Nursing Practice Outcomes   375

Contents

SECTION II　The DNP Project　95

Chapter 5　The Phenomenon of Interest 97

Chapter 6　Developing the DNP Project 121

Chapter 7　Aligning Design, Method, and Evaluation with the Clinical Question . . . 155

Chapter 8　Interprofessional and Intraprofessional Collaboration in the DNP Project 187

Acknowledgments

Our heartfelt thanks go out to the DNP faculty at Madonna University who were there when we started our DNP journey. Your vision, encouragement, and continued support provided us with a wonderful foundation for which we are most grateful. We extend our gratitude to Amanda J. Martin, Jones & Bartlett Learning Executive Editor, for recognizing the value of this project; Rebecca Stephenson, Associate Acquisitions Editor, Nursing; and Anna-Maria Forger, Product Assistant, Nursing & Medicine Division for guidance in completing this project. Finally, we thank Lisa Merriman for enriching our book with her artistic contribution and Evelyn Clingerman, PhD, CNE, RN, FNAP for support and contributions to our scholarship team.

Contributors

Rosanne Burson, DNP, ACNS-BC, CNE, CDE, FAADE
Associate Professor
DNP Program Coordinator
McAuley School of Nursing
University of Detroit Mercy
Doctor of Nursing Practice
    Consultants
Detroit, Michigan

David G. Campbell-O'Dell, DNP, ARNP, FNP-BC
Doctors of Nursing Practice, Inc.
Key West, Florida

Evelyn Clingerman, PhD, CNE, RN, FNAP
Executive Director
The Bonnie Wesorick Center for
    Health Care Transformation
Kirkhof College of Nursing
Grand Valley State University
Grand Rapids, Michigan

Dianne Conrad, DNP, RN, FNP-BC, CDE, FNAP
Associate Professor
Kirkhof College of Nursing
Grand Valley State University
Doctor of Nursing Practice
    Consultants
Grand Rapids, Michigan
Cadillac Family Physicians, PC
Cadillac, Michigan

Shannon Reedy Idzik, DNP, CRNP, FAANP
Associate Professor
Associate Dean, Doctor of Nursing
    Practice Program
University of Maryland School of
    Nursing
Baltimore, Maryland

Karen Kesten, DNP, APRN, CCRN-K, CCNS, CNE, FAAN
Associate Professor
Director of DNP Scholarly Projects
The George Washington University
    School of Nursing
Washington, District of Columbia
Immediate Past Chair, Board of
    Directors,
Certification Corporation, American
    Association of Critical Care Nurses
Aliso Viejo, California

Katherine Moran, DNP, RN, CDE, FAADE
Associate Dean, Graduate Nursing
    Programs
Associate Professor
Kirkhof College of Nursing
Grand Valley State University
Doctor of Nursing Practice
    Consultants
Grand Rapids, Michigan

Patricia Rouen, PhD, FNP-BC
Professor
McAuley School of Nursing
College of Health Professions
University of Detroit Mercy
Detroit, Michigan

Melissa Stec, DNP, APRN, CNM, FACNM, FAAN
Professor
Associate Dean for Evaluation and
    Educational Innovation
SUNY Downstate College of Nursing
Brooklyn, New York

Marisa L. Wilson, DNSc, MHSc, RN-BC, CPHIMS
Associate Professor
University of Alabama at Birmingham
Birmingham, Alabama

Foreword

Lisa Chism, DNP, GNP, BC, NCMP, FAANP

In 1999, the Institute of Medicine (IOM) published a report, *To Err Is Human: Building a Safer Health System.* This report summarized the errors made in health care and estimated the cost of these errors to be between $17 billion and $29 billion per year in hospitals nationwide (Kohn, Corrigan, & Donaldson, 1999). This publication was the catalyst for a substantial shift in the education and preparation of healthcare providers that has dramatically shaped the future direction of nursing education.

In response to this report, the publication *Crossing the Quality Chasm: A New Health System for the 21st Century* was released by the IOM in 2001. This publication focused on how the health system may be reinvented to foster innovation and improve the delivery of care. To assist in achieving this goal, *Health Professions Education: A Bridge to Quality* was published in 2003 (Greiner & Knebel, 2003). This report was instrumental in shaping the recommendations for educating *all* healthcare professionals. Further, *Health Professions Education: A Bridge to Quality* summarized for educators and accreditation, licensing, and certification organizations specific competencies that all healthcare students and professionals should develop and maintain:

- Delivering patient-centered care
- Working as part of interdisciplinary teams
- Practicing evidence-based medicine
- Focusing on quality improvement
- Using information technology (Greiner & Knebel, 2003)

In addition, a report released by the IOM in 2010, *The Future of Nursing: Leading Change, Advancing Health,* recommended that:

- Nurses should practice to the full extent of their education and training.
- Nurses should achieve higher levels of education and training through an improved education system that promotes seamless academic progression.
- Nurses should be full partners, with physicians and other healthcare professionals, in redesigning health care in the United States.
- Effective workforce planning and policy making require better data collection and information infrastructure (IOM, 2010).

To achieve the recommendations of the IOM, it was also recommended that the number of doctorally prepared nurses (practice and research-focused) be doubled by the year 2020 (IOM, 2010).

Nursing responded to the recommendations set forth by the IOM. Dialogue began in 2002 among nursing leaders, healthcare organization leaders, and stakeholders that focused on nursing's response to the immediate needs of health care and nursing education. In 2004, the American Association of Colleges of Nursing (AACN) exhibited true innovation and assigned a task force to develop a new practice doctorate in nursing. This task force resulted in the development and approval of the *Position Statement on the Practice Doctorate in Nursing* (AACN, 2004). This position statement formalized the doctor of nursing practice (DNP) degree as the highest level of preparation for nursing practice, as well as a transition to doctoral-level preparation from traditional master's-level preparation for advanced nursing practice. The year 2015 was set as the target date to complete this transition.

As a result of the recommendations of this task force, AACN published *The Essentials of Doctoral Education for Advanced Nursing Practice* (AACN, 2006). These *Essentials* are reflective of the IOM's recommended competencies for all healthcare students and professionals and are the curriculum standards for the DNP degree.

Through the innovation and leadership exhibited by the AACN, the DNP degree finally took shape. The DNP degree, focusing on *practice,* was developed and instituted a dramatic transition in nursing education. This transition continues as more DNP degree programs are developed and more students enroll.

The Essentials of Doctoral Education for Advanced Nursing Practice (AACN, 2006) have shaped the curriculum standards of DNP programs and are consistent with the recommendations of the IOM. Within the curriculum standards, a DNP project is required of all graduates of DNP programs, and this is perhaps the most daunting requirement for many students. Traditionally, there has been a lack of clarity as to what a scholarly project for a DNP program should include. Consistent themes of DNP project requirements include rigor, the translation of research into practice, and the application of knowledge. The AACN (2006) summarized that "the final DNP project produce a tangible and deliverable academic product that is derived from the practice immersion experience and is reviewed and evaluated by an academic committee" (p. 20). Further, the AACN (2006) related that the final DNP project "documents outcomes of the student's educational experiences, provides a measurable medium for evaluating the immersion experience, and summarizes the student's growth in knowledge and expertise . . . (and) serves as a foundation for future scholarly practice" (p. 20).

However, as stated in the preface of this book, there truly is limited information available to guide students in completing the DNP project. Therefore, this very timely publication has filled a void regarding all aspects of the DNP project. Students from all DNP programs have benefited from this clear, concise, and inclusive text.

This comprehensive guide not only provides a context for the DNP project but also takes the reader on a journey that begins with selecting a phenomenon of interest, the development of a project plan, and finally the culmination and evaluation of the scholarly project. This unique and innovative text thoughtfully describes a *process* designed to help the DNP student succeed in completing a meaningful DNP project. A unique feature of this text is the lived experiences of DNP graduates included in each chapter, which have been updated in this edition. These exemplars provide valuable insights regarding how the scholarly project serves as DNP students' foundation for continued scholarship and contributions to nursing and health care.

The current edition of this text emphasizes the overall value-added impact of the DNP-prepared nurse. Revised chapters include specific sections describing the impact of the DNP-prepared nurse and DNP projects. Attention was also given to the financial implications of completing the DNP project, as well as the potential for project sustainability. This is a timely topic as nurses weigh the feasibility of completing a DNP project and DNP degree. Finally, a new chapter discussing healthcare policy and advocacy was added. This new material provides insights related to advocating for healthcare policy change as this topic relates to the DNP project. Importantly, this new chapter provides examples of how to accomplish this type of work including an exemplar health policy analysis.

Written and edited by DNP-prepared nurses, this updated text is a wonderful resource and exemplar of how DNP graduates are shaping health care and nursing education. The commitment and dedication to transform and improve health care is clearly evidenced by the valuable contributions of DNP graduates in all practice arenas.

▶ References

American Association of Colleges of Nursing (AACN). (2004). *Position statement on the practice doctorate in nursing.* Retrieved from http://www.aacn.nche.edu/publications/position /DNPpositionstatement.pdf

American Association of Colleges of Nursing (AACN). (2006). *The essentials of doctoral education for advanced nursing practice.* Retrieved from https://www.aacnnursing.org/Portals/42 /Publications/DNPEssentials.pdf

Greiner, A. C., & Knebel, E. (Eds.). (2003). *Health professions education: A bridge to quality.* Washington, DC: National Academies Press.

Institute of Medicine (IOM). (2001). *Crossing the quality chasm: A new health system for the 21st century.* Washington, DC: National Academies Press.

Institute of Medicine (IOM). (2010). *The future of nursing: Leading change, advancing health.* Retrieved from http://www.iom.edu/Reports/2010/The-Future-of-Nursing-Leading-Change -Advancing-Health/Report-Brief-Education.aspx

Kohn, L. T., Corrigan, J. M., & Donaldson, M. S. (Eds.). (1999). *To err is human: Building a safer health system.* Committee on Quality of Health Care in America, Institute of Medicine. Washington, DC: National Academy Press.

Preface

Healthcare reform has been on the minds of many individuals across the United States since the introduction of the Patient Protection and Affordable Care Act in 2010. As decisions are made about implementing reform, it is important to thoughtfully consider how we as a nation will meet the healthcare needs of the people. Regardless of the outcome, it is clear that the availability of highly educated nurses to care for individuals is imperative to the health of our nation.

The Institute of Medicine (IOM) and the Robert Wood Johnson Foundation (RWJF) have recognized the need to strengthen the largest component of the healthcare workforce—nurses—to become partners and leaders in improving the delivery of care and the healthcare system as a whole (IOM, 2010, p. ix). Both the IOM and RWJF agree that accessible, high-quality care cannot be achieved without exceptional nursing care and leadership and, as such, have partnered in creating the RWJF Initiative on the Future of Nursing to explore challenges central to the future of the nursing profession (IOM, 2010, p. ix). Two specific recommendations coming from this report that are relevant involve (1) ensuring nurses achieve higher levels of education and training and (2) ensuring nurses become full partners with physicians and other healthcare professionals in redesigning health care.

In 2004, the American Association of Colleges of Nursing (AACN) recognized the need to develop nurses as healthcare leaders and subsequently released a position statement advocating that by 2015, a doctor of nursing practice (DNP) degree be required for advanced practice nurses. Since that time, schools of nursing across the nation have introduced this terminal degree into their respective programs (AACN, 2011).

One universal requirement for any DNP candidate, regardless of the institution attended, is the successful completion of a DNP project that uses evidence-based practice (EBP) for improved delivery of care, patient outcomes, and clinical systems management (AACN, 2004). The requirements for the DNP project are similar to the dissertation requirement for the PhD candidate insofar as both require rigorous scholarly work. The difference is in the focus; for the PhD candidate, the focus is generally on knowledge generation and discovery, whereas the focus for the DNP student is to apply this knowledge in some meaningful way to ultimately serve the needs of society. As mentioned in Chapter 3, Scholarship in Practice, both types of scholars contribute to knowledge generation and are interdependent to fully impact health.

Unfortunately, there are limited comprehensive resources available to guide students in completing the DNP project. Therefore, there is a need for a book that not only explores the journey the student embarks on when completing scholarly work, but also a book that provides a framework for success. For these reasons, this book was designed and written by advanced practice nurses who have an earned DNP degree especially for nurses working toward that end.

Some of the unique features of this book include clearly identified learning objectives at the beginning of each chapter, multiple examples to help illustrate key points, and significant features that are highlighted for easy reference. Where applicable, chapters conclude with impact statements, key messages, and an action plan to help the student through the DNP project development and implementation process.

The authors are proud to include work from DNP scholars across the country that is highlighted in various chapters throughout the book. There is also a chapter dedicated specifically to tools and templates that the DNP student may find useful when embarking on the project process. The authors include an example of a published project manuscript in the appendix after Chapter 15, Disseminating the Results, to encourage students to disseminate their work for the good of nursing and the health of our nation. Ultimately, this book is a demonstration of intraprofessional collaboration of DNP-prepared nurses with PhD and doctor of nursing science (DNSc) colleagues as contributing authors, to produce a resource for enhancing the nursing profession.

▶ References

American Association of Colleges of Nursing (AACN). (2004). *Position statement on the practice doctorate in nursing.* Retrieved from http://www.aacn.nche.edu/publications/position/DNP positionstatement.pdf

American Association of Colleges of Nursing (AACN). (2011). *Fact sheet: The doctor of nursing practice.* Retrieved from http://www.aacn.nche.edu/media-relations/fact-sheets/dnp

Institute of Medicine (IOM). (2010). *The future of nursing: Leading change, advancing health.* Washington, DC: The National Academies Press.

Purpose

The purpose of this book is to provide a road map for DNP students to use on their journey from project conception through completion and dissemination. The goal is to introduce a *process* that will enable DNP students to work through their project in a more effective, efficient manner and will assist in resolving the current variability of DNP projects within DNP programs around the country. This book is not intended to be prescriptive. Rather, it was developed from a broad, inclusive perspective to address the varying needs of DNP students across the country. The authors hope that it will be useful for practical application and that it gives a framework for the scholarly work process.

This book will also serve as an aid to assist faculty who are mentoring, counseling, or coaching students on the process of completing DNP scholarly work. Finally, this resource will assist preceptors and mentors of DNP students in health organizations as many DNP projects are completed within these systems.

SECTION I

The Doctor of Nursing Practice Degree

CHAPTER 1

Setting the Stage for the Doctor of Nursing Practice Project

Katherine Moran

CHAPTER OVERVIEW

The purpose of this chapter is to help the student recognize the value of doctoral education and the practice doctorate and understand the significance of the doctor of nursing practice (DNP) project. This will be accomplished by introducing the student to concepts that will be discussed throughout this text and by highlighting a framework that students can use to complete the DNP project, which reflects attainment of the DNP *Essentials*.

CHAPTER OBJECTIVES

After completing the chapter, the learner will be able to:

1. Describe the DNP-prepared clinical scholar.
2. Conceptualize the evolutionary nature of the DNP project.
3. Discern the purpose of the DNP project.

▶ Taking the Journey

It is well known that the healthcare needs of our nation are becoming more complex, the cost of health care is increasing, and the quality of health care is being questioned. Many Americans are concerned about how these issues will be resolved. Recognizing these challenges, two reports were released from the Institute of Medicine [IOM], *Crossing the Quality Chasm* and the *Future of Nursing*, making an urgent call for fundamental change in healthcare delivery.

In many ways, the DNP degree was designed to help meet these and other challenges within health care. The DNP-prepared nurse possesses *advanced competencies* for increasingly complex clinical, faculty, and leadership roles; enhanced *knowledge* to improve nursing practice and patient outcomes; and enhanced *leadership* skills to strengthen practice and healthcare delivery. In addition, the DNP-prepared nurse gives nursing parity with other health professions, most of which have a doctorate as the credential required for practice (American Association of Colleges of Nursing [AACN], 2004). In essence, DNP-prepared nurses have been called to lead and manage collaborative efforts with other healthcare practitioners to improve health care.

It should be no surprise, then, that the decision to enter a DNP program marks the beginning of what will become a *transformative experience* for many students. The program is both challenging and rewarding. Through the process of personal development, one begins to recognize the need to view the world through multiple lenses, to continue the quest for new nursing knowledge, to apply that knowledge in a practice setting in a meaningful way, and to collaborate with other healthcare practitioners to meet the ever increasing and complex healthcare needs of the nation. It is a journey where the student travels conceptually from one place in his or her clinical practice to a new place in practice. The insight gleaned through the process gives the student a new frame of reference to continue to build a more comprehensive understanding of nursing praxis, which will ultimately benefit nursing as a profession and society as a whole.

It is important to recognize that the DNP degree continues to evolve and that *all DNP-prepared nurses need to influence the outcome*. As the degree continues to mature, the value-added impact of the DNP-prepared nurse on healthcare delivery and health outcomes will be recognized. Therefore, it is essential that DNP students demonstrate that they are prepared for doctoral nursing practice through knowledge synthesis, skill refinement, and the completion of the DNP project. This is a critical point, because completion of the DNP degree is only the beginning; continued practice scholarship is expected from all doctorally prepared nurses. And, the impact from this work will transform health care by addressing policy concerns, costs associated with healthcare delivery, and the quality of care. DNP-prepared nurses (clinical scholars) will need to continue to identify the gaps between the current and the desired state of practice and implement evidence-based solutions. Through these efforts, society will continue to see the impact of practice scholarship and the associated benefit of the practice doctorate.

Soon after the student begins the doctoral program, he or she will start to work

The decision to enter a DNP program marks the beginning of what will become a transformative experience for many students.

on the final program deliverable: the DNP project. Each doctoral-level course provides an opportunity for the student to gain new knowledge that will help him or her complete the project. Through this journey, the student may refine original project ideas, or the student may end up going in an entirely new direction. Be assured that this is part of the process. In the end, the DNP project will be a carefully selected project that not only meets program requirements, but also fulfills the student's professional goals and the organization's goals (where the project is implemented), as well as contributes to the overall goals of the DNP-prepared nurse as a healthcare professional: to *positively influence health care now and in the future.*

As DNP-prepared nurses, the authors have completed multiple scholarly projects and have provided consultation services for many DNP programs across the country that have continued to give us insight and perspective on the DNP-prepared nurse's contribution to health care. The authors want to share their experience and personal insights regarding the topic of the DNP project. Our hopes are to help future DNP students on their journey, to be a guide on the side that lends a helping hand when needed. The goal of this text is to give the student a frame of reference when embarking on the DNP project. However, because there are virtually limitless DNP project ideas being developed, it is impossible to speak to the needs of each of these specifically. Therefore, this text was designed to include the potential requirements for the most comprehensive project even though some DNP projects may not require such detail. This is *not meant to suggest that all projects should mirror the examples* provided; rather, this text is intended to be a reference or a framework that allows the student to choose items that will help inform his or her project and challenges the student to consider new perspectives that foster creativity and the development of innovative ideas. At the same time, it is our hope that doctoral nursing educators, team members, and other healthcare professionals interfacing with DNP students find this text helpful when guiding the DNP student through the scholarly project process.

Developing the DNP project is not a linear process; it is created through a series of explorations that result in a comprehensive, well-thought-out project plan. As such, the student should recognize that although the topics in this text are presented in a stepwise framework to help him or her through the process, some of the work may occur simultaneously because of the evolutionary nature of the project.

Many different DNP programs are available across the United States. All of the programs meet the needs of the community they serve; however, they may accomplish this via different methods. As a result, *program structures will vary*; some may include a formal DNP project team, while others may use a completely different approach. For example, some universities may use a model that requires one faculty advisor and one faculty member from the university who serves as a committee member, while others may include one faculty advisor and one representative from the community. The same is true regarding the final program deliverable requirements. In an attempt to better understand the characteristics of these programs, the

Developing the DNP project is not a linear process; it is created through a series of explorations that result in a comprehensive, well-thought-out project plan.

authors have collaborated with many individuals either providing DNP education in programs throughout the United States or informing DNP education, such as the American Association of Colleges of Nursing (AACN), to better understand the needs of DNP students, faculty, and others working with students to complete the DNP project. We have learned that DNP education and the recommended requirements of DNP projects and teams are continuing to evolve (see Chapter 2, Defining the Doctor of Nursing Practice: Current Trends). Recognizing this, the authors sought to meet the various scholarly requirement needs of these programs by providing a wide variety of options and perspectives for the student to consider and reference where applicable. While there are many examples, templates, and other formats provided as tools for the journey, the intent is to give the student options, not be directive.

▶ The Purpose of the DNP Project

A debate has been ongoing for many years regarding what one should consider as *scholarship*, especially in academe. Many learned individuals have weighed in on this debate over the years, including Ernest L. Boyer, a well-known educator who at one point served as the United States Commissioner on Education. In 1990, Boyer, then president of the Carnegie Foundation for Advancement of Teaching, suggested that for "America's colleges and universities to remain vital a new vision of scholarship is required" (Boyer, 1990, p. 13). It is clear that the scholarship debate began long before the DNP degree; however, since the introduction of this degree, the discussion has shifted to include *practice scholarship*.

In an effort to contribute to the richness of this dialogue, a discussion regarding the evolving scholarship of practice is provided in Chapter 3, Scholarship in Practice.

For the purposes of introduction to the DNP project, it is important to recognize, from a very literal sense, that the term *scholar* is defined as a learned person, who is specialized in an area of knowledge ("Scholar," 2016). Taking this definition and applying it to the DNP project helps one recognize that this project provides the student with a vehicle through which he or she can demonstrate advanced knowledge in a particular area. This is in alignment with AACN, which believes that the final DNP project should demonstrate "synthesis of the student's work" and that it should lay the groundwork for future scholarship (AACN, 2006, p. 20). Certainly, the project should demonstrate the student's achievement of the eight DNP *Essentials of Doctoral Education for Advanced Nursing Practice*, as outlined by the AACN. A detailed discussion regarding these competencies and current trends in DNP education is provided in Chapter 2.

It should be clear that the DNP project is many things: a required program deliverable, the demonstration of doctoral competencies, and a means to achieve professional goals as well as the goals of the organization where the project is implemented. The importance of the impact of this work cannot be overstated. But to realize this impact, DNP students must be focused on

A scholar is a learned person, who is specialized in an area of knowledge (Scholar, 2016).

delivering high-quality, relevant projects that can be sustained.

In addition, it is expected that the project is only the beginning of many future scholarly contributions by the DNP-prepared nurse that lead to improvement in health care and add to nursing knowledge. Therefore, the DNP project plays a very important role in doctoral education; it affords the DNP student an opportunity to *launch into scholarly practice*. The DNP-prepared nurse will have many opportunities to transcend current barriers and positively impact health care in the United States as we know it today—to build a bridge between research and practice, as well as between theory and practice. These are indeed exciting times!

The DNP project plays a very important role in doctoral education; it affords the DNP student an opportunity to launch into scholarly practice.

In many ways, the creation of this text is an example of DNP scholarly work. The authors collaborated with thought leaders in the field, demonstrating the skills attained in *Essential VI: interprofessional collaboration for improving patient and population health outcomes*. Then, using the skills garnered in DNP *Essential III: clinical scholarship and analytical methods for evidence-based practice*, the authors reviewed the current literature and resources available for students on this topic. The authors also collaborated with other practice experts across the United States, considered their personal experiences as DNP-prepared nurses, and determined that a resource designated specifically for the completion of the DNP project would be a useful resource for DNP students, DNP faculty, and members of healthcare organizations.

In essence, the authors formed a *scholarship team* and worked together to meet the perceived needs of DNP students in programs throughout the country to provide the final deliverable, which correlates with DNP *Essential VIII: advanced nursing practice*.

▶ Chapters at a Glance

The reader will note that each chapter begins with an image of Greek Ionic–style columns that symbolize the cumulative doctoral work and overall achievement of the DNP student. The columns represent the eight DNP *Essentials* and corresponding knowledge and skills that are developed or strengthened by completing a practice doctorate program. Finally, the *capstone* that rests on the top of the structure represents the highest point of achievement, when the student successfully completes the final doctoral project.

The DNP *Essentials* are referenced in each chapter where they apply to the chapter discussion. As mentioned in the preface, the student will also note that significant points of the discussion are highlighted throughout the chapter, and *key messages* are reiterated at the end of each chapter. To facilitate learning and to help move the student along in the development of the DNP project, each chapter begins with learning objectives and concludes with an action plan and *helpful resources* (where applicable).

Section I: The Doctor of Nursing Practice Degree

Every good framework begins with a solid foundation. To that end, the focus of the first section of this text is providing an overview of the DNP degree that includes the impetus to the degree, the purpose of the degree, and the current trends, as well as defining the purpose of the DNP project and the current view of potential projects. The student is reminded that both the practice- and research-based doctorate will need to collaborate to impact nursing and health care and that the collaboration between the two doctoral levels of preparation will determine the future of nursing and its impact on health care.

A new chapter on healthcare policy and advocacy (Chapter 4) was added to this edition to showcase how the education, knowledge, and skills that DNP-prepared nurses acquire through doctoral education prepare them to sit at the table where healthcare decisions are being made. The purpose of this new chapter is to help the DNP student understand factors that impact the health of our nation, recognize areas where the student may facilitate change, and utilize methods that can be used to make an impact.

The overall goal of this section is to help the student develop an understanding of the many forms of scholarship as it relates to the practice doctorate, to conceptualize the types of projects that can be and are being considered by DNP students in programs across the United States, to examine potential topics of interest in relation to the appropriate level of scholarship, and to recognize the ultimate significance of the DNP project—*to validate the effectiveness of the DNP-prepared nurse.* To this last point, a recurring theme threaded throughout this new edition relates to the *impact* that DNP students and DNP-prepared nurses are making in their efforts to improve healthcare delivery and health care in the United States.

Section II: The DNP Project

Section II is devoted to guiding the reader through the DNP project process. The complex nature of nursing practice is discussed, as well as how practice provides many opportunities to explore nursing phenomena. The student is introduced to a variety of strategies to help him or her select a phenomenon of interest and to explore the topic comprehensively. The value of identifying a project that will lead to an improvement in clinical practice is stressed. Further, the DNP student is introduced to elements of a scholarly project that need to be considered early in the development phase, including conducting a literature search, writing a literature review to support the value and/or the need to address the phenomenon of interest, performing an organizational assessment, formulating a problem statement, defining the project goal and project scope, developing a project framework, and identifying the appropriate approach to obtain data and the methods used to work with the data received.

Nationally, nurses are being called to actively collaborate within interprofessional teams to improve quality, cost-effective, and efficient care and improve outcomes (IOM, 2003). Therefore, another focus of this section is to help the student understand that (1) the DNP project provides him or her with an opportunity to attain and refine the competencies needed for collaborative team participation and leadership; (2) the DNP student will need additional resources to assist in assessing, planning, implementing, and evaluating the DNP project; and (3) this is best achieved through collaboration.

The student is guided through these and other processes that influence the development and implementation of the DNP project by the faculty mentor and/or project team. Therefore, the composition and roles of the project team, including the faculty mentor and other members, are reviewed. This information is important because project team dynamics, including making the most of team meetings and resources to form a cohesive and collegial team that will work together, is vital to the student's success in completing the DNP project. Further, the point is made that interprofessional, collaborative teams are needed to transform healthcare delivery. Another important component of project development is the project plan. A broad overview of points to consider when preparing for project implementation is provided, such as taking into consideration the client and personnel, monitoring requirements, problem solving/troubleshooting demands, the need to communicate with key stakeholders, and the characteristics and skill set of effective leaders. Samples of a variety of tools are provided for the student to use throughout the DNP project development and implementation cycle to help ensure a successful outcome. Further, the value of the practicum is stressed in this section to help the student recognize (1) how the experience will support the development of DNP competencies and professional scholarly growth and (2) the potential to use the practicum in preparation for and implementation of the DNP project. The benefit of academic practice partnerships is introduced as an effective practicum mechanism to enhance learning for the DNP student and to assist organizations in reaching their strategic goals. The project plan provided as an example is fairly detailed to capture the elements needed in a complex or comprehensive project. However, the student is reminded that *all the elements presented may not be applicable to every potential project.*

Finally, this section concludes with a discussion regarding how the DNP project proposal represents the student's intellectual ability, knowledge in the subject area, and contributions to nursing as a profession. To help the student with the proposal writing process, information is provided to (1) help the student recognize early in the process when he or she may need some additional writing support, (2) introduce the student to the components included in a sample project proposal, and (3) provide a reference for writing the DNP project proposal.

Section III: Doctor of Nursing Practice Outcomes

The last section of this text, Section III, concludes by reaffirming the importance of the DNP project and the need to disseminate the results. Various formats for disseminating the results are reviewed, such as public presentation, a defense of the project, a written manuscript for the university, and a manuscript submission to a scholarly journal. To this point, valuable insight is offered on how to successfully submit a manuscript for publication. The importance of communicating and disseminating the results of the DNP project is stressed not only because it may be a required program deliverable, but also because of the knowledge translation that occurs, benefiting both nursing as a profession and, even more broadly, the health of our nation. The student is reminded that the project is a product of DNP education that reflects the attainment of knowledge and skills that launches the DNP graduate into scholarly practice. The point is made, however, that it is important to recognize the need to evaluate the outcomes of this doctoral degree in nursing for effectiveness in accomplishing the goals of improving the nursing professions and health care, and meeting societal needs. Recognizing that this will be an important focus for the DNP-prepared nurse, an evaluation strategy is proposed using a framework based on the Actualized DNP Model (Burson, Moran, & Conrad, 2016).

Finally, in many of the chapters, there is an excerpt from the perspective of the DNP student regarding the topic of discussion in the specific chapter. For instance, in Chapter 5, The Phenomenon of Interest, a student shares her experience of narrowing the topic related to her clinical expertise, the societal need, data from the organization, and the evidence in the literature.

These examples are included to showcase aspects of the DNP project, to show the potential for the DNP project as a program deliverable, to provide evidence of healthcare transformation, and to illustrate the *impact* of the practice doctorate in nursing. In addition, sustainable projects become the catalyst for ongoing practice change far beyond the original project. Although it is evident that these projects certainly contribute to the health of individual populations, as a whole, they demonstrate that doctorally prepared nurses provide more than protection, promotion, and optimization of health and abilities; these nurses facilitate healing and wellness through human connection. As a result of these efforts, society is beginning to see the impact of practice scholarship and the associated benefit of the practice doctorate.

The first excerpt (see **EXEMPLAR 1-1**), provided by Dr. Deonne Brown Benedict, focuses on her work as a nurse practitioner entrepreneur and the impact that a single nurse practitioner can make in meeting the needs of the community.

DNP-prepared nurses are demonstrating their value to society through practice scholarship that improves healthcare outcomes.

EXEMPLAR 1-1 Nurse Practitioner Entrepreneurship

Deonne Brown Benedict, DNP, ARNP, FNP-BC

My DNP project was a three-pronged undertaking. It evaluated consumer perspectives on nurse practitioners (NPs), interviewed NP entrepreneurs to determine success factors for NP clinic ownership, and studied NP business knowledge. I also evaluated a variety of other local factors for clinic start-up. With these data, I was able to determine many of the components that lead to a successful clinic venture. After completing my DNP degree, I studied several potential clinic models, including free clinics and the "ideal medical practice model." These efforts culminated in the development of a unique hybrid model for my practice, allowing me to meet the needs of both insured clients and uninsured clients who may not be able to afford typical care. This clinic model does not require outside grant support but is able to serve the needs of insured, uninsured, and Medicaid clients, many of whom were previously not receiving adequate care. It also allows for longer visits, valuable time for establishing rapport, educating clients, and living out the philosophy and ideals of NPs.

In 2009, I opened a nurse-owned and managed clinic based on this low-overhead, high-tech, and high-touch model. The clinic paid off its start-up costs in several months and has provided me with a wonderful opportunity to serve my community while maintaining a rewarding job with a reasonable income for many years. However, starting in 2015 I began to notice that several similar clinics had closed their doors. Healthcare reform, while beneficial to many, has resulted in pressure on small clinics with limited administrative and management staff. Since small clinics have difficulty joining Accountable Care Organizations (ACOs), we lost many patients on the state exchange in 2016 and 2017. Without the bargaining power of a group, reimbursements remained stable or lower. The reasons we were given for the lower reimbursement were that we are an NP practice, not part of an ACO, and a small practice. Meanwhile, costs such as administrative reporting requirements, labor, rent, faxing, electronic health record, and supplies have increased.

Previously, I had built my clientele primarily through patient referrals, but in 2017 I realized it was time for a different strategy. Patients continued to appreciate that I spend an hour with new patients and 30 minutes in follow-ups for chronic conditions. I explored options to meet the administrative gaps with virtual assistants and provider group formation (Organizational and Systems Leadership), but I also began to develop a marketing plan based on the niches I thrive in, including genetics and virtual care (Scientific Underpinnings, Information Systems/Technology). Patients who had tired of being seen by a system in 10- to 15-minute increments began to find me! Applying DNP concepts doesn't stop with one's initial progress. I have used the knowledge I gained in the process to consult with NPs across the country and provide tips for getting their own practices started or thriving, and I have spoken to university NP students and NP groups in support of nurse entrepreneurship.

▶ Summary

The journey to the DNP degree may still be via a winding and rugged road; however, given the potential for DNP graduates to improve healthcare outcomes and to positively impact the nursing profession, these authors hope that more and more of our nursing colleagues recognize the value of doctoral education and join us on the journey. For the current DNP student, our hopes are that this text will provide a broad view of the DNP project and shed light on the DNP project journey.

Finally, where healthcare reform is concerned, it is evident that the Institute of Medicine has recognized nurses as valuable players in this process. Therefore, it is time for nurses, especially DNP-prepared nurses, to see health care as something we shape—DNPs are called to lead and manage collaborative efforts with other healthcare practitioners to improve health care.

Do not go where the path may lead, go instead where there is no path and leave a trail.

—Ralph Waldo Emerson

Key Messages

- The decision to enter a DNP program marks the beginning of what will become a transformative experience for many students.
- Developing the DNP project is not a linear process; it is created through a series of explorations that result in a comprehensive, well-thought-out project plan.
- The DNP project is a required program deliverable that demonstrates achievement of doctoral competencies and advanced knowledge in a particular area.
- The DNP project is a means to achieve professional goals and marks the beginning of many future scholarly contributions.
- The *impact* from this work will transform health care by addressing policy concerns, costs associated with healthcare delivery, and the quality of care.

Action Plan—Next Steps

1. Consider the value of the DNP project.
2. Open the mind to a variety of potential project topics.
3. Take advantage of learning opportunities.
4. Enjoy the journey!

References

American Association of Colleges of Nursing (AACN). (2004). *AACN position statement on the practice doctorate in nursing.* Retrieved from http://www.aacn.nche.edu/publications/position/DNPpositionstatement.pdf

American Association of Colleges of Nursing (AACN). (2006). *The essentials of doctoral education for advanced nursing practice.* Retrieved from http://www.aacnnursing.org/Portals/42/Publications/DNPEssentials.pdf

Boyer, E. (1990). *Scholarship reconsidered: Priorities of the professoriate.* Carnegie Foundation for the Advancement of Teaching. New York, NY: John Wiley & Sons.

Burson, R., Moran, K., & Conrad, D. (2016). Why hire a DNP? The value added impact of the practice doctorate. *Journal of Doctoral Nursing Practice, 9*(1), 152-157.

Institute of Medicine (IOM). (2003). *Health professions education: A bridge to quality.* Chapter 3: The core competencies needed for health care professionals. Washington, DC: The National Academies Press. Retrieved from http://www.nap.edu/openbook.php?record_id=10681&page=45

Scholar. (2016). In *American Heritage dictionary of the English language, Fifth Edition.* Copyright © 2016 by Houghton Mifflin Harcourt Publishing Company. All rights reserved. Retrieved from https://www.thefreedictionary.com/scholar

CHAPTER 2

Defining the Doctor of Nursing Practice: Current Trends

Dianne Conrad and Karen Kesten

CHAPTER OVERVIEW

The purpose of this chapter is to define doctoral preparation for nursing and describe nursing practice doctoral education and its role in transforming health care. Current trends in doctor of nursing practice (DNP) education will be explored on how the practice doctorate is evolving to meet the competencies as outlined in *The Essentials of Doctoral Education for Advanced Nursing Practice* (American Association of Colleges of Nursing [AACN], 2006).

CHAPTER OBJECTIVES

After completing the chapter, the learner will be able to:

1. Define "doctor of nursing practice."
2. Describe the state of DNP education.
3. Differentiate between the research and practice doctorate degrees.
4. Discuss how the practice-based doctorate and the research-based doctorate will collaborate to impact nursing and health care.

▶ Defining the Practice Doctorate in Nursing

The time is now for the practice doctorate in nursing. Nursing education has evolved to meet the needs of society in preparing nurses throughout history. The emergence and dramatic growth of Doctor of Nursing Practice (DNP) programs in the United States reflect this country's demand for highly competent providers to improve the health care of its people.

In 2001, the Institute of Medicine (IOM) outlined aims for healthcare improvement in *Crossing the Quality Chasm: A New Health System for the 21st Century,* which included care that is safe, effective, patient centered, timely, efficient, and equitable. To provide that care, the IOM (2003), in *Health Professions Education: A Bridge to Quality,* called for a change in how healthcare providers are prepared to meet these challenges. Healthcare providers in all professions are to attain the following core competencies:

- Provide patient-centered care.
- Work in interdisciplinary teams.
- Employ evidence-based practice.
- Apply quality improvement.
- Utilize informatics.

By 2010, the IOM's report *The Future of Nursing: Leading Change, Advancing Health* responded with these key messages:

- Nurses should practice to the full extent of their education and training.
- Nurses should achieve higher levels of education and training through an improved education system that promotes seamless academic progression.
- Nurses should be full partners with physicians and other healthcare professionals in redesigning health care in the United States.
- Effective workforce planning and policy making require better data collection and information infrastructure.

These important documents reflect the changing societal needs for a highly educated workforce prepared to meet the complex challenges of health care in the 21st century and beyond. Ten years after the *Crossing the Quality Chasm* was released, evaluations of the impact acknowledged the importance of providing the foundation for quality improvement, but the change in the paradigm had to be followed by more tangible outcomes and that change had been glacially slow (Dentzer, 2011; McKinney, 2011). In response to these challenges, nursing as a profession has developed an educational program at

> *The DNP is a degree, not a role.*

the doctoral level to prepare individuals for advanced nursing practice. The purpose of practice-focused doctoral programs is to *prepare experts in specialized advanced nursing practice,* as defined by the AACN (2006). The programs are to *focus heavily on innovative and evidence-based practice, reflecting the application of credible research findings.*

See **TABLE 2-1** for a comparison of IOM recommendations on healthcare improvement, the competencies of healthcare professionals, and practice nursing doctoral preparation *Essentials.*

TABLE 2-1 Comparison of IOM Recommendations on Healthcare Improvement, Competencies of Healthcare Professionals, and Clinical Nursing Doctoral Preparation

Six Aims for Healthcare Improvement (IOM, 2001)	Core Competencies of Healthcare Professionals (IOM, 2003)	*The Essentials of Doctoral Education for Advanced Nursing Practice* (AACN, 2006)
DNP Essential VIII: **Advanced Nursing Practice**		
Safe: Avoid injuries to patients from the care that is intended to help them.	■ Apply quality improvement. ■ Work in interdisciplinary teams.	I. Scientific underpinnings for practice II. Organizational and systems leadership for quality improvement and systems thinking VI. Interprofessional collaboration for improving patient and population health outcomes
Effective: Provide services based on scientific knowledge to all who could benefit, and refrain from providing services to those not likely to benefit.	■ Employ evidence-based practice. ■ Utilize informatics.	I. Scientific underpinnings for practice II. Organizational and systems leadership for quality improvement and systems thinking III. Clinical scholarship and analytical methods for evidence-based practice IV. Information systems/technology and patient care technology for the improvement and transformation of health care V. Healthcare policy for advocacy in health care
Patient centered: Provide care that is respectful of and responsive to individual patient preferences, needs, and values, and ensure that patient values guide all clinical decisions.	■ Provide patient-centered care.	V. Healthcare policy for advocacy in health care VII. Clinical prevention and population health for improving the nation's health

(continues)

TABLE 2-1 Comparison of IOM Recommendations on Healthcare Improvement, Competencies of Healthcare Professionals, and Clinical Nursing Doctoral Preparation *(continued)*

Six Aims for Healthcare Improvement (IOM, 2001)	Core Competencies of Healthcare Professionals (IOM, 2003)	The Essentials of Doctoral Education for Advanced Nursing Practice (AACN, 2006)
Timely: Reduce waits and sometimes harmful delays for both those who receive and those who give care.	▪ Work in interdisciplinary teams. ▪ Apply quality improvement. ▪ Employ evidence-based practice.	II. Organizational and systems leadership for quality improvement and systems thinking VI. Interprofessional collaboration for improving patient and population health outcomes
Efficient: Avoid waste, including waste of equipment, supplies, ideas, and energy.	▪ Work in interdisciplinary teams. ▪ Utilize informatics. ▪ Apply quality improvement.	I. Scientific underpinnings for practice III. Clinical scholarship and analytical methods for evidence-based practice IV. Information systems/ technology and patient care technology for the improvement and transformation of health care V. Healthcare policy for advocacy in health care VI. Interprofessional collaboration for improving patient and population health outcomes
Equitable: Provide care that does not vary in quality because of personal characteristics such as gender, ethnicity, geographic location, and socioeconomic status.	▪ Provide patient-centered care. ▪ Apply quality improvement. ▪ Utilize informatics.	II. Organizational and systems leadership for quality improvement and systems thinking VII. Clinical prevention and population health for improving the nation's health IV. Information systems/ technology and patient care technology for the improvement and transformation of health care

Reprinted with permission from American Association of Colleges of Nursing (AACN). (2006). *The essentials for doctoral education for advanced nursing practice.* Washington, DC: Author; Institute of Medicine. (2003). *Health professions education: A bridge to quality.* Washington, DC: National Academies Press. Retrieved from http://www.nap.edu/openbook.php?record_id=10681&page=45

The practice doctorate for nurses, the DNP, is a *degree*, not a *role*. There are many roles in advanced nursing practice. The AACN (2004) defined advanced nursing practice as:

Any form of nursing intervention that influences healthcare outcomes for individuals or populations, including the direct care of individual patients, management of care for individuals and populations, administration of nursing and healthcare organizations, and the development and implementation of health policy. (p. 2)

Therefore, advanced nursing practice encompasses such roles as nurse practitioner (NP), clinical nurse specialist (CNS), certified nurse-midwife (CNM), nurse anesthetist, nurse administrator, nurse informaticist, and nurse health policy specialist. This list of roles is not inclusive because nursing entrepreneurs continue to pioneer advanced nursing practice roles to meet patient needs in a variety of settings. However, the AACN (2004) has not recognized nursing education as a stand-alone advanced nursing practice specialty for DNP education. The AACN (2004) recommends that both DNP and PhD programs offer additional coursework in pedagogy and practica that would prepare graduates to fill the role of nurse educator.

There is a special definition of the roles of the advanced practice registered nurse (APRN). In 2008, a report titled *Consensus Model for APRN Regulation: Licensure, Accreditation, Certification & Education* was completed through the work of the APRN Consensus Work Group and the National Council of State Boards of Nursing APRN Advisory Committee (APRN Joint Dialogue Group, 2008). This group defined four specific APRN roles—certified registered nurse anesthetist (CRNA), CNM, CNS, and certified nurse practitioner—for the purpose of standardizing licensure language across the country. However, the group acknowledged that

. . . many nurses with advanced graduate nursing preparation practice in roles and specialties (e.g., informatics, public health, education or administration) that are essential to advance the health of the public but do not focus on direct care to individuals and, therefore, their practice does not require regulatory recognition beyond the Registered Nurse license granted by state boards of nursing. Like the four current APRN roles, practice in these other advanced nursing roles requires specialized knowledge and skills acquired through graduate-level education. (p. 5)

Though the APRN consensus document did not specify the practice doctorate as the education level for these advanced practice roles, graduate-level education was a requirement. Any of these roles benefit from education at the doctoral level to prepare nurses for the challenges of today's healthcare arena. These advanced nursing practice roles are oriented toward providing quality care and improving patient outcomes.

The *Essentials of DNP Education* (AACN, 2006) give these doctorally prepared nurses the tools and competencies they need to carry out their role at the highest level (see **FIGURE 2-1**).

The AACN (2004) further delineates the benefits of a practice-focused doctorate to:

- Develop the needed advanced competencies for increasingly complex practice, faculty, and leadership roles.
- Enhance knowledge to improve nursing practice and patient outcomes.
- Enhance leadership skills to strengthen practice and healthcare delivery. (p. 4)

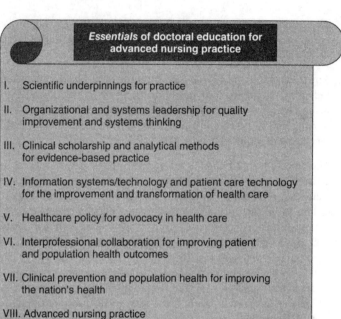

FIGURE 2-1 *Essentials* of doctoral education for advanced nursing practice.

Data from American Association of Colleges of Nursing (AACN). (2006). *The essentials for doctoral education for advanced nursing practice.* Washington, DC: Author.

Most important, the DNP-prepared nurse is able to translate scientific evidence into practice in a timely fashion.

▶ Comparison of the DNP and PhD in Nursing

Doctoral preparation in nursing currently has two paths: the research-based doctorate that began in 1934 at New York University and flourished in the 1970s (Chism, 2019), and the current practice doctorate, the DNP, which has been defined and developed by the AACN since 2002. See Chapter 3, Scholarship in Practice, for a discussion of the evolution of the practice doctorate.

The two doctoral programs, according to the AACN (2006), are different in their goals and in the competencies of their graduates. The practice doctorate (DNP) and the research doctorates (PhD and Doctor of Nursing Science [DNS]) offer complementary, alternative approaches to attaining the highest level of educational preparation in nursing with rigorous and demanding programs of study. The profession of nursing benefits from scholar leaders who are committed to the advancement of the science and practice of nursing.

A comparison of nursing doctoral programs is outlined in **TABLE 2-2**.

The challenges of healthcare delivery in the 21st century will necessitate the collaboration of interdisciplinary teams (IOM, 2003). Partnering of the research

TABLE 2-2 Comparison of Doctoral Nursing Programs

	Practice Doctorate DNP	Research Doctorate PhD/DNS
Common Characteristics	■ Rigorous and demanding expectations ■ Scholarly approach to the discipline ■ Commitment to the advancement of the profession	
Program of Study	■ Prepares leaders at highest level of nursing practice to improve patient outcomes and translate research into practice.	■ Prepares nurses at the highest level of nursing science to conduct research to advance the science of nursing.
Students	■ Commitment to practice career. ■ Oriented toward improving outcomes for patient care and population health.	■ Commitment to research career. ■ Oriented toward developing new nursing knowledge and scientific inquiry.
Program Faculty	■ Practice doctorate in nursing, and expertise in area of teaching. ■ Leadership experience in area of role and population practice. ■ High level of expertise in practice congruent with focus of academic program.	■ Research doctorate in nursing or related field. ■ Leadership experience in area of sustained research funding. ■ High level of expertise in research congruent with focus of academic funding. ■ High level of expertise in research congruent with focus of academic program.
Resources	■ Mentors and/or preceptors in leadership positions across practice settings. ■ Access to diverse practice settings with appropriate resources for areas of practice. ■ Access to financial aid. ■ Access to information and patient-care technology resources congruent with areas of study.	■ Mentors and/or preceptors in research settings. ■ Access to research settings with appropriate resources. ■ Access to dissertation support dollars and financial aid. ■ Access to information and research technology resources congruent with program of research.

(continues)

TABLE 2-2 Comparison of Doctoral Nursing Programs		*(continued)*
	Practice Doctorate **DNP**	**Research Doctorate** **PhD/DNS**
Program Assessment and Evaluation	■ Program outcomes: Healthcare improvements and contributions via practice, policy change, and practice scholarship. ■ Receives accreditation by nursing accreditor.	■ Program outcomes: Contributes to healthcare improvements via the development of new knowledge and scholarly products that provide the foundation for the advancement of nursing science. ■ Oversight by the institution's authorized bodies (i.e., graduate school) and regional accreditors.

Modified from American Association of Colleges of Nursing (AACN). (2014). *Key differences between DNP and PhD/DNS programs.* Retrieved from: http://www.aacnnursing.org/Portals/42/DNP/ContrastGrid.pdf?ver=2017-05-25-113051-180http://www.aacn.nche.edu/dnp/ContrastGrid.pdf

doctorate with the practice doctorate will demonstrate cooperation within nursing that can advance the profession. Lamb (2012) described building collaboration "readiness" with the combination of the PhD and the DNP in nursing. She stated that the PhD in nursing brings:

■ More minds, more tools, and more innovation
■ A broader range of theories and more explanatory theoretical models
■ An expanded toolkit for research design and methods
■ The opportunity for more competitive grants

The DNP in nursing brings the following to the team:

■ Better teamwork, leading to better outcomes
■ The contribution of a broader range of evidence
■ Greater opportunities to accelerate nurse-led and interprofessional practice models

The benefits of interprofessional and intraprofessional collaboration will be discussed further in Chapter 8, Interprofessional and Intraprofessional Collaboration in the DNP Project.

▶ Current Trends in Doctoral Education

IOM Future of Nursing *report calls for a doubling of doctorally prepared nurses by 2020.*

One of the concerns about beginning a practice doctorate for nursing was the ability of the profession to produce doctoral-level graduates. *The Future of Nursing* report (IOM, 2010) called for the doubling of doctorally prepared nurses by 2020. Rapid growth of DNP programs has occurred since the AACN's work on defining and developing the practice doctorate *Essentials* in 2004. The number of DNP programs has increased from 11 in 2005 to 344 in 2017, with many more programs in development (AACN, 2018a). The concern that the practice doctorate would decrease the number of nurses pursuing a research doctorate in nursing appears to be unfounded. The AACN tracks the number of nursing education programs as well as graduates of those programs. The data show that since 2003, the number of PhD students enrolled in the United States has increased from 3,229 to 4,632 in 2017. During the same period, the enrollment in DNP programs increased dramatically—from 70 in 2003 to 29,093 in 2017 in 344 DNP programs across the country (AACN, 2018b). The number of PhD programs in nursing has also increased, from 106 in 2006 to 138 in 2017 (AACN, 2018a) (see **FIGURE 2-2** and **FIGURE 2-3**).

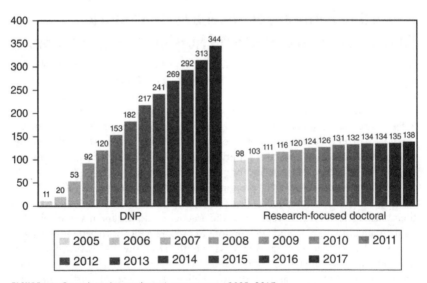

FIGURE 2-2 Growth in doctoral nursing programs: 2005–2017.

Reprinted with permission from American Association of Colleges of Nursing (AACN). (2018a). *Custom report on doctoral program enrollments, 2005–2017.* Washington, DC: AACN Research and Data Services.

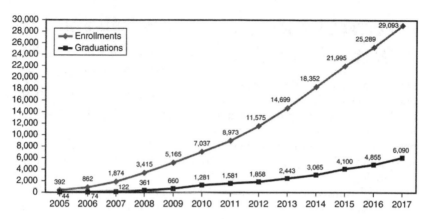

FIGURE 2-3 Doctoral program enrollments and graduations 2005–2017.

Reprinted with permission from American Association of Colleges of Nursing (AACN). (2018a). *Custom report on doctoral program enrollments, 2005–2017.* Washington, DC: AACN Research and Data Services.

▶ Reports Affecting DNP Education

The RAND Corporation Report: The DNP by 2015: A Study of the Institutional, Political, and Professional Issues that Facilitate or Impede Establishing a Post-Baccalaureate Doctor of Nursing Practice Program

In 2004, member schools of the American Association of Colleges of Nursing (AACN) voted to endorse the *Position Statement on the Practice Doctorate in Nursing*, which called for moving the level of preparation necessary for advanced nursing practice from the master's degree to the doctorate by the target year of 2015 (AACN, 2004). Since that time, colleges of nursing have made great strides in moving toward this goal. Currently, the majority of schools with APRN programs (the largest subset of all advanced nursing practice programs) either offer or are planning to offer a DNP at the post-baccalaureate and/or post-master's level.

While the number of DNP programs for APRNs has grown significantly and steadily over this period, not all colleges of nursing have been able to fully transition their master's-level APRN programs to the practice doctorate and many are electing to maintain both master's and DNP options to prepare APRNs. To better understand the issues facing colleges of nursing moving to the DNP, the AACN board of directors commissioned the RAND Corporation to conduct a national survey of nursing schools with APRN programs to identify the barriers and facilitators to offering a post-baccalaureate DNP (Auerbach et al., 2014). The report includes recommendations for next steps that AACN can take to help schools accelerate programmatic change and overcome challenges, including:

1. Conduct, and collaborate with others to conduct, outcome studies of DNP practice to better understand the impact of DNP graduates on patient care.

2. Provide outreach data to help employers and healthcare organizations understand the comprehensive competencies and capabilities of DNP-educated APRNs.
3. Focus on understanding and documenting successful strategies in overcoming barriers to offering BSN-to-DNP programs of departments or divisions within larger universities, since they may face greater hurdles to offering BSN-to-DNP programs.
4. Document and showcase examples of collaborative partnerships between schools and hospitals or other healthcare organizations for the purpose of providing clinical practice sites.
5. Provide greater clarity and guidance related to requirements for the DNP project.
6. Continue with ongoing efforts to assist schools in overcoming challenges to offering the BSN to DNP.

As a response to these recommendations, follow-up and active steps taken by AACN include the formation of two task forces to further improve DNP education: the Implementation of the DNP Task Force and the APRN Clinical Training Task Force. Each task force has produced white papers that address some of the barriers identified in the RAND Corporation study.

To find out more about these task forces and their charges, see www.aacnnursing.org/About-AACN/AACN-Governance/Committees-and-Task-Forces.

AACN Report on APRN Education: The APRN Clinical Training Task Force Report

Much attention has been paid to the Institute of Medicine's (IOM) 2010 *The Future of Nursing* report that APRNs be allowed to practice to "the full extent of their education and training" (p. 29). APRNs have a potential opportunity to contribute to the delivery of care to the additional 16.4 million *newly insured* patients due to healthcare reform (Office of the Assistant Secretary for Planning and Evaluation [ASPE], 2015). Nationwide, APRN education programs are experiencing increased demand for APRN enrollment and many programs report challenges in expanding enrollment to meet this demand. Colleges of nursing cite inadequate numbers and quality of clinical training sites and preceptors for APRN students.

In response to these societal healthcare challenges, the AACN convened the APRN Clinical Training Task Force to develop a white paper regarding clinical education and training for APRNs. The AACN Task Force Report (AACN, 2015a) concluded that the current methods of providing clinical education for APRNs need to be re-envisioned in order to expand the pool of opportunities available to contemporary students and to reduce strictures in the pipeline to educating the APRN workforce in sufficient numbers to meet societal demand for these valuable services. Variability among APRN programs, particularly for nurse practitioners and clinical nurse specialists, exists in the clinical competencies expected at various points throughout the curriculum and evaluation processes and tools. Increasingly, new models of care are emerging with a greater emphasis on interprofessional practice and education. Advances in technology, both within healthcare delivery and education, have created opportunities for APRNs to lead the effective integration of technologies into healthcare delivery. Academic practice partnerships are important to all APRN clinical education programs to ensure that students have access to patients, healthcare professional teams, and current data and experiences. Partnerships are increasingly important when considering interprofessional education, transition to practice for new graduates, implementation of new clinical education models, and the rapid changes that are occurring in healthcare systems. Across higher education, there is an increased interest and emphasis on examination and implementation of competency-based education and assessment models in a variety of disciplines and more specifically in the health professions (Carraccio & Englander, 2013; Carraccio, Wolfsthal, Englander, Ferentz, & Martin, 2002).

The AACN Task Force made the following recommendations:

I. **Simulation should be used to enhance APRN clinical education, and the use of simulation to replace more traditional clinical experiences should be explored.**
    - Seek funding for five demonstration projects that are designed to study the impact of various methods along the continuum of simulation learning approaches as one component of APRN clinical education and assessment.
    - Funding and other resources should be provided at both the national and local levels for the development and use of simulation for learning and assessment, including funding for a national center of faculty innovation and faculty preparation and certification.
    - A national repository should be created and maintained for reliable and valid APRN simulation education materials.
    - Simulations should be developed and tested for assessment of the APRN common competencies.

II. **AACN-American Organization of Nurse Executives (AONE) principles for academic-practice partnerships should be adopted by all APRN programs.**
    - APRN programs, including face-to-face and distance education programs, should implement expectations described in Section II regarding the development and maintenance of APRN clinical experiences and student oversight.
    - Encourage and support the development of innovative partnerships for APRN clinical education as well as the use of a variety of incentives for practice sites and preceptors, e.g., adjunct faculty status, joint appointments, participation on curricular committees, research support, continuing education credits, and academic credit toward graduate degrees.
    - Support the development and testing of innovative APRN academic and practice regional consortia that reflect geographic and institutional diversity.
    - Develop and implement an accessible repository for APRN preceptor orientation materials.

III. **APRN clinical education and assessment should be competency based.**
    - Establish a common language or taxonomy by adopting definitions for competence, competencies, and competency framework that are recognized by APRN organizations and other health professions.

- Identify common, measurable APRN competencies that cross all four roles and build on or reaffirm the APRN core competencies (AACN, 2006).
- Progression of competence or milestones should be identified and defined across each of the common competencies.
- Develop a standardized assessment tool to be available to faculty and preceptors to use for formative and summative evaluation of the common APRN competencies.

IV. **Support the development of alternative or innovative APRN clinical education models.**
- Encourage regulatory bodies to support or allow APRN education programs to develop and test innovative or less traditional clinical models.
- Encourage APRN programs to explore, implement, and test innovative or less traditional clinical models, including interprofessional learning experiences and use of technology.
- Seek funding to support the development and evaluation of alternative or innovative APRN clinical training models.

Common Advanced Practice Registered Nurse Doctoral-Level Competencies: Report from the APRN Competency-Based Education for Doctoral-Prepared APRNs Work Group – 2017

In response to recommendation III from the AACN Task Force Report that APRN clinical education and assessment should be competency based, the AACN commissioned the APRN Competency-Based Education for Doctoral-Prepared APRNs Work Group in 2016. The work group was inclusive of members from each of the four APRN roles and representatives of 25 organizations involved in education, licensure, certification, and accreditation of APRNs. Recognizing that many of the APRN organizations had developed role-specific competencies, the goal of the work group was to develop a *common taxonomy for the doctorally prepared APRN*. Definitions adopted were common to other health professions and included:

- **Competency**: an observable ability of a health professional, integrating multiple components such as knowledge, skills, and attitudes. Since competencies are observable, they can be measured and assessed to ensure their acquisition (Frank et al., 2010).
- **Competence**: the array of abilities (knowledge, skills, and attitudes) across multiple domains or aspects of performance in a certain context. Competence is multidimensional and dynamic. It changes with time, experience, and settings (Frank et al., 2010).

Also recognizing that a common language among all health professions was essential to effective communication in collaborative practice environments, the work group adopted Englander, Cameron, Ballard, Dodge, Bull, and Aschenbrener's (2013) *Toward a Common Taxonomy of Competency Domains for the Health Professions and Competencies for Physicians*. The framework includes eight domains of competence for health professionals, also identified by the Interprofessional Education Collaborative (IPEC). The domains include:

1. Patient Care
2. Knowledge of Practice
3. Practice-based Learning and Improvement
4. Interpersonal and Communication Skills
5. Professionalism
6. Systems-based Practice
7. Interprofessional Collaboration
8. Personal and Professional Development

Each domain identifies competencies for the doctorally prepared APRN at two distinct points during the educational journey, the first when entering the first meaningful clinical experience and finally, competencies expected upon graduation. Access the Competency-Based Education report at www.aacnnursing.org /Portals/42/AcademicNursing/pdf/Common-APRN-Doctoral-Competencies.pdf.

The shift from time-based educational experience to competency-based education for health professional education is further supported by the report from the Josiah Macy Jr. Foundation (2017), *Achieving Competency-Based, Time-Variable Health Professions Education.* The report acknowledges that if the healthcare system is to meet the health needs of our nation, which include an aging population burdened by costly, complex chronic diseases, the pedagogy and curricula in health professional schools must align with the evolving realities of clinical practice. "In a competency-based, time-variable educational system, learners advance when they have demonstrated mastery of all required, previously agreed upon competencies" (p. 9).

Recommendations from the Josiah Macy Jr. Foundation report (2017) include:

1. System redesign: Curricula, learning environments, and faculty development require systematic redesign to achieve a successful competency-based, time-variable health professions education system.
2. Creating a continuum of education, training, and practice: Institutions responsible for health professions education and healthcare delivery as well as those who lead, learn, and work within them should embrace the view of health professions education as a learning continuum that spans formal education, clinical training, and professional practice.
3. Implement a robust assessment system: Leaders in health professions, schools, and their healthcare system partners should champion, develop, and implement a program of assessment that supports competency-based, time-variable training and explicitly links educational programs to improved healthcare outcomes.
4. Enabling technologies: Health professions education and healthcare delivery institutions should develop and use enabling technologies in the implementation of competency-based, time-variable education throughout the professional education continuum of the practitioner.
5. Outcomes evaluation: Competency-based, time-variable health professions education programs should be designed, implemented, and evaluated in relation to preparing their graduates to advance important societal goals, including improved patient care and improved practitioner performance and satisfaction. (p. 10)

Doctoral nursing education is at the forefront of responding to these identified societal needs with expanded doctoral level curricula, based on the AACN (2006), and in developing competency-based language and education in collaboration with other health professions.

The Implementation of the DNP Task Force Report: Current Issues and Clarifying Recommendations

The *AACN Position Statement on the Practice Doctorate in Nursing* (AACN, 2004) changed the course of nursing education by recommending that advanced nursing practice education be transitioned to the doctoral level. A decade later, the DNP degree is widely accepted as the preferred pathway for those seeking preparation at the highest level of nursing practice. Considering the changing landscape in health care and higher education over the last 10 years as well as the dramatic growth of DNP programs, the AACN Board of Directors convened the Implementation of the DNP Task Force to review the current state of DNP programs, and to provide recommendations to clarify curricular and practice expectations as outlined in the *Essentials of Doctoral Education for Advanced Nursing Practice [DNP Essentials] (*AACN, 2006).

Growing evidence exists regarding variability among program requirements for the DNP final scholarly products, including the scope of project, level of implementation, impact on system and practice outcomes, extent of collaborative efforts, dissemination of findings, and degree of faculty mentorship/oversight. Similar to other healthcare professions, nursing is faced with competition for practice sites and preceptors, complex affiliation agreements, and regulatory issues for distance learning modalities when obtaining practice experiences for DNP students. These issues were documented in the RAND report (Auerbach et al., 2014) and thoroughly explored by the task force. The white paper presents clarification as well as new and innovative ways to meet the DNP practice requirements.

The national dialogue reflects an ongoing need for clarification and restatement of the foundational concept of how *advanced nursing practice* is defined.

- *Advanced nursing practice* focuses on the provision of direct care to individual patients or populations, and the provision of indirect care such as nursing administration, executive leadership, health policy, informatics, and population health.
- The task force reaffirms that the discipline of education encompasses an entirely separate body of knowledge and competence (AACN, 2004, p. 13) and is not an area of advanced nursing practice.
- Also, it is important to remember that the DNP is an academic degree and not a role.

Implementation of the DNP Task Force Recommendations:

    I.   **DNP Graduate Scholarship**
- Graduates of both research- and practice-focused doctoral programs are prepared to generate new knowledge.
  - Practice-focused graduates are prepared to generate new knowledge through:
    1. Innovation of practice change
    2. Translation of evidence

3. Implementation of quality improvement processes in specific practice settings, systems, or with specific populations to improve health or health outcomes.

- Organizational and systems leadership knowledge and skills are critical for DNP graduates to:
  - ○ Develop and evaluate new models of care delivery.
  - ○ Create and sustain change at the organization and systems levels.
- The delineations in knowledge generation are not a hierarchical structure of importance; both are types of knowledge-generating methods.
- DNP and PhD graduates have the opportunity to improve health outcomes.

II. **DNP Project**
- The title of the final product is to be "The DNP Project."
- DNP project elements include planning, implementation, and evaluation components.
- All DNP projects should:
  - ○ Focus on a change that impacts healthcare outcomes either through direct or indirect care.
  - ○ Have a systems or population focus.
  - ○ Demonstrate implementation in the appropriate area of practice.
  - ○ Include a plan for sustainability.
  - ○ Include an evaluation of processes and/or outcomes.
  - ○ Provide a foundation for future practice scholarship.
- As mentioned, the discipline of education encompasses an entirely separate body of knowledge and competence; therefore, the focus of a DNP program, including practicum and DNP project, should not be on the educational process, the academic curriculum, or on educating nursing students.
- Integrative and systematic reviews **alone** are not considered a DNP project and do not provide opportunities for students to develop and integrate scholarship into their practice.
- A student's portfolio is not considered a DNP project but rather a tool to document learning.
- Group/team projects are acceptable when the project aims are consistent with the focus of the program.
  - ○ Each member of the group must meet all expectations of planning, implementation, and evaluation of the project, and be evaluated accordingly.
  - ○ Each student must have a leadership role in at least one component of the project and be held accountable for a deliverable.
- Dissemination of the DNP project should include a minimum of an executive summary or a written report that disseminates DNP project outcomes.
- Dissemination of the DNP project could take these forms:
  - ○ Publishing in a peer-reviewed journal, print or online
  - ○ Poster and podium presentations

- ○ Presentation of a written or verbal executive summary to stakeholders and/or the practice site/organization leadership
- ○ Development of a webinar presentation or video
- ○ Submission and publication to a non-refereed lay publication
- ○ Oral presentation to the public at large
- ○ Development and presentation of a digital poster, a grand rounds presentation, and/or a PowerPoint presentation
- The DNP project team should consist of a student or a group of students with a minimum of a doctoral prepared faculty member and a practice mentor.
- The term "DNP Project Team" should be used to minimize confusion between the PhD dissertation committee and the faculty and mentors who oversee the DNP final project.
- Evaluation of the final DNP project is the responsibility of the faculty.
- A digital repository for the DNP final projects should be used to advance nursing practice by archiving and sharing outcomes.

III. **DNP Program Expectations**
- DNP programs should provide evidence of meeting program outcomes delineated in the DNP *Essentials*.
- DNP programs should map student learning objectives to expected program outcomes and DNP *Essentials*.
- A post-baccalaureate full-time program of study should be 3 years in length, including summers, or 4 years on a traditional academic calendar.
- A post-master's program of study should be a minimum of 12 months full-time study to allow for acquisition of the doctoral-level outcomes and completion of the DNP project.
- The programs should be designed with attention to program efficiency.
- Consider new models and processes for implementing DNP project teams that provide efficient use of resources and support student learning.
- Adopt a process that allows for oversight and evaluation of DNP projects that ensures quality and equity of resources.
- Programs should provide faculty development to ensure quality student learning outcomes to include:
  - ○ Curricular design of DNP programs
  - ○ Development of new, innovative teaching strategies
  - ○ Development of innovative, new practice opportunities to support achievement of the DNP *Essentials* learning outcomes
  - ○ Strategies to support and evaluate the DNP project
  - ○ Implementation of quality improvement processes
  - ○ Interprofessional education and practice experiences
- Preparation for the nurse educator role:
  - ○ Requires additional coursework in pedagogies.
  - ○ Is not an area of advanced nursing practice.

IV.   **DNP Practice Hours**
- Practice experiences should prepare the post-baccalaureate and post-master's DNP student with the outcomes delineated in all of the DNP *Essentials*.
- Opportunities to integrate all of the *Essentials* into one's practice are imperative for both post-baccalaureate and post-master's students.
- Faculty are responsible for assessing students' learning needs and designing practice experiences that allow students to attain and demonstrate the DNP *Essentials*.
- Programs are expected to demonstrate the synthesis and application of all DNP *Essentials*.
- All DNP students, including those in post-master's programs, are expected to complete a minimum of 1,000 post-baccalaureate practice hours.
- Practice-immersion experiences afford the opportunity to apply, integrate, and synthesize the DNP *Essentials* necessary to demonstrate achievement of desired outcomes in an area of advanced nursing practice.
- Practice experiences for the DNP student are not intended to be solely direct patient-care focused but should include indirect care practices in healthcare-related environments.
- Programs must demonstrate that graduates have attained all of the DNP *Essential* outcomes.
- Students who have completed more than 1,000 practice hours in their master's program will need to complete additional hours in the DNP program.
- Practice hours spent in master's nursing programs can be counted as post-baccalaureate practice hours, provided they can be verified.
- Practice experiences should have well-defined learning objectives and provide experiences over and above the individual's job responsibilities or activities.
- Schools may credit practice hours to a post-master's DNP student who holds current national certification in an area of advanced nursing practice, as defined in the AACN 2006 DNP *Essentials*, and requires a minimum of a graduate degree.
- Post-master's students must have faculty-supervised practice hours in the DNP program that provide the opportunity for the student to integrate all of the outcomes delineated in the DNP *Essentials*.
- DNP programs should not be preparing the nurse educator; therefore, the focus of the practicum and DNP project should not be on the academic educational process, the academic curriculum, or on educating nursing students. Practice as a nurse educator should not be included in the DNP practice hours.

V.   **Collaborative Partnerships**
- Programs should follow the Academic-Practice Partnership guiding principles developed by the AACN-AONE (2012) Task Force on Academic-Practice Partnerships.
- Programs are encouraged to consider a broad range of academic-practice partnerships (e.g. with school systems, prison systems,

public health departments) that afford students opportunities to engage in the full planning, implementation, and evaluation of a project that impacts healthcare outcomes.

• Academic and practice partners are encouraged to collect outcome data to demonstrate the added value of DNP graduates.

AACN-Manatt Report: Advancing Healthcare Transformation: A New Era for Academic Nursing

In 2016, AACN released a report titled *Advancing Healthcare Transformation: A New Era for Academic Nursing,* which recommended ways to enhance nursing's contributions to improving healthcare delivery and the health of the nation. The report advanced a new definition for academic nursing as:

> . . . [e]ncompassing the integration of practice, education, and research within baccalaureate and graduate schools of nursing. Faculty engaged in academic nursing demonstrate a commitment to inquiry, generate new knowledge for the discipline, connect practice with education, and lead scholarly pursuits that improve health and health care. (AACN, 2016)

As the need for academic and clinical partnerships has intensified, so has the demand for doctoral education for advanced practice and nursing scholarship. The paradigm shift to a broader definition ensures that academic nursing scholarship is at the highest level of scholarly endeavor. Access the report at www.manatt.com /getattachment/d58fee3a-2eb1-4490-82d5-94b94d0d5331/attachment.aspx.

Defining Scholarship for Academic Nursing Task Force

In 1999, AACN's membership voted to endorse a position statement on *Defining Scholarship for the Discipline of Nursing,* which focused on four aspects of scholarship that are salient to academic nursing—discovery, teaching, applications in clinical practice, and integration of ideas from nursing and other disciplines. Given the changes that have occurred within health care and higher education since 1999, and in light of the new definition of academic nursing contained in the AACN-Manatt report, this landmark AACN position statement was revisited to ensure that it fully captures contemporary expectations related to nursing scholarship.

This AACN *Defining Scholarship for Academic Nursing Task Force* was charged to:

- Evaluate AACN's 1999 *Position Statement on Defining Scholarship for the Discipline of Nursing.*
- Propose a definition of scholarship as related to education, research, and practice that accounts for trends in new research methods, concerns for improving health, and multiple ways of knowing.
- Differentiate how nurses prepared in research-focused and practice-focused doctorates operationalize scholarship.
- Describe the integration of scholarship across institutional missions and how scholarship is promoted via improvement science, participatory action research, team science, and big data, and how it is translated to practice.

Defining Scholarship for Academic Nursing Task Force Recommendations

Colleges and universities across the nation are continually evolving to ensure that they meet the healthcare needs of the public by educating the next generation of nurses. The task force recommendations account for many contemporary issues such as the trends in new research methods, concerns for improving health, increasing demands and complexity of health care, and multiple ways of knowing.

Recommendations related to scholarship in the task force report include definition and examples of:

- Scholarship related to education, research, and practice
- Policy scholarship threaded throughout the document
- Integration of scholarship across institutional missions
- Definition of scholarship:

> Nursing scholarship is the generation, synthesis, translation, application, and dissemination of knowledge that aims to improve health and transform health care. Scholarship is the communication of knowledge generated through multiple forms of inquiry that inform clinical practice, nursing education, policy, and healthcare delivery. Scholarship is inclusive of discovery, integration, application, and teaching (Boyer, 1990). The hallmark attribute of scholarship is the cumulative impact of the scholar's work on the field of nursing and health care. (AACN, 2018b, p. 2)

This broader definition of scholarship supports recognition and value for scholarly contributions by nursing scholars in practice, service, teaching, or research. The paradigm shift expands the definition of scholarship to ensure that academic nursing is at the highest level of scholarly endeavor to improve health and transforms health care. For more detailed information on the impact of the AACN *Defining Scholarship for Academic Nursing Task Force* recommendations on the Doctor of Nursing Practice–prepared nurses, see Chapter 3, Scholarship in Practice.

▶ Trends in Support for DNP Requirement for APRN Educational Preparation

AANA Support of Doctorate for Entry into Nurse Anesthesia Practice by 2025

The American Association of Nurse Anesthetists (AANA) supports doctoral education for entry into nurse anesthesia practice by 2025. The AANA recognizes that the educational standards for nurse anesthesia programs have grown to meet the required knowledge and skills for entry into practice and doctoral education is essential to meet the extraordinary changes in today's healthcare environment. The AANA strongly supports doctoral education that includes technological and pharmaceutical advances, informatics, and evidence-based practice systems approaches to quality improvement along with other subjects that shape the future for nurse anesthetists and their patients (Doctorate of Nurse Anesthesia Practice [DNAP], 2009).

National Association of Clinical Nurse Specialists Endorses the Doctor of Nursing Practice Degree as Entry into Practice for Clinical Nurse Specialists by 2030

While the National Association of Clinical Nurse Specialists (NACNS) has consistently supported both master's and DNP preparation for entry into the clinical nurse specialist (CNS) role, considering the complex needs of patients and the future direction of nursing practice, NACNS believes that DNP preparation for practice in the CNS role will better position the CNS to meet the demands of an evolving healthcare system. Consistent with the strategic recommendations proposed to facilitate healthcare transformation, NACNS believes it is imperative to increase the number of doctoral-prepared advanced practice registered nurses (APRNs), which will increase the number of doctoral prepared nurses overall (Benner, Sutphen, Leonard, & Day, 2009; IOM, 2010). As a result, NACNS endorses the DNP degree as an important opportunity for CNS education and supports the need to increase doctoral preparation for nursing practice (IOM, 2010). See the endorsement from NACNS at www.nacns.org/advocacy-policy/position-statements /position-statement-on-the-doctor-of-nursing-practice/.

National Organization of Nurse Practitioner Faculty Support of DNP by 2025

In May 2018, the National Organization of Nurse Practitioner Faculty (NONPF) announced the support of DNP education for nurse practitioners by 2025. The organization not only committed to move all entry-level nurse practitioner (NP) education to the DNP degree by 2025, but also supports a seamless, integrated DNP curriculum without a master's exit point as preparation for entry to the NP role. NONPF has been a leader in nurse practitioner education and asserts that DNP degree reflects the rigorous education that NPs receive to lead and deliver quality health care (NONPF, 2018). See the NONPF position statement at https://c.ymcdn.com/sites /www.nonpf.org/resource/resmgr/dnp/v3_05.2018_NONPF_DNP_Stateme.pdf

▶ Summary of Trends

In summary, the trends identified confirm that DNP education is evolving, and change has occurred rapidly in recent years. The major trends relating to the practice doctorate identified are as follows:

- DNP programs are rapidly growing and changing. However, DNP student enrollments are not negatively affecting enrollment in research-focused PhD programs in nursing.
- There is a shift from programs offering only a post-master's level to DNP option to more programs adding the BSN-to-DNP option.

- The roles identified by DNP students are not only the traditional APRN clinical roles; students are also choosing a focus on nonclinical (indirect care) advanced nursing practice roles, such as nurse executive, health policy specialist, and informaticist.
- In response to the variability in DNP education, the AACN commissioned several task forces, including the Implementation of the DNP Task Force (2015b), to outline recommendations to define and clarify various aspects of DNP education.
- Most DNP programs are becoming accredited by organizations such as the Commission on Collegiate Nursing Education (CCNE), which ultimately should decrease variability in program standards.
- Academic rigor and scholarship continues to be defined for the practice doctorate because the definition of rigor and scholarship can be different from that applied to research- focused doctorates.
- Health professional education, including doctoral-level nursing education, is moving to competency-based, time-variable evaluation to produce graduates prepared for the realities of the rapidly changing practice environment.
- The move to DNP level education for APRNs is endorsed by national APRN organizations.

▶ Summary

The demands of providing health care in our country to an increasingly complex population of patients require higher levels of nursing education and practice. The practice-based doctorate in nursing, the DNP, has emerged to address the competencies that healthcare providers must have in order to apply evidence-based practice in the provision of high-quality, patient-centered care in interdisciplinary teams, using such tools as information technology. There is an emerging model of generation of knowledge by both the research and practice nursing doctorates working in teams to develop clinical knowledge and translate that knowledge into practice in a timely fashion. Nonclinical roles (indirect care) for advanced nursing practice and the traditional roles of clinical advanced nursing practice benefit from the competencies attained through doctoral-level education.

With the rapid growth of DNP programs since 2004, standardization of DNP education is emerging along with an increased number of accredited programs. In response to variability in certain aspects of DNP programs, the AACN commissioned the Implementation of the DNP Task Force to clarify recommendations regarding the DNP project, DNP educational program characteristics, and DNP practicum hour requirement, and to encourage collaborative partnerships between academia and practice. Because the DNP project is the demonstration of attainment of the *Essentials of Doctoral Education for Advanced Nursing Practice* outcomes, these guidelines from the AACN are necessary to promote high-quality and rigorous standards.

To recognize major contributions to the profession from doctoral level work, the AACN has established awards annually for outstanding research dissertations and DNP projects. In 2017, Dr. Erin Downey received the AACN Outstanding DNP Project Award for her DNP Project "Implementation of a Patient Agreement for Opioids and Stimulants in a Primary Care Practice" (see **EXEMPLAR 2-1**).

EXEMPLAR 2-1 Implementation of a Patient Agreement for Opioids and Stimulants in a Primary Care Practice

Erin Downey, DNP, MSN, MPA, BSN, RN

The dramatic increase in the consumption of controlled substances across the nation has resulted in a public health crisis with epidemic levels of medication diversion, misuse, abuse, unintentional overdose, and death. Primary care providers are often the first-line source for potentially harmful medications. Consensus is that patient agreements reduce provider risk and promote patient safety. Lack of a patient agreement places the patient, prescriber, practice, and public at risk.

My project responded to a timely practice dilemma and involved implementation of a Schedule II controlled substance patient agreement and prescribing policy in a small primary care practice. The project demonstrated that a controlled substance policy was feasible and adherence to the policy was excellent over a 7-month period. In March 2016, the Centers for Disease Control and Prevention (CDC) issued the Guideline for Prescribing Opioids, www.cdc.gov/mmwr/volumes/65/rr/rr6501e1.htm. The protocol implemented includes almost all aspects of the guideline, which increases the probability of associated costs being covered by insurance. All these factors enhance the project's sustainability. The cost of implementation was not measured directly but has proven to be minimal. In North Carolina, the prescription monitoring program is state funded with free access to registered users. All project-associated tasks such as presentation and explanation of the patient agreement and urine collection are completed within the normal workday and do not require additional man hours. All providers in the practice continue to follow the policy and are initiating patient agreements for new patients as well as following all aspects of the protocol. Monitoring for adherence is ongoing.

Dissemination of the project work included publication of a manuscript in the *Journal of Family Medicine and Primary Care* in January 2017. The journal audience is family practice providers who frequently struggle with the complexity of prescribing controlled medications. The project results were shared at an evidence-based research conference in September 2016 at UCLA. The project was presented nationally at the AACN's Doctoral Education Conference in January 2017 and received the Outstanding DNP Project Award.

The DNP program I completed requires students to design *and* implement a quality improvement project. Implementation was the key to understanding how a proposed project is translated to practice and how potential barriers can affect project implementation. The process of designing and implementing a prescription policy and patient agreement also introduced me to the intricacies of the Institutional Review Board process. Working through the implementation process allowed me to experience the importance of interdisciplinary team work, analyze data, and measure outcomes. This process provided knowledge and experience that will enhance my ability to successfully implement future projects as a DNP prepared nurse.

Key Messages

- The DNP is a degree, not a role.
- Current educational preparation for the DNP is evolving but still reflects the *Essentials* of DNP education.
- The DNP is the practice-based doctorate.

- The PhD in nursing and the DNS are the research-based doctorates.
- The collaboration between the two doctoral levels of preparation will determine the future of nursing and its impact on health care.
- The definition and education of the DNP will continue to evolve, and the DNP graduate will be a part of the evolution.
- Nurses must have an understanding of the definition of the DNP and be able to clearly articulate it.
- The *Essentials* are intertwined within DNP education, and the DNP project is the culmination/demonstration of the DNP final product/skill set.

References

American Association of Colleges of Nursing (AACN). (2004). *AACN position statement on the practice doctorate in nursing.* Washington, DC: Author.

American Association of Colleges of Nursing (AACN). (2006). *The essentials of doctoral education for advanced nursing practice.* Retrieved from http://www.aacnnursing.org/Portals/42/Publications /DNPEssentials.pdf

American Association of Colleges of Nursing (AACN). (2014). *Key differences between DNP and PhD/DNS programs.* Retrieved from http://www.aacnnursing.org/Portals/42/DNP/ ContrastGrid.pdf?ver=2017-05-25-113051-180

American Association of Colleges of Nursing (AACN). (2015a). White paper: *Current state of APRN clinical education.* Retrieved from http://www.aacnnursing.org/News-Information/APRN -Clinical-Training-Task-Force-Report-Brief

American Association of Colleges of Nursing (AACN). (2015b). *The doctor of nursing practice: Current issues and clarifying recommendations.* Retrieved from http://www.aacnnursing.org /Portals/42/News/White-Papers/DNP-Implementation-TF-Report-8-15.pdf

American Association of Colleges of Nursing (AACN). (2016). *Advancing healthcare transformation: A new era for academic nursing.* Retrieved from https://www.manatt.com/getattachment/ d58fee3a-2eb1-4490-82d5-94b94d0d5331/attachment.aspx

American Association of Colleges of Nursing (AACN). (2017). *Common advanced practice registered nurse doctoral level competencies.* Retrieved from http://www.aacnnursing.org/Portals/42 /AcademicNursing/pdf/Common-APRN-Doctoral-Competencies.pdf

American Association of Colleges of Nursing (AACN). (2018a). *Custom report on doctoral program enrollments, 2005–2017.* Washington, DC: AACN Research and Data Services.

American Association of Colleges of Nursing (AACN). (2018b). *Defining scholarship for academic nursing.* Task Force Consensus Position Statement. Retrieved from http://www.aacnnursing .org/Portals/42/News/Position-Statements/Defining-Scholarship.pdf

American Association of Colleges of Nursing-American Organization of Nurse Executives (AACN-AONE) Task Force on Academic-Practice Partnerships. (2012). *Guiding principles to academic-practice partnerships.* Retrieved from http://www.aacnnursing.org/Academic -Practice-Partnerships/The-Guiding-Principles

APRN Joint Dialogue Group and the National Council of State Boards of Nursing (NCSBN) APRN Advisory Committee. (2008). *Consensus model for APRN regulation: Licensure, accreditation, certification & education.* Retrieved from https://www.ncsbn.org/Consensus_Model_for _APRN_Regulation_July_2008.pdf

Auerbach, D., Martsolf, G., Pearson, M., Taylor, E., Zaydman, M., & Muchow, A., . . . Dower, C. (2014). *The DNP by 2015: A study of the institutional, political, and professional issues that facilitate or impede establishing a post-baccalaureate doctor of nursing practice program.* Retrieved from http://www.aacnnursing.org/Portals/42/DNP/DNP-Study.pdf?ver=2017-08-01-105854-190

Benner, P., Sutphen, M., Leonard, V., & Day, L. (2009, December 9). *Educating nurses: A call for radical transformation.* San Francisco, CA: Jossey-Bass.

Boyer, E. (1990). *Scholarship reconsidered: Priorities of the professoriate.* Carnegie Foundation for the Advancement of Teaching. New York, NY: John Wiley & Sons.

Carraccio, C., & Englander, R. (2013). From Flexner to competencies: Reflections on a decade and the journey ahead. *Academic Medicine, 88*(8), 1067–1073.

Carraccio, C., Wolfsthal, S. D., Englander, R., Ferentz, K., & Martin, C. (2002). Shifting paradigms: From Flexner to competencies. *Academic Medicine, 77,* 361–367.

Chism, L. A. (2019). *The doctor of nursing practice: A guidebook for role development and professional issues. 4th edition.* Burlington, MA: Jones & Bartlett Learning.

Dentzer, S. (2011). Still crossing the quality chasm—or suspended over it?" *Health Affairs, 30(4),* 554–555. doi:10.1377/hlthaff.2011.0287

Doctorate of Nurse Anesthesia Practice (DNAP) (2009). *AANA announces support of doctorate for entry into nurse anesthesia practice (DNAP) by 2025.* Retrieved from http://www.dnap.com/

Englander, R., Cameron, T, Ballar, A. J., Dodge, J, Bull, J, & Aschenbrener, C. A. (2013). Toward a taxonomy of competency domains for health professions and competencies for physicians. *Academic Medicine, 88(8),* 1088–1094.

Frank J. R., Snell, L. S, Cate, O. T., Holmboe, E. S., Carraccio, C., & Swing, S.R., . . . Harris, K. A. (2010). Competency-based medical education: Theory to practice. *Medical Teacher, 32(8),* 638–645.

Institute of Medicine (IOM). (2001). *Crossing the quality chasm: A new health system for the 21st century.* Washington, DC: National Academies Press. Retrieved from http://www .nationalacademies.org/hmd/~/media/Files/Report%20Files/2001/Crossing-the-Quality -Chasm/Quality%20Chasm%202001%20%20report%20brief.pdf

Institute of Medicine (IOM). (2003). *Health professions education: A bridge to quality.* Washington, DC: National Academies Press. Retrieved from http://www.nap.edu/openbook.php?record_id =10681&page=45

Institute of Medicine (IOM). (2010). *The future of nursing: Leading change, advancing health.* Washington, DC: National Academies Press.

Josiah Macy Jr. Foundation (2017). *Achieving competency-based, time-variable health professions education.* Retrieved from http://macyfoundation.org/publications/publication/conference -summary-achieving-competency-based-time-variable-education

Lamb, G. (2012, January). *Interprofessional initiatives in doctoral nursing education: The ASU experience.* Presented at the AACN Doctoral Conference, San Diego, CA.

McKinney, M. (2011, February 21). About that quality chasm. *Modern Healthcare.* Retrieved from http://www.modernhealthcare.com/article/20110221/MAGAZINE/110219950

National Association of Clinical Nurse Specialists (NACNS) (2016). *Position statement on the doctor of nursing practice.* Retrieved from http://nacns.org/advocacy-policy/position-statements /position-statement-on-the-doctor-of-nursing-practice/

National Organization of Nurse Practitioner Faculties (NONPF) (2018). *The doctor of nursing practice degree: Entry to nurse practitioner practice by 2025.* Retrieved from https://c.ymcdn .com/sites/www.nonpf.org/resource/resmgr/dnp/v3_05.2018_NONPF_DNP_Stateme.pdf

Office for the Assistant Secretary for Planning and Evaluation (ASPE). (2015). *Health insurance coverage and the affordable care act, September 2015.* Retrieved from https://aspe.hhs.gov /pdf-report/health-insurance-coverage-and-affordable-care-act-september-2015

CHAPTER 3

Scholarship in Practice

Rosanne Burson

CHAPTER OVERVIEW

To appreciate the doctor of nursing practice (DNP) project, there must be an understanding of both practice and scholarship. This chapter reveals the history of scholarship as it supports the developing nature of the practice doctorate and knowledge generation. The purpose of the DNP project is defined, and the current view of potential projects is presented. Several exemplars highlight the process of developing the DNP project and the impact of the process on the DNP student. Finally, recommended action steps are offered in considering project topics.

CHAPTER OBJECTIVES

After completing the chapter, the learner will be able to:

1. Define scholarship as it relates to the practice doctorate.
2. Explore the historical underpinnings that have evolved nursing's view of knowledge generation.
3. Critique the evolution of practice scholarship and its impact on the DNP project and health outcomes.
4. Review the current state of DNP projects.
5. Conceptualize the types of projects that can be and are being considered.
6. Begin to examine potential topics of interest in relation to the appropriate level of scholarship.

▶ What Is Scholarship?

An investigation of scholarship as it relates to history, and specifically to nursing practice, contributes to the understanding of the DNP project as practice scholarship. Scholarship is defined in *Merriam-Webster's Learner's Dictionary* as "serious formal study or research of a subject" ("Scholarship," 2018, para. 2). Evidence from the nursing literature confirms that scholarship is a critical feature of our continuing survival and implies a unique knowledge base (Bunkers, 2000; Fawcett, 1999). Magnan (2019) identified "three recurring themes in the literature regarding nursing scholarship as (a) breadth and depth of knowledge within a defined area, (b) innovation and creativity, and (c) exposure of the scholarly project to public scrutiny and peer review" (p. 103–104). As the DNP student considers topics for scholarly work, an assessment of the topic in relation to these themes will assist in ensuring a project that meets the expectations of scholarly work.

Scholarship is the mechanism that provides knowledge development within a discipline. Knowledge production is measured according to its contribution to improved outcomes rather than its contribution to generalizable knowledge (Rolfe & Davies, 2009). The development of the clinical scholar in knowledge generation in the practice setting is continuing to evolve. (American Association of Colleges of Nursing [AACN], 2015a, National Organization of Nurse Practitioner Faculties [NONPF], 2016; Rolfe, 2018). This is validated by the complexity of evidence-based practice and the need for practice inquiry (Brown & Crabtree, 2013). What this means for the DNP student is that the work that is done in relation to improving outcomes for patients and healthcare systems is increasingly viewed as *new* knowledge that is important and will be accrued and shared to produce further improvements. This is a big change in what historically has been accepted as knowledge generation.

Ferguson-Pare predicted in 2005 that future nurses would be practice scholars driven by emerging trends in patient-centered care. She stated, "This is the time for nursing to embrace scholarly activities and to engage in continuous teaching-learning, research, and scholarly inquiry in our practice. The emergence of practice scholars in nursing will assure a future for the profession" (p. 120). That future is here, driven by forces internal and external to nursing that are demanding nursing's full contribution to improving health. It is a time of opportunity and potential.

Important external forces have contributed to the movement of incorporating practice more deeply in scholarship. As has been discussed in earlier chapters, the Institute of Medicine (IOM) has been a key driver to instrumental change in health care. The IOM reports have identified the lack of quality and safety within our health systems and a need for fundamental change that supports a redesigned system focused on quality outcomes that use evidence, information technology, organizational support, and the alignment of payment policy (IOM, 1999, 2001, 2012). In 2010, the IOM produced the report *The Future of Nursing*, which stated that nurses should practice to the full extent of their training and be full partners in redesigning health care. Evidence-based care, high-quality outcomes, and cost containment are required

> *Scholarship is the mechanism that provides knowledge development within a discipline.*

components of healthcare reform and transformation. While these concepts are applied to populations, systems, and policy, the individual patient must also be considered in expert practice. Precision nursing that incorporates the genomic patterns, lifestyle, and social determinants of health needs to be considered to provide a unique patient experience as well as great potential for nursing practice scholarship. The practice scholar balances the individual, specific approach of each patient with population- and system-based needs to create a healing, efficient environment.

It is time to expand the nursing repertoire to incorporate a broader base of knowledge that includes, but reaches beyond, the clinical focus.

Nursing's expertise and input are critical at this time but must be provided at an appropriate level of scholarship to be an optimal and valued contribution. It is time to expand the nursing repertoire to incorporate a broader base of knowledge that includes, but reaches beyond, the clinical focus. In 2006, Kitson reflected on her 1999 article regarding scholarship in practice in the *Journal of Advanced Nursing*: "But what we need now is the political and business acumen to improve and integrate our academic and practice infrastructures to enable nursing scholarship and nursing innovation to flourish" (p. 545). The *Essentials* of DNP education serve to further drive the nature of the practice doctorate to lead healthcare

The ability to develop innovations specific to health incorporates all the components of DNP practice, including collaboration, informatics, business, and political aspects.

systems. Each of the DNP *Essentials* contributes by strengthening the student's core knowledge skill set. The ability to develop innovations specific to health incorporates all the components of DNP practice, including collaboration, informatics, business, and political aspects. As the doctoral student develops a DNP project, identifying the specific *Essentials* that will be demonstrated in the project can confirm evidence of doctoral-level work.

The demonstration of doctoral work is important to the validation of the educational degree, the potential for leadership, and effective knowledge development that affects healthcare outcomes.

▶ History of Scholarship and Nursing Practice

Nursing has explored and struggled with critical aspects of practice as they relate to scholarship over many years. The doctor of nursing science (DNSc) was presented in 1970 with an emphasis on advanced clinical practice and was an early effort to give nursing parity with other disciplines. The DNSc required both clinical competence *and* demonstrated ability to perform scholarly research. In 1979, the doctor of nursing (ND) degree emerged. Again, parity with other health professional doctoral programs, such as medicine, dentistry, optometry, and others, was sought. However, the ND focused exclusively on the advanced clinical aspects rather than research (AACN, 2004). *The doctorate of nursing practice (DrNP)* evolved to also focus on advanced clinical expertise and was geared

> *Societal needs are driving scholarship to develop knowledge that affects outcomes.*

toward preparing *nurse practitioners* for independent primary care roles. Today, the DNP-prepared nurse concentrates on evidence-based practice (EBP) for improved delivery of care, patient outcomes, and clinical systems management (AACN, 2004) within unique organizations that are served. The DNP is considered a practice doctorate and is *inclusive* of all advanced nursing practice roles: nurse practitioner, nurse-midwife, nurse anesthetist, and clinical nurse specialist, as well as nurse administrator, nurse informaticist, and nurse policy expert.

Over the years, there have been many barriers to full implementation of the practice doctorate. One barrier was the lack of a broader view of scholarship beyond generalizable knowledge. Previously, it had been assumed that knowledge generation could only be elicited from a quantitative research process. However, today, societal needs are driving scholarship to develop knowledge that affects outcomes. The current healthcare environment is in need of leaders that demonstrate ability and effectiveness to transition current health systems to patient-centered, cost-effective systems. The DNP-prepared nurse is equipped with the skill set to take on this challenge (Reed and Brewer, 2018; Terharr and Sylvia, 2016). This demonstration begins with the DNP project and will expand as the DNP-prepared nurse continues to impact practice.

▶ Scholarship Evolution

It is important for the DNP-prepared nurse to have an understanding of the evolution of scholarship. Many brilliant minds have paved the way for this progression. The significance of this evolution has been critical to the current state of the practice doctorate in nursing and the ability to have an impact on population outcomes.

During the early to middle part of the 20th century, empirical science was viewed as the only way to generate knowledge. Quantitative research was regaled as the highest level of truth. This had been demonstrated in the hierarchy of types of research and in the predominance of quantitative research. However, the scientific/laboratory view of controlling for variables has been difficult to transition to practice. This separation of research and practice has limited our ability to integrate new knowledge into practice and for practice to have an important influence on research. Increasingly, it is understood that the complexities of health care cannot always be explained via a single model of research. Nursing's holistic history implores a view of knowledge through multiple lenses.

A broadening of the view of scholarship has occurred over the last quarter century. For example, qualitative research added to the understanding of many phenomena and became more relevant and accepted as a format to generate new knowledge. One of the most significant contributions to the broadening of scholarship was developed by Ernest Boyer. In his classic book, *Scholarship Reconsidered:*

Priorities of the Professoriate (1990), Boyer established an inclusive view of scholarship consisting of discovery, teaching, practice, and integration. He asked, "How can the role of the scholar be defined in ways that not only affirm the past but also reflect the present and adequately anticipate the future?" (p. 75). This reflective quote should guide scholars in respecting knowledge generation of the past. At the same time, the scholar should be encouraged to develop and accept new methods to meet the needs of new knowledge generation. Boyer suggested moving beyond the usual way of looking at scholarship in a narrow view of original research and to consider *how useful the work is for society*. It is no longer enough to develop knowledge for knowledge's sake; now the requirement is to investigate how the scholarship relates to the world.

New ideas are evolving about this relationship between theory and practice that defines truth for a discipline (Reed & Shearer, 2018). The outcome of scholarship and knowledge generation should be a positive result for society. Scholars with a variety of strengths and perspectives will be required to participate in these more complex approaches, using each other's strengths as in a network.

In 1999, the AACN published the position paper *Defining Scholarship for the Discipline of Nursing*. The paper confirms a view of the evolution of scholarship to include discovery, teaching, application in clinical practice, and integration of ideas. The report identified that the four areas of scholarship developed by Boyer were important to the values of the profession of nursing. These values include a commitment to scientific advancement and recognition of its significance for society. This argument is very applicable in nursing because of the demands of practice and the commitment to the public to incorporate the latest research in the delivery of care. In addition, these values highlight the integrated relationship between theory, research, and practice. This view was confirmed and expanded in 2018 with the completion of the AACN task force report, *Defining Scholarship for Academic Nursing*. In this report, a broader definition of scholarship was described to be inclusive of all nursing scholars.

> *"How can the role of scholar be defined in ways that not only affirm the past but also reflect the present and adequately anticipate the future?" (Boyer, 1990, p. 75).*
>
> *Scholars with a variety of strengths and perspectives will be required to participate in these more complex approaches, using each other's strengths as in a network.*

> Nursing scholarship is the generation, synthesis, translation, application, and dissemination of knowledge that aims to improve health and transform health care. Scholarship is the communication of knowledge generated through multiple forms of inquiry that inform clinical practice, nursing education, policy, and healthcare delivery. (AACN, 2018, p. 2)

Over the last decade, differentiation between the research scholar and practice scholar was defined in the following manner. As the research scholar (PhD) defines and tests new theories that are generalizable to populations, the practice scholar (DNP) will apply them within a local context and measure their applicability within settings (translation and implementation science). The PhD-prepared nurse generates external evidence through rigorous research to extend science and theory and guide practice. The DNP-prepared nurse generates internal evidence through outcomes management, quality improvement, and EBP projects that translate external evidence into practice and policy to improve care and outcomes (Melnyk, 2013). However, these distinctions are blurred with the collaboration of PhD/DNP teams that inform discovery and progress to application, integration, engagement, and optimization in the context of the organization or population served (Velasquez, McArthur, & Johnson, 2018). Both types of scholars contribute to knowledge generation and are interdependent to fully impact health. The worth of the contribution and collaboration of both practice and research are increasingly understood and valued (National League of Nurses [NLN] Board of Governors, 2018). There is a developing understanding that both practitioner and scientist play a role in research and theory development. Neither is exclusive of the other and both contribute to knowledge development from their specific perspective (Velasquez, McArthur, & Johnson, 2018).

This new approach to knowledge generation is a critical feature of how the doctorally prepared nurse will move forward. "The practice doctorate in nursing has helped stimulate movement away from strict adherence to traditional methods of research with new models of clinical knowledge generation and practice being envisioned" (Reed & Shearer, 2018, p. 49). Practice scholarship demonstrates that new knowledge is built on both sides of the bridge. Implementation science is highlighted in the scholarship of the DNP-prepared nurse. DNP scholarship generates new knowledge through practice change innovation, translation of evidence, and quality improvement processes that may be transferable to other contexts but not generalizable. PhD scholarship generates new knowledge through research and statistical methodologies that may be broadly applicable (AACN, 2015a). Convergence of the concepts of research from both the practice and science realms is expected to move forward to impact health.

All areas of knowledge generation need to support each other in order to have an impact on science advancement and society. Reed and Shearer (2018) discussed the relationship between theory and practice, stating that "theory will not so much be applied or disseminated from research to practice as it will emerge from scholarly thinking in practice, and then continue to be transformed as practice contexts change" (p. 40). **FIGURE 3-1** visually captures the integration of knowledge generation

FIGURE 3-1 The relationship among theory, research, and practice.

Modified from McEwen, M., & Wills, E. M. (2018). *Theoretical basis for nursing*. Philadelphia, PA: Wolters Kluwer Health/Lippincott Williams & Wilkins.

through research, practice, and theory. Note that all aspects affect the others and are affected by each other. This depiction suggests that various types of scholars need to interact at their highest level of skill to allow the network to function at its highest capacity and have the greatest societal impact.

▶ Types of Scholarship

Boyer (1990) defined the scholarship of *discovery* as original research. Discovery scholarship typically reflects the historical view of knowledge generation of research and theory development, which has been the work of the PhD research nurse. Four phases of knowledge development have been described by Velasquez, McArthur, and Johnson (2018) in an effort to qualify all aspects of scholarly activity within the doctoral work of both PhD and DNP. The first two phases tease out different aspects of discovery. The *exploration phase* incorporates knowledge discovery in both quantitative and qualitative avenues. This terminology aligns with AACN's (1999, 2018) applied definition of discovery scholarship to include empirical and historical research, theory development, methodological studies, and philosophical inquiry and analysis. The term *explication* is described as theory evaluation, also identified by AACN within the discovery component of scholarship. The first two phases of knowledge development fit well with the definition of discovery scholarship and suggest an overlap between practice and research nursing doctorates.

The scholarship of *integration* (Boyer, 1990) is "serious, disciplined work that seeks to interpret, draw together, and bring new insight to bear on original research" (p. 19). Within nursing, the scholarship of integration includes interfaces between nursing and other disciplines. Some products of this level of scholarship include integrative reviews of the literature, analysis of health policy, development of interdisciplinary educational programs and service projects, studies of systems in health care, original interdisciplinary research, and integrative models or paradigms across disciplines (AACN, 1999, 2018). Nursing's history as a collaborator and team player makes scholarship of integration a natural fit. Nursing's understanding of theory based in multiple disciplines also contributes to this fit. However, nursing will need to continue to step up to the table, using higher levels of analysis to be considered a *team leader* who can fully develop as the IOM has envisioned.

The scholarship of integration refers to writings and other products that use concepts and original works from nursing and other disciplines in creating new patterns. Integration places knowledge in a larger context and illuminates data in a more meaningful way. The scholarship of integration emphasizes the interconnection of ideas and brings new insight to bear on original concepts and research (Boyer, 1990). Original work in the scholarship of integration

> *Nursing's history as a collaborator and team player makes scholarship of integration a natural fit. Nursing will need to continue to step up to the table, using higher levels of analysis to be considered a team leader.*

takes place between two or more disciplines. Integration combines knowledge in new creative applications that change paradigms and offer keen insights to solve problems. The scholarship of integration has great potential to be a key aspect of practice scholarship because of its collaborative nature and outcome focus.

The scholarship of *application* focuses on these questions: "How can knowledge be applied to consequential problems? How can it be helpful to individuals as well as institutions? Can social problems themselves define an agenda for scholarly investigation?" (Boyer, 1990, p. 22). Thoun (2009) encouraged a look beyond Boyer's work in defining practice scholarship and suggested, "This pattern of scholarship involves systematic inquiry of professional practice that is imaginative, artistic, and resourceful" (p. 555).

Application scholarship is related to practice issues. Some of the works included in application scholarship are analysis of patient or health services outcomes, reports of clinical demonstration projects, and policy papers related to practice. Other examples include the measurement of quality-of-life indicators, the development and refinement of practice protocols and strategies, the evaluation of systems of care, and the analysis of innovative healthcare delivery models (AACN, 1999, 2018).

Velasquez, McArthur, and Johnson (2018) further described levels of knowledge development that can be identified with integration and application. The terms used to describe aspects of knowledge development related to integration and application are *engagement* and *optimization*. Engagement incorporates implementation, evaluation, and dissemination of knowledge. Types of work within engagement include program evaluation and quality improvement. Optimization is described as a revising and refinement of interventions. Within the conceptual model of knowledge generation, there is an understanding that overlap and mutual support will exist within doctoral scholarship. Knowledge generation is not hierarchal but is shared with contributions from practice and research.

Within the conceptual model of knowledge generation, there is an understanding that overlap and mutual support will exist within doctoral scholarship.

Knowledge generation is not hierarchal but is shared with contributions from practice and research.

Scholarship activities will continue to develop within integration and application and will begin to converge because both aspects are needed in a scholarly practice environment.

Scholarship activities will continue to develop within integration and application and will begin to converge because both aspects are needed in a scholarly practice environment. The complex nature of health systems as they affect patient outcomes will require an integrated, interdisciplinary approach within the application of practice. The DNP-prepared nurse, focused in these areas of scholarship, is expected to participate within this environment.

▶ Practice Scholarship and Nursing Theory

Practice scholarship has been infused in nursing throughout nursing history. Early nursing scholars include Florence Nightingale, who used data in her clinical explanations to improve patient care. "Nurses such as Virginia Henderson brought nursing education and practice closer by concentrating on the relationship between nurses and patients rather than on the intricacies of procedures and manual skills" (Fairman, 2008, p. 4). Scholarship has been intricately woven with societal needs as well. Nursing knowledge continued to be framed by clinical experience. Patients who would not have survived previously began to suffer from chronic diseases. "Much of the practice scholarship that emerged in the 1950s through the 1970s was . . . a response to nurses' demands for knowledge to safely care for patients, experientially based to organize the complexity of clinical situations" (Fairman, 2008, p. 4).

In the past few years, clinical inquiry has become a first step in development toward evidence-based practice. Clinical inquiry identifies knowledge gaps. Expert nurses ask questions that relate to patient outcomes. This process involves questioning and evaluating. "In the EBP paradigm, clinical expertise is combined with best scientific evidence, patient values and preferences and the clinical circumstance" (Salmond, 2007, p. 114). The value of this distinction is the unique contribution of the practice expert to understand both the

Practice is a key source of knowledge application and knowledge development.

evidence and the individual patient. It is clear that links among practice, nursing theory, and research need to be further developed and that practice is a key source of knowledge application and knowledge development.

Reed and Brewer (2018) explained strategies for theorizing that include concepts such as guerilla theorizing, bricoleur, and improvisation. *Guerilla theorizing* is making something that is innovative, flexible, and impermanent, derived from the practitioner's inspiration and knowledge, ethical concern, and interaction with the immediate world. The practice scholar knows that understanding the context of the care delivery directly affects the impact on outcome. Consideration of each unique situation creates a specific plan of action that is inclusive. *Bricoleur* is creating a new coherent structure from what is at hand. Drawing on knowledge and experiences, the practice scholar considers multiple sources to create an innovation that improves care delivery. *Improvisation* is creation out of existing elements in the moment. Just as the jazz musician improvises in the moment to create a beautiful sound, the practice scholar creates a strategy from known elements to effect success within a local context. These strategies are rooted in the scholarship of integration and application and are examples of knowledge generation within practice. Nursing practice has often used strategies to affect outcomes. However, there is newfound power in the description of the processes that occur in practice-based knowledge generation. The scholarly nature of this application also demands dissemination of the local knowledge. Dissemination will be further discussed in Chapter 15, Disseminating the Results.

TABLE 3-1 shows combined similar descriptions of types of scholarship and knowledge generation in an effort to assist the DNP student in considering types of scholarship for the DNP project and differentiating PhD scholarship.

TABLE 3-1 Types of Scholarship and Knowledge Generation

Types of Scholarship/ Knowledge Generation	Definition	Examples
Discovery	■ Original research	■ Empirical and historical research
Exploration	■ Quantitative/qualitative	■ Theory development and testing
Explication	■ Theory testing	■ Methodological studies ■ Philosophical inquiry and analysis
Integration	■ New insight on original research ■ Interfaces between nursing and a variety of disciplines ■ Creating new patterns, placing knowledge in a larger context, or illuminating the data in a more meaningful way	■ Integrative reviews of the literature ■ Analysis of health policy ■ Development of interdisciplinary educational programs and service projects ■ Studies of systems in health care, including program development and evaluation
Bricoleur	■ Creating knowledge or combining knowledge in applications that offer new paradigms and insights	■ Original interdisciplinary research ■ Integrative models or paradigms across disciplines

Types of Scholarship/ Knowledge Generation	Definition	Examples
Application	■ Related to practice issues and outcomes ■ Knowledge applied to problems	■ Analysis of patient or health services ■ Outcomes reports of clinical demonstration projects
Engagement	■ Implementation/ evaluation dissemination of knowledge	■ Policy papers related to practice ■ Assessment and validation of patient-care outcomes
Optimization	■ Revising and refinement of interventions	■ Measurement of quality indicators
Guerilla theorizing	■ Local interaction to make something innovative and flexible	■ Development and refinement of practice protocols/strategies ■ Evaluation of systems of care
Improvisation	■ Creating something new in the moment out of preexisting elements	■ Analysis of innovative healthcare delivery models ■ Program evaluation ■ Quality improvement ■ Clinical inquiry ■ Translation of EBP
Teaching	■ Centers on student learning ■ Entices future scholars ■ Dissemination of existing knowledge ■ Creation of new knowledge through interaction	■ Research related to teaching methodology or learning outcomes ■ Learning theory development ■ Development or testing of educational models or theories ■ Successful applications of technology to teaching and learning ■ Design of outcome studies or evaluation/assessment

Data from concepts in AACN, 1999, 2018; Boyer, 1990; Melnyk, 2013; Reed & Shearer, 2018; Velasquez, McArthur, & Johnson, 2018.

To demonstrate the ability of the DNP student in using clinical expertise, EBP, and the *Essentials* of DNP education to create an innovation, the following project is described.

Two DNP students proposed an innovation of care within the primary care arena for patients with diabetes. This short story illustrates how the students progressed in the development of the DNP project. Their extensive clinical background as advanced practice nurses, diabetes program managers, and certified diabetes educators (CDEs) had given them a deep understanding of diabetes care, education, and management. The skill set at their disposal included knowledge of the scope and standards of care of diabetes education and care; proven competencies as diabetes educators; years of team interdisciplinary collaborations; experiences in the field around the country observing the primary care environment; and finance and management skills from experience in industry, entrepreneurial efforts, and management. Personal experiences with diabetes and family members also added to the conglomeration of strengths.

As the two students progressed through doctoral education, they continued to build on their original strengths and developed new skills, particularly in the areas of data mining, implementation science, outcome management, and policy. They continued to examine their phenomena of interest through multiple, varied lenses, and they explored their topic of interest within the literature. The students began to integrate (connect the dots) all of what they knew and were continuing to learn. Gaps and needs were identified that could support a primary care innovation that had the potential for clinical and cost-effectiveness. All the pieces of the intervention were built from known parts but redesigned in a new way.

The DNP project was titled *Exploring the Cost and Clinical Outcomes of Integrating the Registered Nurse–Certified Diabetes Educator in the Patient-Centered Medical Home* (Moran, Burson, Critchett, & Olla, 2011).

The type of scholarship described is one of integration and application. It was interdisciplinary and focused on practice outcomes that included financial and clinical viability. The project interfaced nursing with multiple disciplines and exemplified teamwork and collaboration. Multiple theories were used to build the framework of the innovation. These included chaos theory, caring science, and Donabedian's quality improvement model. The project was specific to practice issues and outcomes reporting on a multiplicity of clinical and psychological measures, as well as cost features. The term *bricoleur* accurately explains this process of combining knowledge applications to offer new paradigms and insights. The success of this project moved the scholarship team into an entrepreneurial business venture to further expand and develop the innovation.

It is important to understand that this process occurred over 2 years of study. The DNP student will bring personal strengths and experiences to the table and will expand the possibilities through new knowledge, skill sets, and views. The process takes time, and ideas will change and develop as the scholarly project takes shape. Patience and

> *The DNP student will bring personal strengths and experiences to the table and will expand the possibilities through new knowledge, skill sets, and views.*

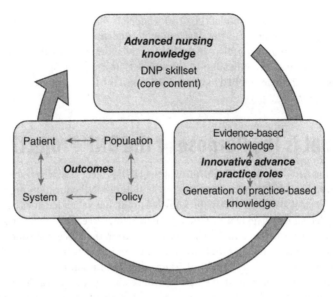

FIGURE 3-2 Actualized DNP model.

Reproduced from Burson, R., Moran, K. J., & Conrad, D. (2016). Why hire a DNP prepared nurse? The value-added impact of the practice doctorate. *Journal of Doctoral Nursing Practice, 9*(1), 152–157.

perseverance are important characteristics of the DNP student as doctoral education is experienced and transforms the student.

The previous exemplar can be reviewed in the context of the Actualized DNP model (see **FIGURE 3-2**). The Actualized DNP model explores how the unique skill set of the nurse prepared with a practice doctorate is able to apply advanced practice knowledge in existing and new nursing roles that lead to achievement of healthcare outcomes (Burson, Moran, & Conrad, 2016).

Advanced nursing knowledge refers to achievement of the DNP *Essentials* that prepares experts in advanced nursing practice and implementation science and leaders in applying research in order to improve practice (AACN, 2006; Burson, Moran, & Conrad, 2016; Cary & George, 2011; Levin & Slyder, 2012). Clinical knowledge includes leadership abilities, a focus on nursing theory, clinical management, coordination of care, information technology utilization, interprofessional collaboration, and business and policy acumen (Burson, Moran, & Conrad, 2016; Draye, Acker, & Zimmer, 2006; Swanson & Stanton, 2013).

In enacting advanced nursing roles incorporating this unique skill set, the practice doctorate uses an EBP application component that generates new knowledge in practice (practice-based evidence) (Burson, Moran, & Conrad, 2016). Implementation science is used to promote the integration of research science and evidence into healthcare policy and practice (National Institutes of Health, 2015).

As the DNP-prepared nurse functions within organizations using a unique skill set and advanced knowledge bases, data are used to drive innovation and measure outcomes, not only for individuals and populations but also systems and policy outcomes. This demonstrates practice scholarship achieving healthcare reform goals to improve healthcare quality while decreasing costs (Burson, Moran, & Conrad, 2016).

The Actualized DNP model (Figure 3-2) depicts the DNP project, demonstrating many of the *Essentials* in the development, implementation, and evaluation of the project. Note that each sphere identifies the collaborative work that was required for this project and its connection to the appropriate *Essential*. See more about the Actualized DNP model applied to various aspects of the DNP-prepared nurse's practice in Chapter 16.

▶ What Is the Purpose of the DNP Project?

In 2006, the AACN defined the purpose of the DNP project as a deliverable of accumulation of knowledge and summative evaluation of DNP education process. The scholarly project also adds to nursing knowledge and has value that goes beyond the program deliverable. The DNP curriculum contributes to each of the competencies that are then demonstrated in the DNP project. Within the process of education and knowledge synthesis, the *Essentials* are integrated and demonstrated (AACN, 2006). The *Essentials* exemplify a thoughtful contribution and roadmap of the competencies the nursing scholar must exemplify to have an impact on health care from a nursing perspective. The DNP *Essentials* are presented and described in Chapter 2, Defining the Doctor of Nursing Practice: Current Trends, and are listed in **TABLE 3-2**. Doctoral coursework supports the DNP *Essentials* and the development of the new knowledge and skill set for the DNP student. The coursework also offers the student an opportunity to explore his or her topic of interest within each of the *Essentials*.

TABLE 3-2 Doctor of Nursing Practice *Essentials*

I	Scientific Underpinnings for Practice
II	Organizational and Systems Leadership for Quality Improvement and Systems Thinking
III	Clinical Scholarship and Analytical Methods for Evidence-Based Practice
IV	Information Systems/Technology and Patient Care Technology for the Improvement and Transformation of Health Care
V	Health Care Policy for Advocacy in Health Care
VI	Interprofessional Collaboration for Improving Patient and Population Health Outcomes
VII	Clinical Prevention and Population Health for Improving the Nation's Health
VIII	Advanced Nursing Practice

Data from American Association of Colleges of Nursing (AACN). (2006). *The essentials of doctoral education for advanced nursing practice*. Retrieved from http://www.aacnnursing.org/Portals/42/Publications/DNPEssentials.pdf

Taking the preceding example, the patient-centered diabetes project, to the next step demonstrates the connection to the DNP *Essentials*. See **FIGURE 3-3**, which depicts the DNP project plan and the facilitation of multiple team collaborations. In the center is the patient, depicting patient-centered chronic disease management related to DNP *Essential* I: Scientific Underpinnings for Practice. This *Essential* drove the development of the intervention based on empirical knowledge of disease process, educational principles, and caring science. This core also incorporates DNP *Essential* VIII: Advanced Nursing Practice. The DNP connects the dots among practice, organizational, population, fiscal, and policy issues to develop the intervention.

The DNP Essentials *exemplify a thoughtful contribution and roadmap of the competencies the nursing scholar must exemplify to have an impact on health care from a nursing perspective.*

The top icon, Physician Health Organization (PHO), illustrates multiple *Essentials*. Within this collaboration, the DNP demonstrates organizational and systems leadership in order to develop the innovation (*Essential* II: Organizational and

Care Delivery Innovation

FIGURE 3-3 Model of DNP scholarly project *Essentials*.
PHO: Physician Health Organization; CDE: Certified Diabetes Educator; MODE: Michigan Organization of Diabetes Educators.

Systems Leadership for Quality Improvement and Systems Thinking). It was also at this level that *Essential* IV: Information Systems/Technology was used to assess data before and after intervention, as well as population health data that were used specific to each practice (*Essential* VII: Clinical Prevention and Population Health for Improving the Nation's Health).

Moving clockwise, health plan collaboration occurred to evaluate the current reimbursement and revenue-generating contributions that could assist in making the project viable in the long term (*Essential* II). Collaboration also occurred with CDEs, primary care providers, and staff within the primary care setting using *Essential* VI: Interprofessional Collaboration for Improving Patient and Population Health Outcomes. The Michigan Organization of Diabetes Educators (MODE) was a part of the networking that occurred to identify interest in and the knowledge base of CDEs in the patient-centered medical home (PCMH) strategies.

Of course, the process of developing the proposal, achieving Institutional Review Board (IRB) status, and analyzing the data is evidence of *Essential* III: Clinical Scholarship and Analytical Methods for Evidence-Based Practice. Advanced nursing practice (*Essential* VIII) was demonstrated in mentoring registered nurses and the office staff, as well as the providers, in transforming care within the practice.

Seven of the eight *Essentials* were identified in this project plan. The completion of the project and the knowledge derived could then be used to promote *Essential* V: Health Care Policy for Advocacy in Health Care. Although not every project will exemplify all the *Essentials*, the student should consider the elements that will be used in order to effectively develop and implement the DNP project. It is the systems approach—focused on data, outcomes, finance, and clinical measures—that will promote both the skills of the DNP-prepared nurse and attainment of healthcare transformation.

The DNP project incorporates practice and scholarship. There is an emerging realization that scholarship requires the integration of practice in a practice discipline. The defining feature of practice is that it incorporates an intervention that influences an outcome. The expansive view of the AACN definition of nursing practice allows for the full impact of contributions from all avenues of advanced practice in order to positively influence the nation's health system. The AACN (2004) definition of *advanced nursing practice* is

> any form of nursing intervention that influences health outcomes for individuals or populations, including the provision of direct care or management of care for individual patients or management of care populations, and the provision of indirect care such as nursing administration, executive leadership, health policy, informatics and population health. (p. 2)

Advanced nursing practice includes nurse practitioners, clinical nurse specialists, nurse anesthetists, nurse-midwives, nurse administrators, policy specialists, and informaticists.

Earlier discussion in this chapter focused on the critical nature of scholarliness in contributing to the knowledge base of nursing from a practice perspective. It becomes clear that the DNP project is much more than a mere demonstration of what the student has learned; it is a demonstration of how practicing scholarly nurses can build new knowledge. The DNP project is an effort to build the bridge between research and practice, narrowing the gap that has existed there. This gap has prevented nursing from contributing fully to the body of knowledge that is desperately needed to achieve the clinical effectiveness and fiscal benefits so sorely needed in our healthcare system. The DNP project is a demonstration of how practicing scholarly nurses can build new knowledge.

The DNP project contributes to the DNP's understanding of practice knowledge generation by the lived experience. The experience of the DNP project fulfills the transformation of the student to adopting a scholarly way of thinking. The transformed student approaches issues with a new and developed view that incorporates a broad skill set. It is practice scholarship that is embraced in the DNP project.

> *The DNP project is a demonstration of how practicing scholarly nurses can build new knowledge.*

▶ What Qualifies as a DNP Project?

The DNP project should encompass multiple aspects of the DNP *Essentials*. The project should be broadly practice based (refer back to the AACN definition of "practice"). A few topic examples include a project based on a population, health system, or policy issue. Some formats for the DNP project include quality improvement, demonstration projects, clinical inquiry, or translation of EBP and program evaluation. The DNP student should reflect on life experiences, both professionally and personally, to understand the strengths and the passions that are already owned and can be used in building a strong scholarly project. Developing an understanding of the needs of the stakeholders within the context of an organization must also be considered (see information on conducting an assessment in Chapter 6, Developing the DNP Project).

The DNP project has been reviewed in the literature and within various venues. The variability of projects has been noted, with the developing understanding that DNP projects must incorporate evidence synthesis, leadership, and measurement of outcomes (Brown & Crabtree, 2013; Grey, 2013; Kirkpatrick & Weaver, 2013; Roush & Tesoro, 2018; Terharr & Sylvia, 2015).

There has been further inquiry by the AACN in the development of appropriate criteria for DNP scholarship that will include particular aspects of practice knowledge generation and DNP accountability. In response to the variability in DNP education, the AACN commissioned the Implementation of the DNP Task Force (2015a) to outline recommendations for the DNP project (see Chapter 2, Defining the Doctor of Nursing Practice: Current Trends). DNP project elements, including planning, implementation, and evaluation components, must be considered in order to have the desired impact. Projects should focus on changes that impact healthcare outcomes either through direct/indirect care with a system or population focus. Implementation should be demonstrated in an appropriate area of practice and include an evaluation of processes and/or outcomes and a plan for sustainability (AACN, 2015a). As the student considers development of the DNP project, it is helpful to have consistent criteria applied. Waldrop, Caruso, Fuchs, and Hypes (2014) suggest an acronym of "EC as PIE" for criteria that include Enhancing outcomes (health/practice/policy), Culmination of practice inquiry, Partnership engagement, Implementing evidence, and

Evaluation of outcome. The results of the work from the AACN task force on the DNP project have given new direction to the criteria of the project, which serve to clarify consistency and rigor without strangling creativity (AACN, 2015a).

Practice scholarship encompasses all aspects of the delivery of nursing interventions to have a direct impact on outcomes. If the DNP project is to have an impact on our healthcare system and the quality of care, it must be done within the context of outcomes. In considering projects worthy of such study, several questions can be asked: Is there a contribution to comprehensive quality health care? Are there specific benefits for a group, population, community, or policy? Does the project advance nursing practice at the local, state, and national levels? Is the project sustainable and cost effective? See Chapter 16, The Rest of the Story—Evaluating the Doctor of Nursing Practice, for a framework for evaluation of the DNP degree and outcomes.

▶ Current Views of the DNP Project

Rigor of the DNP Project

Rigor can be defined as a "systematic, logical, and thorough approach to the design and implementation of a project that addresses a significant problem and includes an evaluation process based on appropriate metrics, collected and analyzed using methods that provide a valid and reliable determination of project outcomes" (Roush & Tesoro, 2018, p. 2). Ongoing evaluation of DNP projects will shed light on the evolving educational needs that faculty must address in developing the DNP-prepared nurse.

In addition, there is new clarity with what the project is called. Previously, it was recognized that programs called the DNP project a variety of names that exemplified variability in focus (Moran et al., 2014). Nineteen project titles were identified (N = 39). The AACN (2015a) has recommended that the title of the DNP scholarly project be "DNP Project." Each of these steps forward serves to bring us toward consensus and continued evolution.

It is clear that DNP knowledge generation and scholarship are in the early stages of development and will continue to evolve in response to society's needs. As students contemplate the significance of the project for themselves, they should also consider the work that has been done to get nursing to this important crossroad. The DNP project not only will contribute to the student's successful transition but also will add to the knowledge base of nursing and impact nursing's work from now and into the future.

▶ Scholarship Beyond the DNP Project

DNP student enrollment and graduation rates continue to increase (AACN, 2018). With the increase in DNP graduate numbers, we are now at a point in the DNP degree trajectory where society is beginning to see the impact of practice scholarship and the associated benefit of the practice doctorate. Therefore, defining the practice scholarship of the DNP is critical to ensure the impact of the work in clinical, political, administrative, and academic venues.

The DNP project is the beginning of the work that will be continued by the DNP graduate. Because the DNP-prepared nurse is becoming part of the fabric of systems within organizations, universities, and entrepreneurial efforts, practice scholarship will need to be further developed in the multiple arenas where the DNP graduate interfaces.

The DNP-prepared nurse is becoming part of the fabric of systems within organizations, universities, and entrepreneurial efforts.

The DNP-prepared nurse within organizations is beginning to drive scholarship to implement institutional policy change, funnel EBP to the bedside, and direct practice-based evidence to research. This DNP graduate works in teams and employs high-level interdisciplinary competencies to improve health systems and populations. Roles will continue to evolve to incorporate the knowledge and skill set that the DNP-prepared nurse brings to quality efforts within organizations. It is crucial that the DNP-prepared nurse demonstrate the ability to successfully impact outcomes related to leading system change, implementing policy change, and management of persons with multiple chronic conditions across sites and that the impact is evaluated (Brown & Crabtree, 2013; Redman, Pressler, Furspan, & Potempa, 2015). In addition, the DNP-prepared nurse within health policy scholarship is beginning to enhance the vision of emerging healthcare systems. The rigor of practice scholarship gives credibility to the DNP-prepared nurse and influences policy.

The DNP-prepared nurse within academia is beginning to incorporate a practice model that influences tenure track (see Chapter 16, The Rest of the Story–Evaluating the Doctor of Nursing Practice). The scholarship of integration and application is becoming a part of this model. As more and more of these DNP-prepared faculty members encounter organizational appointments and are asked to provide consultation services, there will be a need to balance competing priorities.

An emerging approach to engage both healthcare organization and academic practitioners and researchers is the academic-practice partnership (APP). APPs are formalized relationships between an academic nursing program and care setting and may include other professionals, corporations, government entities, and foundations. Some examples of academic-practice partnerships include those between schools of nursing and acute care settings, community-based settings, and long-term care facilities (AACN, 2018). There is a need for alignment and integration of academic nursing with practice settings to advance health, health care, and transformation. Academic and practice leaders can accelerate dissemination of shared knowledge, scientific inquiry, translational research, and policy advocacy that affect health. Research conducted on successful partnerships reveals that they have shared vision, common goals, ongoing commitment, shared knowledge, clear communication, and mutual respect (AACN-AONE, 2012). APPs are an important mechanism to strengthen nursing practice and help nurses to become well-positioned to lead change and advance health, thus addressing the recommendations of the IOM *Future of Nursing* report. Both DNP students and graduates can benefit from the development of the APP. For students, a supporting organization with identified strategic goals that align with the DNP project can strengthen and sustain the project. For DNP graduates, ongoing practice scholarship can be supported for DNP-prepared nurses in practice or academia that ultimately benefit patients and systems.

Dr. Amy Manderscheid describes her experience implementing her DNP project between the academic and practice settings (see **EXEMPLAR 3-1**).

EXEMPLAR 3-1 Leveraging Interprofessional Collaboration between Academia and Practice Settings to Impact a Pediatric Quality and Safety Improvement Imperative

Amy Manderscheid, DNP, RN, CMSRN

The power of a collaborative partnership among academia and practice settings offers staggering outcomes when promoting a culture of high reliability, quality, and safety in a leading Midwestern pediatric hospital. This unique relationship is an exemplar of an innovative role of a DNP-prepared nurse who chose to engage with an interprofessional team of healthcare providers and leaders to address quality-based processes and communication gaps in preparation of seasonal high patient volumes. The purpose was to assess nursing perspectives regarding confidence, teamwork, communication, and elements attributing toward a culture of safety, while leveraging in situ simulation to mitigate respiratory decline with interprofessional teams of nurses, physicians, and respiratory therapists.

The setting for this work occurred in a large Midwestern academic children's hospital on an acute care medical-surgical 24-bed unit. This children's hospital is part of a large health system and is a level one trauma center. Specifically, the patient population on this nursing unit consists of fairly complex medical patients with diagnoses including, but not limited to, respiratory syncytial virus (RSV), bronchiolitis, and pneumonia. Two pediatric interprofessional teams conduct bedside rounds, where providers openly discuss concerns, progress, and questions in partnership with patients and families as appropriate. Team members are primary responders when rapid response teams are notified to quickly assess a deteriorating patient, and participants in our team-based simulations.

Because of the organizational commitment to safety and training, this initiative entailed use of the on-site pediatric simulation program with use of fully functional, advanced audiovisual equipment, computers, and software. Participants worked in patient rooms with equipment and supplies as three clinical simulations were offered to teams of nurses, respiratory therapists, and physicians. Simulations were offered twice per week across 8 weeks, timed specifically prior to the seasonal peak of respiratory illness. This design led to opportunities to enhance application of safety culture principles through simulation training, identification of opportunities to eliminate risks, enhancing strategies as highly functioning interprofessional teams, and increasing proficiency in multiple unit (or specialty)–based scenarios.

This approach is consistent with evidence-based practice, as simulation can lead to increases in the effectiveness of teamwork and communication, which can result in a reduction in errors, cost, and mortality rates (Merchant, 2012). Furthermore, Bultas, Hassler, Ercole, and Rea (2014) examined the use of high-fidelity simulation in the Pediatric Emergency Assessment Recognition Stabilization course. In this study, participants were able to maintain or increase their ability to recognize the deteriorating patient and felt more confident in their ability to recognize and treat the deteriorating patient (Bultas, Hassler, Ercole, & Rea, 2014). The utilization of an early warning system, along with the timely delivery of interventions, is crucial in the prevention of patient deterioration (Murray, Williams, Pingataro, & Volpe, 2015). The delay in the recognition and treatment of the deteriorating pediatric patient is a recognized cause of preventable cardiac arrest and mortality (Panesar et al., 2014).

Through use of the Plan-Do-Study-Act (PDSA) model (Associates in Process Improvement, 2018), in tandem with the Clinical Practice Model framework (Elsevier CPM Resource Center, 2011), respiratory-based pediatric simulations, and questionnaires with physician, nursing, and respiratory therapist teams, outcomes suggest a strong impact on recognizing clinical signs of patient deterioration while promoting safety culture principles, team-based assessments, and communication standards. Questionnaires included the Agency for Healthcare Research and Quality (AHRQ) Patient Safety Culture Survey, in addition to an assessment of safety behaviors and use of organizational tools, including the Pediatric Early Warning System (PEWS). Response rates exceeded 60%, indicating committed, engaged interprofessional providers as the project was implemented.

Positive outcomes resulted in eight distinct pre- and post-measurement areas, indicating a positive shift in the areas of nursing confidence and performance, teamwork, and communication standards consistent with safety culture principles. Length of stay and number of transfers to the pediatric intensive care unit continue to be monitored. Secondary gains were highly valuable, including capturing candid moments of peer support and education, nursing and medical student observations, executive leadership support, as well as simulation debriefs led by attending physicians, nurse educators, and the simulation specialist to discuss evidence-based practice and safety culture principles.

In conclusion, collaborations among practice and academia professionals may result in impactful patient and system outcomes as relationships are formed, patient care processes are examined, and action plans are implemented and evaluated. The *Doctor of Nursing Practice Essentials* (AACN, 2006) are imperative to apply and maximize healthcare outcomes, from both clinical and administrative aspects. Furthermore, the return on investment with high-impact interventions, learning, teamwork, and recognition of safety culture principles and behaviors may be palpable as patients, leaders, and teams experience changes in care standards, reimbursement models, and positive culture transformations in sustainment of being recognized as a high-reliability organization.

▶ Recommendations

It is critical that the outcome-focused nature of practice scholarship be recognized as an effective means of knowledge development that contributes to the changes needed in our healthcare system. To reach these goals, utilization of all skill sets of DNP-prepared nurses is needed to affect change in populations, healthcare organizations, and policy. A word of caution is exercised in focusing too heavily on one advanced practice role or another. The strengths of nurse practitioners, nurse midwives, clinical nurse specialists, nurse anesthetists, nurse administrators, informaticists, and policy experts will be required to meet the challenges that are before us.

There will be ongoing challenges to continue scholarship after attainment of the DNP degree to continue to impact health care. The DNP-prepared nurse will need to more clearly define practice scholarship for organizations and academia to carve out time for scholarship in his or her clinical role—which ultimately is the purpose of the DNP-prepared nurse.

There is a need to develop ways to categorize our knowledge development to further disseminate and build on practice-based knowledge. This work is already under way and is further discussed in Chapter 16, The Rest of the Story—Evaluating the Doctor of Nursing Practice.

There is great value in the work of teams. PhD- and DNP-prepared nurses working together in scholarship teams will continue to evolve to advance the profession of nursing. Interdisciplinary and intradisciplinary relationships will be required to impact complex issues. Development of scholarship teams will increase creativity, impact, and production. There is movement in group and team models for DNP projects. Each member of the group must meet all expectations of planning, implementation, and evaluation of the project and have a leadership role in at least one component of the project and accountability for a deliverable (AACN, 2015a). Working closely with PhD colleagues to further the work of scientific inquiry will build a nursing repository of knowledge that can be used to solve issues and is further discussed in Chapter 8, Interprofessional and Intraprofessional Collaboration in the DNP Project.

Impact

The DNP nurse is prepared to answer the charge from the IOM for nurses to take their place at the decision-making table and to collaborate with other healthcare professionals to improve the health and health care of our nation. Practice scholarship is the driving force that will disseminate practice-based evidence and support the developing success of the practice doctorate to close the gap between research and practice, thereby meeting societal needs of improved health for our populations. Dissemination of outcomes related to DNP-prepared nurses' work will propel the influence and the impact forward. This dissemination is an obligation of the DNP-prepared nurse to society and results in a positive effect on health care.

Key Messages

- Scholarship is the mechanism that provides knowledge development within a discipline.
- A broadening of the view of scholarship includes integration and application.
- Practice scholarship embodies all aspects of nursing interventions that affect outcomes in individuals, populations, systems, and policy.
- The DNP project integrates and demonstrates the *Essentials* of DNP education.
- DNP project elements include planning, implementation, and evaluation components that impact healthcare outcomes.
- The DNP project is also a demonstration of the effectiveness of the DNP-prepared nurse.

Action Plan—Next Steps

1. Which DNP *Essentials* could be demonstrated in your idea for a DNP project?
2. Does your project idea consist of breadth and depth of knowledge within a defined area?

3. Is there the potential for innovation and creativity to affect an outcome?
4. Will you be able to expose the DNP project to public scrutiny and peer review?
5. What type of scholarship is evidenced within your project idea—discovery/integration/application?
6. What aspects of practice are you focused on—individual, population, system, policy?
7. Is there a contribution to comprehensive quality health care? Are there specific benefits for a group, population, community, or policy? Does the project advance nursing practice at the local, state, and national levels? Is the project sustainable and cost effective?
8. Is this topic of interest a need at the organizational level? What organizations are potential project implementation sites?
9. Is there a planning, implementation, and evaluation component?
10. How will this project impact healthcare outcomes?
11. What areas of expertise and passion do you bring that you can build on?
12. What skill sets do you need to develop in order to successfully implement your DNP project?

References

American Association of Colleges of Nursing (AACN). (1999). *American Association of Colleges of Nursing position statement: Defining scholarship for the discipline of nursing.* Retrieved from https://www.professionalnursing.org/article/S8755-7223(99)80068-4/pdf

American Association of Colleges of Nursing (AACN). (2004). *Position statement on the practice doctorate in nursing.* Retrieved from http://www.aacnnursing.org/DNP/Position-Statement

American Association of Colleges of Nursing (AACN). (2006). *The essentials of doctoral education for advanced nursing practice.* Retrieved from http://www.aacnnursing.org/Portals/42/Publications/DNPEssentials.pdf

American Association of Colleges of Nursing (AACN). (2015a). *The doctor of nursing practice: Current issues and clarifying recommendations.* Retrieved from https://www.pncb.org/sites/default/files/2017-02/AACN_DNP_Recommendations.pdf

American Association of Colleges of Nursing (AACN). (2015b). *DNP fact sheet.* Retrieved from http://www.aacnnursing.org/News-Information/Fact-Sheets/DNP-Fact-Sheet

American Association of Colleges of Nursing (AACN). (2018). *Defining scholarship for academic nursing.* Retrieved from http://www.aacnnursing.org/News-Information/Position-Statements-White-Papers/Defining-Scholarship-Nursing

American Association of Colleges of Nursing-American Organization of Nurse Executives (AACN-AONE). (2012). *Guiding principles to academic-practice partnerships.* Retrieved from http://www.aacnnursing.org/Academic-Practice-Partnerships/The-Guiding-Principles

Associates in Process Improvement (API). (2018). PDSA Cycle. Retrieved from http://www.apiweb.org

Boyer, E. (1990). *Scholarship reconsidered: Priorities of the professoriate.* Carnegie Foundation for the Advancement of Teaching. New York, NY: John Wiley & Sons.

Brown, M. A., & Crabtree, K. (2013). The development of practice scholarship in DNP programs: A paradigm shift. *Journal of Professional Nursing, 29*(6), 330–337. doi:10.1016/j.profnurs.2013.08.003

Bultas, M., Hassler, M., Ercole, P. & Rea, G. (2014). Effectiveness of high-fidelity simulation for pediatric staff nurse education. *Pediatric Nursing, 40*(1), 27–42.

Bunkers, S. S. (2000). The nurse scholar of the 21st century. *Nursing Science Quarterly, 13*(2), 116–123.

Burson, R., Moran, K., & Conrad, D. (2016). Why hire a DNP? The value-added impact of the practice doctorate. *Journal of Doctoral Nursing Practice, 9*(1), 152–157.

Cary, A. H., & George, G. (2011). The doctor of nursing practice (DNP). *Oregon State Board of Nursing Sentinel, 30*(1), 10–11.

Draye, M., Acker, M., & Zimmer, P. (2006). The practice doctorate in nursing: Approaches to transform nurse practitioner education and practice. *Nursing Outlook, 54,* 123–129. doi:10.1016/j.outlook.2006.01.001

Elsevier CPM Resource Center. (2011). The CPM Framework™: Culture and professional practice for sustainable healthcare transformation [Brochure]. Grand Rapids, MI: Author.

Fairman, J. (2008). Context and contingency in the history of post World War II nursing scholarship in the United States. *Journal of Nursing Scholarship, 40*(1), 4–11.

Fawcett, J. (1999). The state of nursing science: Hallmarks of the 20th and 21st centuries. *Nursing Science Quarterly, 12*(4), 311–315.

Ferguson-Pare, M. (2005). What is a community of scholars in the practice environment? *Nursing Science Quarterly, 18*(2), 120. doi:10.117/0894318405275863

Grey, M. (2013). The doctor of nursing practice: Defining the next steps. *Journal of Nursing Education, 52*(8), 462–465. doi:10.3928/01484834-20130719-02

Institute of Medicine (IOM). (1999). *To err is human: Building a safer health system.* Washington, DC: National Academies Press.

Institute of Medicine (IOM). (2001). *Crossing the quality chasm.* Washington, DC: National Academies Press.

Institute of Medicine (IOM). (2010). *The future of nursing: Leading change, advancing health.* Washington, DC: National Academies Press.

Institute of Medicine (IOM). (2012). *Best care at lower cost: The path to continuously learning healthcare in America.* Washington, DC: National Academies Press. Retrieved from http://www.nationalacademies.org/hmd/Reports/2012/Best-Care-at-Lower-Cost-The-Path-to-Continuously-Learning-Health-Care-in-America.aspx

Kirkpatrick, J. M., & Weaver, T. (2013). The doctor of nursing practice capstone project: Consensus or confusion? *Journal of Nursing Education, 52*(8), 435–441. doi:10.3928/01484834-20130722-01

Kitson, A. (1999). The relevance of scholarship for nursing research and practice. *Journal of Advanced Nursing, 29*(4), 773–775.

Kitson, A. (2006). From scholarship to action and innovation. *Journal of Advanced Nursing, 56*(5), 435–572.

Levin, R. F., & Slyder, J. (2012). Evidence-based practice on the DNP. *Research and Theory for Nursing Practice: An International Journal, 26*(1), 6–9.

Magnan, M. A. (2019). The DNP: Expectations for theory, research and scholarship. In L. Chism (Ed.), *The doctor of nursing practice: A guidebook for role development and professional issues* (4th ed., pp. 97–124). Burlington, MA: Jones & Bartlett Learning.

McEwen, M., & Wills, E. M. (2018). *Theoretical basis for nursing.* Philadelphia, PA: Wolters Kluwer Health/Lippincott Williams & Wilkins.

Melnyk, B. M. (2013). Distinguishing the preparation and roles of doctor of philosophy and doctor of nursing practice graduates: National implications for academic curricula and health care systems. *Journal of Nursing Education, 52*(8), 442–443.

Merchant, D. (2012). Does high-fidelity simulation improve clinical outcomes. *Journal for Nurses in Staff Development, 28*(1), E1–E8.

Moran, K., Burson, R., Critchett, J., & Olla, P. (2011). Exploring the cost and clinical outcomes of integrating the registered nurse–certified diabetes educator in the patient-centered medical home. *The Diabetes Educator, 37*(6), 780–793.

Murray, J., Williams, L. A., Pingantaro, S., & Volpe, D. (2105). An integrative review of Pediatric Early Warning System scores. *Pediatric Nursing, 41*(4), 165–174.

National Institutes of Health (NIH). (2015). *Fogarty International Center: Advancing science for global health.* Retrieved from https://www.fic.nih.gov/Pages/Default.aspx

National League of Nurses (NLN) Board of Governors (2018*). Doctoral faculty collaboration in nursing education.* Retrieved from http://www.nln.org/docs/default-source/default-document-library/dnp_2018.pdf?sfvrsn=2

National Organization of Nurse Practitioner Faculties (NONPF). (2016). *The doctor of nursing practice nurse practitioner: Clinical scholar.* Retrieved from https://c.ymcdn.com/sites/www.nonpf.org/resource/resmgr/docs/ClinicalScholarFINAL2016.pdf

Panesar, R., Polikoff, L. A., Harris, D., Mills, B., Messina, C., & Parker, M. (2014). Characteristics and outcomes of pediatric rapid response teams before and after mandatory triggering by an elevated Pediatric Early Warning System (PEWS) score. *Hospital Pediatrics, 4*, 135–140. doi:10.1542/hpeds.2013-0062

Redman, R. W., Pressler, S. J., Furspan, P., & Potempa, K. (2015). Nurses in the United States with a practice doctorate: Implications for leading in the current context of health care. *Nursing Outlook, 63*, 124–129.

Reed, P. G., & Brewer, B. B. (2018). Generating knowledge in practice: Philosophical and methodological considerations. In Reed, P. G., & Shearer, N. B. C. (Eds.) *Nursing knowledge and theory innovation: Advancing the science of practice*. New York, NY: Springer Publishing Company.

Reed, P. G., & Shearer, N. B. C. (2018). *Nursing knowledge and theory innovation: Advancing the science of practice*. New York, NY: Springer Publishing Company.

Rolfe, G. (2018). Practitioner-centered research: Nursing praxis and the science of the unique. In Reed, P. G., & Shearer, N. B. C. (Eds.), *Nursing knowledge and theory innovation: Advancing the science of practice* (pp. 63–81). New York, NY: Springer Publishing Company.

Rolfe, G., & Davies, R. (2009). Second-generation professional doctorates in nursing. *International Journal of Nursing Studies, 46*, 1265–1273.

Roush, K., & Tesoro, M. (2018). An examination of the rigor and value of final scholarly projects completed by DNP nursing students. *Journal of Professional Nursing*. In press. http://www.doi .org/10.1016/j.profnurs.2018.03.003

Salmond, S. W. (2007). Advancing evidence-based practice: A primer. *Orthopaedic Nursing, 26*(2), 114–123.

Scholarship. (2018). *Merriam-Webster's Learner's Dictionary*. Retrieved from http://www .learnersdictionary.com/definition/scholarship

Smith, M. J., & Liehr, P. (2005). Story theory: Advancing nursing practice scholarship. *Holistic Nursing Practice, 19*(6), 272–276.

Swanson, M., & Stanton, M. (2013). Chief nursing officers' perceptions of the doctorate of nursing practice degree. *Nursing Forum, 48*(1), 35–44. doi: 10.1111/nuf.12003

Terharr, M. F., & Sylvia, M. (2016, January). Scholarly work products of the doctor of nursing practice: One approach to evaluating scholarship, rigour, impact and quality. *Journal of Clinical Nursing, 25*, 163–174. doi: 10.1111/jocn.13113

Thoun, D. S. (2009). Toward an appreciation of nursing scholarship: Recognizing our traditions, contributions, and presence. *Journal of Nursing Education, 48*(10), 552–556.

Velasquez, D. M., McArthur, D. B., & Johnson, C. (2018). Doctoral nursing roles in knowledge generation. In Reed, P. G., & Shearer, N. B. C. (Eds.), *Nursing knowledge and theory innovation: Advancing the science of practice* (pp. 47–62). New York, NY: Springer Publishing Company.

Waldrop, J., Caruso, D., Fuchs, M. A., & Hypes, K. (2014). EC as PIE: Five criteria for executing a successful DNP final project. *Journal of Professional Nursing, 30*(4), 300–306.

CHAPTER 4

Healthcare Policy and Advocacy

Katherine Moran

CHAPTER OVERVIEW

The goal of health policy is to find equilibrium between the competing forces in health care to produce an optimal system (Bodenheimer & Grumbach, 2016). The healthcare system in the United States (U.S.) has been in a state of unrest for years. The discontent lies primarily in the polarizing views of the predominant political parties. Finding a balance between achieving a basic level of equity for health services and paying for these services remains at the center of the polarity. Yet, managing these polarities is critical, as the outcome will ultimately shape the health of our nation.

Doctor of nursing practice (DNP)–prepared nurses have the education, knowledge, and skills to sit at the table and actively participate in the discussions where healthcare delivery and population health decisions are being made. These practice scholars have advanced competencies in practice improvement, development of new innovations, testing interventions and care delivery models, evaluation of healthcare outcomes, expertise to inform health policy, and leadership in establishing clinical excellence (American Association of Colleges of Nursing [AACN], 2004). DNP-prepared nurses and students have the potential to impact policy change at both the local and population level. DNP students with an interest in this work should consider a policy-focused project as a foundation for ongoing policy scholarship. The purpose of this chapter is to help the DNP student understand factors that impact the health of our nation, recognize areas where the student may facilitate change, and develop methods that can be used to make an impact.

CHAPTER OBJECTIVES

After completing the chapter, the learner will be able to:

1. Identify key factors that impact the health of our nation.
2. Compare and contrast approaches to addressing disparities in health and healthcare delivery in organizations (micro level), communities (meso level), and beyond (macro level).
3. Acknowledge ways that the DNP student may facilitate change.

▶ Health Policy Historical Perspective

The complexity of the U.S. healthcare system, as it is known today, has been years in the making. Political decisions that impacted the health of the country date back to the early 1900s. Therefore, to fully appreciate the multitude of factors that have impacted the health of the nation, one must consider the broad healthcare landscape; that begins with the *macro* level view. For example, in 2010 the Patient Protection and Affordable Care Act (ACA) was enacted into law with a goal of providing "numerous rights and protections that make health coverage more fair and easy to understand, along with subsidies (through 'premium tax credits' and 'cost-sharing reductions') to make it more affordable" (HealthCare.gov, n.d., para 1). There were numerous controversies that surfaced since the implementation of the ACA—for example, the constitutionality of the individual mandate and Medicaid expansion. The important point to note is that prior to the implementation of the ACA, as a country, the U.S. was not realizing the health outcomes one would expect given the amount of money spent on health care annually; therefore, a concerted effort was made to improve outcomes.

This was not the first attempt to reform health care in the U.S.—and will likely not be the last. The U.S. has had multiple failed attempts to reform health insurance programs over the course of history. For example, Theodore Roosevelt's proposal for national health insurance in 1912; Franklin Delano Roosevelt's proposal for universal health insurance, which was dropped to win support for Social Security; Lyndon B. Johnson's unsuccessful effort toward gaining a universal plan that would include all Americans; Richard M. Nixon's proposal for universal health insurance that would have required employers to offer affordable coverage to all; and Senator Ted Kennedy's attempt to gain support for his single-payer health insurance plan. The reforms that paved the way for the ACA include Johnson's mandate for his Great Society reforms in 1964 and, in 1965, the establishment of Medicare (a federal health insurance program for people who are 65 years old or older, certain younger people with disabilities, and people with end-stage renal disease) and Medicaid (a state and federally funded health insurance program for low-income individuals and families); and finally, in 1997, the Children's Health Insurance Program (CHIP) (a federal program that provides matching funds to states for health insurance to families with children) (Lavarreda & Brown, 2014).

Unfortunately, the cost-sharing provisions of Medicare have posed significant financial barriers for the elderly and disabled beneficiaries. Medicare has also had limited effectiveness because of the absence of long-term care services and prescription drug coverage. An attempt to address lack of prescription drug coverage was initiated in 2006 with the development of the Medicare Prescription Drug, Improvement, and Modernization Act of 2003 (MMA), which established the prescription drug benefit, Medicare Part D (Lavarreda & Brown, 2014).

Medicaid has also had its share of controversy. For example, some believe that because of Medicaid there has been a substantial increase in use of health services among low-income individuals. But, this does not mean that there is *equity* in access among socioeconomic classes. Access issues among low-income individuals remain, primarily due to the variability across states as it relates to the population covered by Medicaid (eligibility requirements) and the benefits offered (even though Medicaid is federally regulated, the states have significant latitude in administration). Budget cuts and Medicaid reform (Personal Responsibility and Work Opportunity Reconciliation Act of 1996) have contributed to this phenomenon (Lavarreda & Brown, 2014).

Moving forward, it will be critical that DNP-prepared nurses focus on systematically analyzing and evaluating the factors that impact access to care, the cost of care, health behaviors, and outcomes of care. However, to address the most pressing needs of society, an intentional effort is needed to understand and ultimately address the "social determinants of health." The social determinants of health include genetic as well as lifestyle and environmental factors, such as the availability of resources to meet daily needs such as housing, food markets, job opportunities, access to health services, and education (Shi & Singh, 2019). These factors have a huge impact on the health of our nation.

Population Health Perspective

Having a clear understanding of the social determinants of health can shed light on how multiple social factors impact health and health care. Ponce & Ko (2014) indicate that the social determinants of health that have the most impact are those that cause stratifications in social position; for example, income/income inequality, social status, race/ethnic composition, segregation, political power, and favorable environmental exposures and assets provide advantages in some communities, but unfortunately, create disadvantage and produce inequities for others. It is important to note that these "disadvantages" accumulate over time and prevail over generations, and are, therefore, intractable without policy solutions (Ponce & Ko, 2014).

Income disparity contributes to health both at an individual and community level. People with a higher income tend to live in a desired neighborhood, have access to better health care, and live in areas where there are more physicians and larger healthcare systems. Lower-income people tend to have fewer choices for specialty physicians and less access to care. Higher-income people also have more choices in health insurance and more options for where they would like to receive their care. These individuals tend to have higher social status and political power and have a direct influence on how healthcare dollars are spent (Ponce & Ko, 2014).

The social processes and subsequent varying levels of social capital (aspects of social life that promote working together to achieve shared objectives) found within a community have an impact on income inequality and segregation. Further, they can in turn lead to inequities in social class and position and, ultimately, different levels of community assets and opportunities. As noted by Ponce and Ko (2014), there is a potential for social capital to improve access to care by linking disadvantaged populations and healthcare resources. But they go on to say that this process could also augment the advantages more privileged groups already possess. They conclude that "government-level macroeconomic and social policies that reduce structural inequities may be more appropriate" (p. 149).

Two important indicators of health status, morbidity and mortality rates, should also be reviewed to gain an understanding of the health of a population, especially vulnerable populations. Yancey, Banstani, and Glenn (2014) purport that minorities experience higher rates of morbidity and mortality. There has been a plethora of research around the experiences of racial and ethnic minorities in the United States that have been described in reports from the Institute of Medicine (IOM): *Unequal Treatment: Confronting Racial and Ethnic Disparities in Health Care* (Smedley, Stith, & Nelson, 2003) and *Crossing the Quality Chasm* (IOM, 2001).

Even with the spotlight on ethnic disparities in the U.S., there is still a long way to go to address these concerns, especially as it relates to overall health and life expectancy. For example, African Americans' overall health and life expectancy are impacted the most. Contributing factors include the historical, political, policy, and social treatment of people of color and/or ethnic backgrounds; socioeconomic status (SES); behavioral risk factors; physical environmental influences; and socioenvironmental influences. This is particularly important to note when considering that disease burden has shifted from communicable to chronic diseases. Since chronic conditions are primarily self-managed, and the ability to successfully self-manage is impacted by the above-mentioned factors, it should be no surprise that as a result of this shift, inequality in chronic disease burden is now evident. Of note, obesity is identified as a major driver of chronic disease disparities. Here again, "lower SES is associated with obesity, but higher socioeconomic status is less protective against obesity for African Americans than for Latinos and whites" (Yancey, Banstani, & Glenn, 2014, p. 84).

Socioeconomic status has the largest impact on racial and ethnic disparities. A lower SES (poverty) determines where a person lives, the amount of food available, the types of food available, the type of insurance a person has, whether a person will have access to health care, and the quality of the health care that is available in the community. As previously mentioned, African Americans are the most disadvantaged—reflecting centuries of exploitation and oppression, forced immigration, enslavement, and subjugation (Yancey, Banstani, & Glenn, 2014).

In addition to SES position, other factors also have an impact on racial/ethnic differences in health status. For example, the cumulative effects of prolonged exposure to individual stressors, long-term effects of an early childhood/prenatal environment of deprivation, and the reaction to macrosocial factors (i.e., marketing to children and adolescents that increases a desire for goods and services, enjoyed by affluent whites, that are beyond the means of working and middle-class families) (Yancey, Banstani, & Glenn, 2014). As noted by Bustamante, Morales, and Ortega (2014), addressing racial and ethnic disparities in health care is of growing importance. Keep in mind that because the U.S. is ethnically diverse, one can expect to see suboptimal health status for a substantial portion of the population if disparities in health care (i.e., a difference in care that is not accounted for by a difference in access to care, personal preference, clinical need, or clinical appropriateness) continue in these populations. This could include discrimination at the system level (influenced by the structure of healthcare systems and the legal and regulatory environment), discrimination at the patient-provider level (prejudice or unconscious stereotyping), or even patient factors that could have an impact on outcomes (perception of health status or psychosocial constructs, such as readiness for change or perceived self-efficacy).

The Cost and Quality of Health Care

Other important factors that contribute to healthcare outcomes are the cost and quality of health care. According to Claxton, Rae, Levitt, and Cox (2018), healthcare prices in the U.S. have increased (21.6%) more rapidly than general economic inflation (17.3%), especially for the privately insured. In fact, Squires and Anderson (2015) from The Commonwealth Fund report that the U.S. spends more on health care compared to 12 other industrialized countries (see **FIGURE 4-1**).

Further, there is wide variation in the prices paid for the same services based on geographic location in the U.S. (Claxton et al., 2018, para 1). For example, inpatient care costs have risen approximately 13% for patients with private insurance, compared to a 3% increase for patients with Medicare or Medicaid (Claxton et al., 2018). Also note that these increases are found in some common inpatient procedures, such as inpatient laparoscopic appendectomy prices and full knee replacements,

* 2012.
Notes: GDP refers to gross domestic product, Dutch and Swiss data are for current spending only, and exclude spending on capital formation of health care providers.
Source: OECD Health Data 2015.

FIGURE 4-1 The Commonwealth Fund report on healthcare spending.

which have risen 136% and 78% (respectively) between 2003 and 2016 for large employer plans. This growth has been faster than general price increases (28%) over the same period.

There is also significant variation in the average price paid for these same procedures in the U.S. According to Claxton et al. (2018), the average price paid by large employers for an admission for a full knee replacement in 2016 was $34,063; however, this ranged from $24,734 or less (approximately 25% of admissions) to $52,181 or more (approximately 10% of admissions). The same was true for laparoscopic appendectomies. The average cost in 2016 was $20,192, ranging from $12,088 (approximately 25% of admissions) to over $35,308 (approximately 10% of admissions). And these costs varied across markets. For example, the national average was $34,063 for a full knee replacement in the U.S. in 2016. However, in the New York City area the cost was $50,000, which was more than twice the price of the same procedure in the Louisville, Kentucky area ($23,000). These price increases are not unique to the inpatient setting. Escalation in costs was also seen for outpatient office visits (69% increase) and lower back magnetic resonance imaging (MRI) costs (14% increase) during the same time period (Claxton et al., 2018, para 8). The reasons for these wide variations are multifaceted; for example, some of the variation may be due to geographic differences in insurance coverage or even cost of living.

Another healthcare cost concern relates to the need to control pharmaceutical costs while assuring access and measuring health-related quality of life (HRQL). Where pharmaceutical costs are concerned, Schweitzer and Comanor (2014) suggest that there needs to be a better understanding of (1) the relationship between drug price and quality, (2) how the quality of a drug is determined, and (3) the extent of competition in the pharmaceutical marketplace, including the breadth of these markets.

Prices to date have been positively affected by a drug's efficacy and therapeutic advance, but to what degree has yet to be determined. For example, most consumers are aware that some of the increase in expenditures is likely related to pharmaceutical companies' desire to recoup the costs associated with research and development. However, expenditures have also grown in part because of how integral pharmaceuticals have become to medical care (for preventing hospitalizations, improving outcomes, etc.), but currently no one has been able to account for quality improvement as it relates to price increases. Regarding quality control, the U.S. Food and Drug Administration (FDA) used a crude measure of improvement score in the past when a drug was seeking market approval. Now, the FDA does not use that mechanism; in fact, there is currently no "agreed-upon" measure of therapeutic improvement needed for new drugs. Finally, as pharmaceutical companies continue to consolidate in the marketplace, one must consider how competition will impact the market to determine the best course of action for creating public policies in this industry (Schweitzer & Comanor, 2014).

Overall quality of healthcare delivery also varies widely nationally. As noted in two landmark reports from the IOM (1999, 2001), poor quality is a concern in the U.S. healthcare delivery system. To give context to this concern, consider the report from The Commonwealth Fund (Davis, Stremikis, Schoen, & Squires, 2014) that ranked the U.S. last in measures of quality, equity, access, efficiency, and health lives when compared to 11 industrialized countries (see **FIGURE 4-2**). While the overall results are dismal, there are efforts underway to improve the quality of care in the U.S. For example, chronic disease management, primary care coordination, and health

Exhibit ES-1. Overall Ranking

	AUS	CAN	FRA	GER	NETH	NZ	NOR	SWE	SWIZ	UK	US
Overall ranking (2013)	4	10	9	5	5	7	7	3	2	1	11
Quality care	2	9	8	7	5	4	11	10	3	1	5
Effective care	4	7	9	6	5	2	11	10	8	1	3
Safe care	3	10	2	6	7	9	11	5	4	1	7
Coordinated care	4	8	9	10	5	2	7	11	3	1	6
Patient-centered care	5	8	10	7	3	6	11	9	2	1	4
Access	8	9	11	2	4	7	6	4	2	1	9
Cost-related problem	9	5	10	4	8	6	3	1	7	1	11
Timeliness of care	6	11	10	4	2	7	8	9	1	3	5
Efficiency	4	10	8	9	7	3	4	2	6	1	11
Equity	5	9	7	4	8	10	6	1	2	2	11
Healthy lives	4	8	1	7	5	9	6	2	3	10	11
Health expenditures/capita, 2011**	$3,800	$4,522	$4,118	$4,495	$5,099	$3,182	$5,669	$3,925	$5,643	$3,405	$8,508

Country rankings

■ Top 2*
■ Middle
□ Bottom 2*

Notes: * Includes ties. ** Expenditures shown in SUS PPP (purchasing power parity): Australian $ data are from 2010. Source: Calculated by the Commonwealth Fund based on 2011 International Health Policy Survey of Sicker Adults; 2012 International Health Policy Survey of Primary Care Physicians; 2013 International Health Policy Survey; Commonwealth Fund National Scorecard 2011; World Health Organization and Organization for Economic Cooperation and Development, OECD Health Data, 2013 (Paris: OECD, Nov. 2013).

FIGURE 4-2 The Commonwealth Fund healthcare quality and cost comparison.

Reproduced from Davis, K., Stremikis, K., Squires, D., & Schoen, C. (2014). *Mirror, mirror on the wall. How the performance of the US Health care system compares internationally.* New York: CommonWealth Fund with permission.

information technology (HIT) have shown promise in improving healthcare quality (Brennan et al., 2009). The United States must capitalize on its strengths and implement strategies to improve healthcare quality among all sectors of healthcare delivery.

▶ The Potential Impact of the DNP-Prepared Nurse

The gravity of the overall condition of our nation's health and the status of the healthcare delivery system can be overwhelming to consider; yet as a DNP student, there are things that can be done to address disparities in health and healthcare delivery in healthcare organizations (micro level), the community (meso level), and beyond (macro level). Healthcare professionals must use an unbiased lens to recognize differences between communities, and as a community, take up the initiative to help others gain access to valuable resources.

To begin, the DNP student should ask him or herself a few simple questions: How well is (are) the healthcare system(s) in the community doing delivering the care needed for the population it (they) serve? What services should be provided that are currently not available? Are there issues related to access to care in the community? Do all the individuals in the community have healthcare coverage? Do the individuals in the community understand what they can do to improve and/or maintain their health? Then, the student should think about what is within his or her sphere of influence and advocate for a change. For example, many agree that education and primary prevention are key to the health of our nation. And, that healthcare organizations should encourage families within the communities they serve to maintain a healthy lifestyle and provide education via a variety of innovative formats, such as at a health-oriented grocery store or through vegetable vans in urban areas. This micro-level approach is an example of an initiative that the DNP student could take to address healthcare concerns at the local level. DNP students can take the lead in introducing this type of advocacy work within organizations.

> *Remember, all change begins with one person.*

Other examples include: working with the local health department (meso level) to address the disparities in the community by gearing the care that is provided to those who are underserved (e.g., a DNP project to begin an immunization clinic within a homeless shelter) or focusing on community health resources that incorporate education to teach young children about health and wellness. For example, Food Corps (2018) incorporates agricultural education to demonstrate how growing fresh fruits and vegetables allows families a resource to cook healthy meals; this promotes nutrition using natural resources in the heart of the city. This national (macro-level) initiative can be used as an exemplar to improve the health of the population in cities across the United States. Another example of a macro-level initiative includes development of an evidence-based toolkit to inform teachers, staff, coaches, bus drivers, and other school professionals how to safely and effectively care for a child with diabetes in the school setting. This initiative began as a state effort, but was also adapted at the national level.

These examples illustrate the work that has been done to date, but also suggest that there is still much work to be done. Healthcare policies not only need to address access to care but must support and enhance communities to evolve into places for all residents of the community to live healthy, active, and safe lives. But, to be successful in this endeavor, the nation must be able to identify, understand, and monitor progress in addressing disparities.

To this end, healthcare professionals should advocate for vulnerable populations and urge politicians to change this system. The DNP student should think about these policies through multiple lenses; this is a complex issue that requires a multi-system approach. Consider "noncompliant" patient behavior as an example. What does the evidence show regarding noncompliant behavior? Can it be said that patients that do not comply with treatment do not care about their health? Or, could a reason for their noncompliance be related to the social determinants of health? According to Ponce and Ko (2014), the link between the social determinants of health and health outcomes is poorly understood because it is difficult to track outcomes over a person's lifetime (where he or she lives/works), because some things are difficult to observe (capacity to cope with social stressors) and because it is yet to be determined how/if the availability and quality of health care links the social determinants of health with health outcomes. The point is, policy should be viewed through a *broad lens* and one should consider what the evidence reveals. To do this effectively, advances in available data will be required and *individual-level data* will need to be linked with *administrative data* to determine how social determinants interact with the health system. At the end of the day, policy changes must be focused on evidence (as limited as it may be) rather than political opinion.

▶ Evidence-Based Health Policy

Evidence-based public policymaking is a topic of increasing interest today; especially, as it relates to how it will (or should) be used in the decision-making process. The term *evidence-based policy* refers to the process "whereby policy decisions are informed by rigorously established objective evidence" ("Evidence-based policy," 2018, para 1). While as healthcare professionals it makes sense to base decisions on evidence, the use of evidence in the policy-making process is not as straightforward. For example, policies involve multiple social concerns that may have different *evidence bases* relevant to each one; therefore, the act of policymaking requires political reasoning. There are also inherent political biases that ultimately drive how evidence is interpreted and used (Parkhurst, 2017). Nevertheless, one should not reject the importance of evidence; instead, move forward to overcome these challenges and include evidence in the *policy-making process* to meet societal goals.

To accomplish this, Parkhurst (2017) suggests building systems to guide the use of evidence in the policy-making process to promote the *good governance of evidence*. In other words, the DNP student must "ensure that rigorous, systematic and technically valid pieces of evidence are used within decision-making processes that are inclusive of, representative of and accountable to the multiple social interests of the population served" (p. 8). This requires a two-prong approach. First, the DNP student must realize that policy decisions require *trade-offs* between the competing interests. From this perspective, evidence serves as a tool of measurement by identifying who will benefit from different decisions that are made or what groups may accrue (or lose) benefits over time. Parkhurst aptly points out that evidence cannot dictate the right choice. As mentioned above, to determine what is right or wrong requires political reasoning. The second approach involves the consideration of the contextual structures where all political decisions take place. These structures have the potential to direct or constrain the range of policy choices and/or decisions.

This two-prong approach aligns perfectly with the advanced skills and competencies that all DNP-prepared nurses acquire during their doctoral studies. These advanced skills and competencies can be used to assure that evidence is critically analyzed and that perspectives from consumers, nursing, other health professions, and stakeholders with competing values are included in the policy-making process.

The nature of DNP work requires the recognition of the context of the problem and assessment of facilitators and barriers to achieving a desired state. This includes engagement of stakeholders, collaboration, and negotiation. DNP-prepared nurses are perfectly suited to establish the good governance of evidence.

▶ DNP *Essential* Core Competencies Used to Advocate for Healthcare Policy Change

The core competencies for healthcare policy for advocacy in health care are embedded in DNP *Essential* V, but competencies from many of the DNP *Essentials* are also applicable. For example, as mentioned above, healthcare professionals must advocate for low-income individuals and urge politicians to change the current system. This is consistent with *Essential* V-7 that specifically calls for the DNP-prepared nurse to advocate for social justice, equity, and ethical policies within all healthcare arenas. When considering evidence, DNP-prepared nurses are adept at analyzing scientific data related to individual, aggregate, and population health (*Essential* VII-1) and critically appraising existing literature and other evidence to determine and implement the best evidence (*Essential* III-1). And when linking *individual-level data* with *administrative data* to determine how social determinants interact with the health system, the DNP-prepared nurse uses the competencies acquired in *Essential* IV-2 to first analyze the data within the healthcare information and patient care technology systems, then informs key stakeholders what critical elements are necessary to the selection, use, and evaluation of this information (AACN, 2006).

▶ The DNP Project and Health Policy

The following health policy analysis is an example of how one could advocate for a change to address a population health problem. In this example, Dr. Sonya Kowalski addresses a food insecurity problem within a local community using Bardach and Patashnik's (2016) *Practical Guide for Policy Analysis: The Eightfold Path to More Effective Problem Solving* (see **EXEMPLAR 4-1**).

EXEMPLAR 4-1 Policy Analysis for Michigan Food Bank Food and Operations Support Funding

Sonya Kowalski, DNP, APRN, ACNS-BC

Economists declared an end to the "Great Recession" in the summer of 2009, yet over 60% of the employment shortfall that was caused by the recession remains, which requires a greater amount of government safety net spending (Fieldhouse 2014). The persistent problem with unemployment and underemployment has led to an increase in food insecurity, which has been identified as a health problem nationally (Murthy, 2016). Food insecurity is categorized as low food security, which is the experience of insufficient food quality, variety, and desirability, or very low food security, which is described as disrupted eating patterns and reduced food intake by the U.S. Department of Agriculture (USDA, 2016). The state of Michigan food insecurity rate in 2014 was 15.7% and the food insecurity rate for Wayne County was 22% (Gundersen, Dewey, Crumbaugh, Kato, & Engelhard, 2016).

In February of 2017, the Michigan jobless rate was 5.3% compared to the U.S. jobless rate of 4.7% (Michigan Department of Technology, Management & Budget, 2017). In 2014, the percentage of Michigan residents living in poverty was 16.2%, compared to the national poverty rate of 15.5% (Wisely & Tanner, 2015). The same year, the child poverty rate in Michigan was 22.6%, compared to the national child poverty rate of 21.7% (Wisely & Tanner, 2015). A poverty rate that is much higher than the unemployment rate indicates that Michigan has a higher number of working poor families compared to the national average, and these numbers have not been improving. The poverty rates for African American children have been as high as 47% in Michigan, with over 30% of Hispanic and Native American children, 15.6% of white children, and 13.7% of Asian American children living in poverty (Ruark, 2015). These numbers indicate a greater number of people working but still in poverty among ethnic minorities.

The majority of families who utilize food banks are considered the working poor. The working poor are employed but do not make enough money to pay all of their expenses. According to the Food Bank Council of Michigan (2015), "When families have to choose between paying for childcare, medications, housing, and food, food is usually the first budget that gets cut" (para 2). The greatest factors that drive people into emergency feeding programs are housing, heating, and health care (Zimet, 2017). This indicates that, in addition to the working poor, homeless, disabled, ill, and elderly persons are also at high risk for food insecurity. Rent increases in areas with gentrification lead to food insecurity among people with limited incomes (Whittle et al., 2015). Female-headed households have been found to have 75% greater chance of being food insecure than male-headed households (Jung, de Bairros, Pattussi, Pauli, & Neutzling, 2017). University students have been found to have between 12.7% and 46.5% incidence of food insecurity (Hughes, Serebryanikova, Donaldson, & Leveritt, 2011). Veterans who served from 1975 and after have been found to be at high risk for food insecurity (Miller, Larson, Byrne, & DeVoe, 2016). Food insecurity is also a problem in 14.1% of households with an active duty service member, with 4.7% reporting very low food security (Wax & Stankorb, 2016). Food insecurity is an important issue for multiple populations in Michigan and the U.S.

Negative health outcomes are associated with food insecurity, such as increased rates of asthma, hypertension, hyperlipidemia, diabetes, birth defects, mental illness, depression, suicidal ideation, and premature aging (Gundersen & Ziliak, 2015). These negative health outcomes, related to food insecurity, resulted in estimated direct healthcare costs and indirect lost productivity costs of $160.07 billion in 2014. Additionally, an estimated $18.85 billion was spent in special education and school dropout costs related to food insecurity (Cook & Poblacion, 2016).

Food insecurity in Michigan has recently increased due to the 2014 federal Farm Bill. The Farm Bill covered both agriculture and nutrition programs and changes led to reduction in the Supplemental Nutrition Assistance Program (SNAP) in states like Michigan that did not increase funding into the federal Heat and Eat program. Some senior citizens saw their nutrition benefits drop to $16 per month (Tower, 2016). The state of Michigan recently allocated $6.8 million to restore approximately $76 per month for nutrition to these low-income families in the 2018 budget (Snyder, Calley, & Pscholka, 2017). The average SNAP benefit is $126 per person per month (Center on Budget and Policy Priorities, 2016). SNAP benefits are available to persons who are at or below 130% of the federal poverty level.

In addition to the SNAP program, some programs to combat hunger provide cash assistance, such as Temporary Assistance to Needy Families (TANF), which has a 4-year limit; Supplemental Security Income; and federal and state earned income tax credits. Other nutrition programs include the national school lunch program and the Special Supplemental Nutrition Program for Women, Infants, and Children (WIC) (Schmidt, Shore-Sheppard, & Watson, 2015). However, in the U.S., 45% of the food insecure

(continues)

EXEMPLAR 4-1 Policy Analysis for Michigan Food Bank Food and Operations Support Funding *(continued)*

are above the SNAP threshold and 26% are above the threshold for other nutrition programs (Gundersen, Dewey, Crumbaugh, Kato, & Engelhard, 2016). In Wayne County, Michigan, 17% of adults and 33% of children who are food insecure are above eligibility requirements for nutrition programs (Wayne Metropolitan Community Action Agency, 2016). Many of these people with food insecurity utilize local food pantries and food banks to alleviate hunger (Feeding America, 2011).

The local food pantries and food banks are unable to meet the needs of the food insecure. The Michigan Department of Education has requested more community organization support for the summer food service program to help feed a half-million children over the summer (Ackley, 2016). Local food pantry operators indicate inadequate resources to expand their services. Local and regional nutrition support agencies have a mission to reduce food insecurity, but resource barriers prevent getting the food to the needy at a local, neighborhood level. A state grant program could help to alleviate some of the resource barriers of the food banks and pantries and allow for a greater distribution of food as a community health initiative.

Literature Review

A literature review was conducted utilizing the Cumulative Index to Nursing and Allied Health Literature (CINAHL). The search terms used were policy, food insecurity, populations, interventions, strategies, best practices, government funding, and risk factors. The search was limited to the last 5 years and articles were chosen for review based on likelihood of similarity to U.S. and Michigan populations, such as U.S., Canadian, and Australian populations. Food insecurity articles from poverty-stricken nations such as Ethiopia were not included for this policy analysis.

In addition to the CINAHL database, Google was also searched for information related to recent political events that would not likely yet be available in research journals. The websites of known hunger political action groups, such as the Michigan League for Public Policy, and food resource providers such as Gleaners Food Bank and The Food Bank Council of Michigan were also searched. The review of literature revealed a large amount of information based on the populations and numbers of people affected by food insecurity, such as children and ethnic minorities with poverty rates from 13% to 47% (Ruark, 2015), the working poor (Food Bank Council of Michigan, 2015), university students with poverty rates from 12.7% to 46.5% (Hughes, Serebryanikova, Donaldson, & Leveritt, 2011), and active duty military families with 4.7% very low food security rates (Wax & Stankorb, 2016).

The review of literature also revealed the reasons for food insecurity, such as issues dealing with housing, heating, and health care (Zimet, 2017) and the health outcomes that result from inadequate nutrition, such as increased rates of asthma, hypertension, hyperlipidemia, diabetes, birth defects, mental illness, depression, suicidal ideation, and premature aging (Gundersen & Ziliak, 2015). The food provider websites provided details regarding what is being done to combat hunger, such as retrieving usable and previously discarded food and assisting with the harvest of food that may have gone to waste and donating food to emergency food providers (Forgotten Harvest, 2017); they also gave opportunities for donations and volunteer services (Forgotten Harvest, 2017; Gleaner's Community Food Bank, 2017). There was very little information about comparison of effectiveness of interventions or adequacy of government policies that promote relief of hunger. There was no indication of best practices or benchmarks for hunger alleviation.

Alternative Solutions to Address the Problem

The first alternative would be to do nothing. If the existing programs continue without intervention, then the poorest community members would still be provided with SNAP, limited TANF funds, and WIC. The working poor could continue to try to obtain food from available resources. The rate of food insecurity would likely remain the same unless more high-paying jobs are created. This solution would prevent a greater tax burden on those employed in higher wage jobs. The poor may be encouraged to work more, or obtain higher education. What is likely to happen is an increase in the adverse health effects that impact the food insecure and an increased demand on the healthcare system in the decades to come. The increased health-related costs due to food insecurity will likely rise from the 2014 $160 billion estimate.

Another alternative could be to direct resources into the creation of higher paying jobs. At the national level, President Barack Obama created 22.3 million jobs from the worst part of the recession until the end of his presidency, which is the second greatest number of jobs created by any U.S. president (Amadeo, 2017). Although the number of jobs increased, the number of food insecure remains high. It is possible that this is because the populations who remain food insecure may be too young, too old, too ill to work; may be disabled and unable to work; or may lack the education or child care resources necessary to participate in the labor market.

A third alternative would be to increase both federal and state funding for food assistance programs. Data from 2012 indicated that SNAP benefits lifted 10.3 million people out of poverty and 5.2 million people out of deep poverty in the U.S. (Sherman & Trisi, 2015). An increase in funding could lift even more people out of poverty. According to the President's 2018 budget (Trump, 2017), the funding for U.S. food security programs, including WIC, will remain stable, while funding for foreign food aid will be decreased. According to Governor Snyder's 2018 budget (Snyder, Calley, & Pscholka, 2017) the state funding that had been reduced for the SNAP program in 2015 will be reinstated for qualifying Michigan residents in 2018. At this time, there are no budget appropriations for an increase in SNAP benefits, and since 2014 the average benefits per person have declined (USDA, 2017).

In addition to lifting an increased number of people out of poverty, additional unexpected benefits of an increase in SNAP funding include: every $5 in new SNAP benefits generates $9 in total community spending; every additional dollar of SNAP benefits generates 17 to 47 cents of new spending on food; and $1 billion in retail food demand by SNAP recipients generates about 3000 farm jobs (USDA, n. d.).

The final and recommended solution to the food insecurity problem is an implementation of policy that would allow for improved organization and utilization of existing resources. An analysis of local food providers indicated that the availability of food is not always consistent, convenient, or transparent. Food banks are available regionally, such as Forgotten Harvest and Gleaner's Community Food Bank. These food banks serve the population of food insecure and assist in supplying the local food pantries; however, transportation has been identified as a significant barrier (Wayne Metropolitan Community Action Agency, 2016). Community stakeholders recommend a collaborative effort to meet families where they are and the utilization of community-wide philanthropy and community mapping of available resources (Wayne Metropolitan Community Action Agency, 2016). A survey of the local food pantry operators reveals a reluctance to participate in a collaborative effort such as a coalition to increase food visibility and accessibility for the food insecure. The fear is that demand that will greatly exceed supply and rapidly overwhelm the available resources of food, storage space, and volunteers.

(continues)

EXEMPLAR 4-1　Policy Analysis for Michigan Food Bank Food and Operations Support Funding　*(continued)*

This problem is not unique to the local area. In the state of New York, the Hunger Prevention and Nutrition Assistance Program (HPNAP) has advocated for policy and funding to increase access and improve infrastructure to get food to the hungry (Zimet, 2017). The HPNAP has provided funding to the Food Bank of Central New York, who provide food and operations support in the form of grants to local food pantries. The local food pantries have used the grant money to purchase freezers, refrigerators, and shelving that support their food distribution efforts. This model has been suggested to be "a model for the nation" (IOM, 2011, p. 121). A similar policy for grant funding could help to improve food access for Michigan food pantries.

Analysis of Recommended Solution

According to Zimet (2017), "Hunger, the lack of affordable housing, homelessness, and lack of access to health care are all interconnected and must be addressed in a comprehensive manner" (p. 4). A policy for grant funding to assist food pantries in providing food to the hungry would only address the hunger aspect for the food insecure, which would be a weakness of the program. A strength of the policy would be that it makes use of existing resources and the grant costs would be significantly less than the healthcare-associated costs of doing nothing or the costs of increased SNAP benefits.

The support of the local food banks would be a preferable solution than the solution to increase higher paying jobs because it would provide a more rapid benefit to the hungry and provide for those who are too young, too old, too sick, or disabled and unable to participate in the work force. The grant funding could help the local communities meet their mission goals and ethically provide needed assistance. In the HPNAP program, the grant awards are up to $3000 or, if used for the purchase of food service equipment only, may be up to $6000. The equipment must be transferred to the central food bank if the organization stops providing emergency food assistance. Eligible organizations are nonprofit, tax-exempt organizations that provide emergency food without cost to recipient to all persons in need without discrimination. Grant money may be used for direct service worker staff costs, food storage utility costs, dedicated space costs, supplies necessary for food provision, transportation costs to deliver food to the pantries, and food service equipment necessary for operations such as refrigerators, freezers, shelves, stoves, and cabinets, with prices based on two actual quotes for nonsale prices. The over $1 million dollars utilized for the program between 2004 and 2011 in New York averaged about $150,000 per year in budget allocation (IOM, 2011).

This policy has a relatively low-cost, simple structure and reasonable administrative burden and would be administratively feasible to implement in Michigan. Community stakeholders would benefit from the addition of infrastructure resources. The resources would allow for existing money to go towards food, which would increase availability for the food insecure. The resources would encourage collaboration, as the various food pantries could alternate the acquisition and transportation of low-cost food from the regional food banks, which would conserve both money and volunteer time. The availability of more food locally would benefit the food insecure unable to obtain transportation to the regional food banks.

The grant monies could also be used to fund a small stipend for pantry workers, which may be appreciated and encourage participation in some organizations. Food insecure people who utilize food banks with adequate storage and refrigeration will benefit from a maximization of resource allocation through increased food choices compared to the limited canned and boxed food that is available without the resources. Increased access to fresh fruits, vegetables, and milk may promote a healthier diet among the food insecure. Given the association between food insecurity and numerous poor health outcomes such as diabetes, obesity, depression, and hypertension, the cost of the grant program may more than pay for itself in reduced healthcare costs.

Conclusion

Food insecurity has continued to be a public health issue, years after the end of the "Great Recession." Food insecurity affects many populations, including children, the elderly, the disabled, the ill, immigrants, military veterans, and military families. Food insecurity leads to numerous health conditions and increased healthcare costs. Racial and ethnic minorities have a greater risk of food insecurity, which leads to greater health disparities. Policies that reduce food insecurity have been successful in the state of New York and have the potential to be successful in Michigan.

The policy to award grant money to organizations that supply emergency food is an example of a policy that can be adopted to maximize the use of existing resources without great expense. Assistance provided to community stakeholders can help to remove barriers to reducing food insecurity such as transportation and equipment costs. Available refrigeration and improved storage facilities can help food providers to improve both quality and quantity of available food, which may lead to improved population health outcomes and reduced health disparities. The policy to provide grant funding to organizations that provide emergency food is a good one, both ethically and financially.

▶ Your Health Policy Journey

Why did you first become a nurse? Why did you want to become a DNP-prepared nurse? Many chose nursing as their life's work because they want to "make a difference" in the lives of their patients; they are "called to the profession." There is no doubt that through one's nursing education many things are learned, but what often stand out most are those things that didn't come from a textbook: that there is something sacred in the relationship between the patient and the nurse; that nurses do more than provide protection, promotion, and optimization of health and abilities—nurses facilitate healing and wellness through that human connection. And, with this trusted relationship comes responsibility, especially related to advocacy.

There are many opportunities for DNP-prepared nurses to promote change in health care through advocacy, leading inter- and intraprofessional collaboration efforts, engaging stakeholders, transforming systems to improve care, analyzing policies—and, there are numerous paths the DNP-prepared nurse could take to make an impact. Where healthcare reform is concerned, the IOM has recognized nurses as valuable players in this process. It is time for nurses, especially DNP-prepared nurses, to see policy as something we shape. There will be challenges; however, the good news is we are now at a point in the DNP degree trajectory where we are beginning to see the impact of practice scholarship, and therefore, the associated benefit of the practice doctorate. Those nursing-specific improved healthcare outcomes that have been demonstrated by DNP scholars not only validate the value of the practice doctorate, but also elevate the science-based practice skill set of the nursing profession. That is why it is important for DNP students to explore opportunities and expand their horizons as it relates to healthcare policy and the role of the DNP-prepared nurse.

A Call to Action

Advocacy is "a method by which patients, their families, attorneys, health professionals, and citizen groups can work together to develop programs that ensure the availability of high-quality health care for a community" ("Advocacy," 2018, para 2). Advocacy is a core principle of the nursing profession. Nurses engage in advocacy as part of the role and responsibility of the nurse to advocate on behalf of those whom nurses have been contracted (by society) to provide care at the individual, family, community, or population level (Lewenson & Nickitas, 2016). Certainly, all nurses know the work of Florence Nightingale, the founder of nursing education programs, and perhaps Lillian Wald, who established public health nursing. These revolutionary nursing scholars set the stage for nursing advocacy work for years to come. Today, nurses remain uniquely positioned to advocate for the health of the populations they serve.

In 2017, nurses again topped the Gallup poll for the most trusted profession (American Organization of Nursing Executives [AONE], 2018). With this honor comes the responsibility to act. Nurses, especially DNP-prepared nurses, possess scientific nursing knowledge and experience that can be used to influence policy decisions (Porche, 2019).

We are called to lead and manage collaborative efforts with other healthcare practitioners to improve healthcare delivery and the health of the populations we serve.

DNP-prepared nurses must use the skills and competencies acquired in doctoral study to lead system change to improve patient outcomes, critically analyze health policy proposals, advocate for social justice, and demonstrate leadership as they sit at the table with other healthcare professionals to positively impact healthcare reform.

▶ Advocacy Opportunities

DNP-prepared nurses can begin by advocating for the good of the nursing profession. For example, by addressing workforce issues, the increased need for minority representation in nursing, and title protection, to name a few. The plea to advocate is noted in the American Nurses Association's (ANA) (2010) document, *Nursing Scope and Standards of Practice*, as well as the ANA (2001) *Code of Ethics*, where the ANA calls for professional nurses to advocate for safe healthcare environments. These efforts will ultimately positively impact the care nurses are able to provide to their patients.

As mentioned, nurses are uniquely equipped to advocate for patient populations. Nurses can advocate to address disparities in healthcare access, for better healthcare quality, lower costs, and even extended healthcare insurance coverage. For example, nurses testified in Michigan on behalf of patients to expand Medicaid. Betty O'Connor-Rogers was one of the registered nurses that testified. She shared the following experience with the Michigan Competitiveness Committee in 2013:

> *I took care of a patient who had always been very self-sufficient. He ate right, exercised, never smoked—he took care of himself. He was a trucker whose employer didn't offer health insurance, but he figured he was healthy and could do without.*
>
> *Then, he started having trouble breathing and when he finally went to the doctor he learned he had a genetic form of lung cancer. If they'd found it sooner, they might have been able to do something. During treatment he went through his entire savings to pay his bills, but when he had nothing left he stopped his chemo and passed away. It's one of the hardest things I've ever had to work through. And Medicaid expansion would have helped him.* (Smith, 2013, para 5)

This is just one example of many testimonies from nurses that ultimately pushed the Michigan legislators forward to expand Medicaid.

The opportunities to advocate are virtually limitless. There are also multiple approaches to advocacy. The DNP student could attend a legislator's local town hall meeting, a health policy advocacy day, or a legislative hearing where expertise as a healthcare provider could be shared. Advocacy opportunities also exist via professional organizations. For example, the American Association of Nurse Practitioners (AANP) has an Advocacy Center on their website where members can keep abreast of healthcare issues and legislation and assist with advocacy efforts through submission of expedited form letters that can be sent to legislators at the state and national level (see www.aanp.org for more information). The DNP student should check to see if there is a need for volunteers to sit on the policy or advocacy committee, or attend a march at the state capitol. Or, consider going to Capitol Hill in Washington, D.C. to champion a piece of healthcare legislation with a senator or representative!

Legislators want to hear from their constituents. The following tips are provided to help the DNP student prepare for a health policy advocacy experience.

Calling a Representative

- The DNP student should begin by introducing him- or herself and letting the representative or senator know that he or she is a constituent.
- The student should tell the staffer that he or she is a nurse.
- Then, the student should tell the representative about his or her main concern and share any support from the literature that speaks to the significance of the issue.
- Take the time to share a personal or professional story that relates to the concern. A story gives the problem context and will help illustrate the main point.
- It is important to share one's vision. Tell the representative what is working or is not working, and what he or she could do to address the problem.
- Always remember to thank the representative and his or her staff for their time (ANA, 2017a).

Meeting with a Representative

Setting up the Meeting

- Call the senator or representative's office. Request a meeting with the representative or his or her staff at the nearest district office and inform him or her about the topic of concern.
- The staffer will provide the location for the closest district office. While an appointment may not be necessary, it will assure that there is someone available during the requested meeting time.

Preparing for the Meeting

- The DNP student should prepare with background work before the meeting to find out where the representative stands on the issue of concern. This information may be found on the representative's website or through online press releases.
- Write down an introduction plan. For example, the DNP student could include his or her background in nursing, perhaps the types of patients that he or she sees or the classes he or she teaches, etc. This information will be helpful for the staffers.
- It may be helpful for the DNP student to write down his or her "number-one" concern. It is best to focus the discussion around what is most important; do not feel compelled to speak to every issue.
- The representative probably does not know much about health care, so be ready for questions.
- Again, make sure to thank the representative and staff for their time (ANA, 2017b)!

Speaking at a Town Hall Meeting

- Before attending the meeting, try to get an idea of what the tone of the event will be. To do this, contact the policymaker's district office to see who is expected to attend and if anyone is expected to give a presentation. This will give the DNP student an idea for how to prepare his or her remarks.

- As mentioned above, the DNP student should prepare with background work before attending the meeting. This includes having accurate, timely, and relevant information to share with the group and a plan to introduce his or her position as early in the meeting as possible.
- Share information about the meeting with others and encourage them to attend to show community support for the initiative. The goal is to get as many advocates to attend the meeting as possible.
- The DNP student should be prepared to present his or her views with concise points and support from the literature. These facts will help those attending the meeting understand and remember the main points.
- Remember to practice your message! The goal is to be as comfortable and confident as possible when sharing concerns at the meeting.
- Finally, it is a good idea for the DNP student to leave written copies of his or her position with the policymaker, staff, and others who attend the meeting (American Public Health Association [APHA], n. d.).

Writing a Letter to the Editor

Writing a letter to the editor is a great way to shed light on an issue or concern. For example, the DNP student could address the editor to clarify facts or correct misstatements, to oppose or support current or proposed legislation, or to simply to gain support from the community. Consider the following recommendations when writing a letter to the editor.

- Be strategic in the timing of the letter. The editor of a newspaper will be cognizant of topics that are currently in the news.
- Review the paper guidelines related to word count, format, contact information, and delivery methods (email, etc.). The DNP student should follow these important requirements to assure his or her work is included in its entirety.
- When writing a letter, provide brief, but sufficient background information so that the readers understand the significance of the issue and how it may affect their lives and communities.
- If the DNP student is responding to a previously published editorial, he or she should make sure to include this information in the letter. And, conclude the letter with his or her name and credentials, so that the editor (and audience) recognizes that the student is a healthcare provider.
- The letter should be specific to a circulation area. Do not send the same letter to multiple papers within the same geographic area (ANA, n. d.).

Writing an Opinion Editorial

An opinion editorial (op-ed) is different than a letter to the editor. First, it is generally longer than a letter and is published in a specific section of the paper reserved for opinions. Consider the following information when preparing to write an op-ed.

- Begin with the end in mind! Since papers receive hundreds of submissions a week, the DNP student will want to start early and do his or her homework before submitting the op-ed.

- The DNP student should first check with the newspaper to see if they accept opinion pieces. For example, he or she should call the newspaper, introduce him- or herself, and tell the editorial page editor that he or she would like to submit op-ed.
- Like a letter to the editor, it is important to follow any specific guidelines the newspaper may have for these types of pieces (e.g., word limit [usually around 650 words], how to submit the piece, the format, etc.). When the DNP student submits the op-ed, he or she should consider including a message to remind the editor about their conversation and why it is an important topic for their readers.
- Finally, the DNP student should remember to include his or her name, credentials, and perhaps a brief description of his or her area of expertise so that the editor recognizes the student's level of knowledge on the topic.
- If the student doesn't hear anything after about a week, he or she should reach out again to confirm the editorial page editor received the op-ed (APHA, 2016).

Writing a Policy Brief

A policy brief synthesizes "existing research knowledge on a policy or practice issue of importance. . . and is written in language an interested non-expert would find accessible" (National Education Policy Center, n. d., para 1). It is a helpful tool that uses evidence to influence policy and practice.

As the term "policy brief" implies, the paper should be short (only two to four pages in length) and include a description and context of a problem and the recommended action. There are a variety of policy brief formats that can be used, but many include:

- An introduction that includes a description of the problem and background
- The aim of the brief
- Potential approaches and solutions
- A conclusion
- The recommended option and implications

The goal of a policy brief is to communicate the right message to the right people at the right time; therefore, writing a policy brief requires use of the essential communication skills and competencies attained in doctoral education. Like writing a scholarly paper, the goal of a brief is to share the information. However, simply sharing the information doesn't mean that it will be used in practice. So, the focus of a policy brief is to communicate information in a way that will be understood by those who read it, and subsequently used to make a change. For example, it could be a change in local regulations or state law; it could involve funding priorities, organizational practices, or even program implementation (Johns Hopkins Bloomberg School of Public Health, n. d.).

Since the focus is on clear communication, it is important to know the audience. Before embarking on a policy brief, the DNP student should ask him- or herself the following questions: What do you know about the audience? Are they aware of the problem? Will they be open or resistant to change? This information will help the student identify the best message to use to engage and motivate them for change.

Consider the following from Johns Hopkins Bloomberg School of Public Health (n. d.) when writing a policy brief.

- Begin by writing the aim of the policy brief, because everything in the brief should directly relate to the aim. The aim should include one or two sentences.
- Next focus on describing the problem and why it is relevant to the reader. Use data to describe the extent of the problem. When writing a policy brief it is important to give the right amount of background information to engage the reader, but not overburden him or her with information that is not directly related. So, unlike a scholarly paper where one might include an exhaustive literature review, with a policy brief only include information that is relevant and necessary to make the case.
- In the next section, talk about solutions that have already been implemented and the effectiveness of the solutions.
- Then, the DNP student should describe a few options that he or she is recommending for change with the pros and cons of each option; remember, not doing anything can be an option.
- In the final section, describe your recommendation. It will be important for the DNP student to do his or her homework before writing this section—reach out to the stakeholders to get feedback and gain support for the recommendation. The student's recommended option should be backed by evidence and flow logically from his or her argument. It should be very specific and clearly describe the action the student recommends and the anticipated effect; don't be vague and leave it to the audience to interpret. The audience should clearly understand what the student proposes they do, as this may be the only part of the policy brief that someone reads.
- Once the brief is written, the student will need to come up with a title that is both engaging and informative. The title is very important. It should not only tell the reader what the brief is about, but also *why* he or she should read it.

Remember, a policy brief is intended to be read quickly and should provide the reader with information about the problem, the aim, and recommendation without unnecessary verbiage. With this in mind, structure the brief to highlight key points and make it easier to read, e.g., separate text into sections with headings, use bullet points, bar graphs, and figures where possible, use callout boxes, bold or italicized font, and plenty of white space (Johns Hopkins Bloomberg School of Public Health, n. d.).

Performing a Policy Analysis

The *purpose* of a policy analysis is to "critically appraise the context in which an agenda, issue, or policy exists" (Porche, 2019, p. 189). The policy analysis *process* involves interpretive analysis and the historical context of the policy from the macro-level (focusing on broad influencers, e.g., economics), meso-level (focusing on implementation and individuals and groups that develop policy), and micro-level (focusing on engagement between constituents and policymakers, including the beliefs and values that impact the process) perspectives. The policy analysis *product* reflects the level of focus, purpose, and intent for conducting the analysis, and should include a clear description of the problem, potential solutions, courses of action and expected outcomes, and contextual understanding of the problem and policy (Porche, 2019).

There are multiple approaches that can be used as a guide to conduct a policy analysis (see Chapter 6, Developing the DNP Project for examples of policy analysis approaches). The following policy analysis framework from Bardach and Patashnik (2016) is used to illustrate the process. It is not necessary to follow these steps in order or to include all steps in every analysis. However, the authors point out that although this is an iterative process, *defining the problem* is a good place to start and *telling the story* is generally the ending point.

1. Define the Problem

This is where the problem is defined in quantitative terms; it is where the reason for the work is described. This baseline information should give the reader a sense of the magnitude of the problem and direction. The authors suggest beginning by thinking in terms of deficits and excess. For example, *there are too many people dying in motorcycle accidents* (a public problem) or *the need for primary care practitioners in rural communities is growing faster than our ability to educate practitioners* (indicating a potential breakdown in the education system, an equity concern for rural communities, or both).

As mentioned, it is important for the DNP student to quantify how big the problem is to the best of his or her ability. In some cases, he or she may need to estimate the magnitude of the problem using a metric that provides a reference for the reader. The example above, "too many people are dying in motorcycle accidents, is a concern, but how big of a concern? To quantify this statement one could say, "too many people between 16 and 19 years of age are dying from motorcycle accidents," or to further define it one could say, "there are more people between 16 and 19 years of age who died from motorcycle accidents in the past year than in the past 10 years combined." This provides further context that will be beneficial later in the analysis.

Finally, Bardach and Patashnik (2016) offer a word of caution: Do not define the solution into problem (a problem statement that includes the solution) and to be skeptical about causal claims (in other words, evaluate the evidence carefully).

2. Assemble Evidence

This step in the process requires an investment of time to gather data, but also time to reflect on the meaning of the data collected. Both are time-consuming processes. It is better to *think* before *collecting*, so that the student is sure that the data he or she collects are useful. In other words, the student will need data that are first a source of information (data with meaning), but with the potential to eventually become evidence (information that affects existing beliefs). This can be accomplished through a literature review, by surveying other best practices, or by using analogies from similar programs (e.g., comparing public to private sector, etc.). Finally, take the time to reach out to potential supporters, but also to potential critics to gain their perspectives. It is important that the student doesn't ignore those who disagree with his or her view!

3. Construct Alternatives (Policy Options that Can Be Used to Mitigate the Problem)

Start with a broad, comprehensive list of potential options. For example, the DNP student could start with the options that are currently being discussed, come up with a few on his or her own, and consider letting *the present trend continue*—meaning, to continue with the status quo. Once the student is satisfied with the list of alternatives, he or she will need to narrow the list down to a few best options. With any "new" alternative, it is good practice to run it by a few interested stakeholders, so that the student is sure he or she is on target.

4. Select the Criteria

In this section the DNP student should think about value judgments. In other words, the student needs to determine if the *projected outcome* of an alternative (this distinction is important to keep in mind) would be good or bad for the population, and therefore, whether it would or would not be considered desirable.

Examples of evaluation criteria that are important to consider include efficiency criteria, such as cost effectiveness. Equity criteria may also be used to evaluate fairness across the populations and/or social justice. In addition, there are a variety of freedom criteria that may be considered, such as freedom to choose (e.g., to wear a helmet when riding a motorcycle), privacy, security, etc. Other practical criteria that may be used in the evaluation process include the legality or the political acceptability of a policy, and the degree of opposition and/or lack of support.

Finally, Bardach and Patashnik (2016) point out that, to the extent that is possible, the criteria chosen should be characterized both conceptually and operationally (typically quantitatively). To do this, specify the metrics that will be used to evaluate the criteria. For example, a qualitative metric may be to *maximize the use of helmets when riding a motorcycle*. The quantitative metric may be to *reduce the death rate by 50% in individuals between 16 and 19 years of age dying in motorcycle accidents in the next 12 months*.

5. Project Outcomes

Projecting the outcomes for each of the alternatives is the next step. Here are a few things to consider when projecting outcomes:

- Be as realistic as possible; it is impossible to be completely sure about what the future will bring, but avoid being overly optimistic.
- Combine models and evidence to develop useful projections (e.g., a social science model is used to determine whether something is "smart" practice).
- Choose a base case (common reference mark). For example, let's say that there are currently 1500 teens dying annually from motorcycle accidents. Based on alternative one, one could say that it is reasonable to expect this number to decrease by 750 (based on a 50% reduction proposed earlier).
- Determine what a break-even estimate would be (e.g., 100,000 helmets need to be donated by the end of the first year of the program to assure success).
- Reflect on scenarios that could cause the proposal to fail (think about the political [and other] dangers associated with the implementation process).

- Think about potential "undesirable side effects" (for example, if a policy is initiated that mandates helmet use but then leads to overregulation in other areas).
- Use an outcomes matrix to compare the policy alternatives.

6. Confront Trade-offs

Confronting the trade-offs involves looking at the projected outcomes for each alternative, then, determining which offers the best "trade-off" for the good of the population. The best way to do this is to establish commensurability across the established criterion. Money is often used for this metric. While it is best to quantify trade-offs whenever possible, sometimes it is not possible. In these cases, using rank order may help in the decision-making process. It goes without saying that this should be a thoughtful process, as the trade-offs may include some moral and/or ethical components.

7. Decide

It is now time to make a decision! Which of the alternatives is the best option to solve the problem? What will it take to get it adopted? Remember to consider potential resistance from stakeholders who are happy with the status quo or the possibility that there is no one willing to step up to see this option through.

8. Tell Your Story

It is now time for the DNP student to tell his or her story to the identified stakeholders. To be effective, the student should make sure he or she knows the audience and can easily tell his or her story using simple, down-to-earth terms. Then, choose a method to deliver the information that is appropriate for the identified stakeholders (e.g., oral or written form, such as the example provided earlier).

▶ Summary

As a practice scholar, the DNP-prepared nurse must bring evidence to practice to positively influence healthcare outcomes. This can be accomplished through advocacy efforts at the micro, meso, or macro levels. As mentioned at the beginning of this chapter, DNP students with an interest in this work should consider a policy-focused project as a foundation for ongoing policy scholarship. Ultimately, DNP-prepared nurses are leaders of the nursing profession; therefore, they should consider policy/advocacy work as part of their role.

Impact

- DNP-prepared nurses have the education, knowledge, and skills to sit at the table and actively participate in the discussions where healthcare delivery and population health decisions are being made.

- As the most trusted profession, nurses (especially DNP-prepared nurses) will be heard when they advocate for patients and populations at the local, state, national, and international levels.
- It is critical that DNP-prepared nurses continue to focus on systematically analyzing and evaluating the factors that impact access to care, the cost of care, health behaviors, and outcomes of care.

Key Messages

- Political decisions that impacted the health of the country date back to the early 1900s.
- To address the most pressing needs of society, an intentional effort is needed to understand and ultimately address the "social determinants of health."
- Healthcare policies not only need to address access to care but must support and enhance communities to evolve into places for all residents of the community to live healthy, active, safe lives.
- Even with the spotlight on ethnic disparities in the U.S., there is still a long way to go to address these concerns, especially as it relates to overall health and life expectancy.
- Other important factors that contribute to healthcare outcomes are the cost and quality of health care.
- The term evidence-based policy refers to the process "whereby policy decisions are informed by rigorously established objective evidence" ("Evidence-based policy," 2018, para 1).
- DNP-prepared nurses are adept at analyzing scientific data related to individual, aggregate, and population health and critically appraising existing literature and other evidence to determine and implement the best evidence; therefore, they are perfectly suited to establish the *good governance of evidence.*
- DNP-prepared nurses are called to lead and manage collaborative efforts with other healthcare practitioners to improve healthcare delivery and the health of the populations that are served.
- Advocacy is a core principle of the nursing profession; therefore, DNP-prepared nurses should advocate for social justice, equity, and ethical policies within all healthcare arenas.

Action Plan—Next Steps

1. Consider how to address disparities in health or healthcare delivery in an organization (micro level), community (meso level), or beyond (macro level).
2. Determine which method to use to engage in the advocacy process (meet with a legislator, write a letter to the editor, write a policy brief, or perform a policy analysis).
3. Do your homework (gather the evidence).
4. Analyze the evidence.
5. Engage stakeholders—advocate to address disparities and urge politicians to change the system.

References

Ackley, M. (2016). *More partners needed to help feed Michigan's hungry children.* Michigan Department of Education. Retrieved from http://www.michigan.gov/mde/0,4615,7-140-37818_34785-377583--,00.html

Advocacy. (2018). *The Free Dictionary.* Retrieved from https://medical-dictionary.thefreedictionary.com/advocacy

Amadeo, K. (2017). *Which president created the most jobs?* Bureau of Labor Statistics. Retrieved from https://www.thebalance.com/job-creation-by-president-by-number-and-percent-3863218

American Association of Colleges of Nursing (AACN). (2004). *Position statement on the practice doctorate in nursing.* Retrieved from http://www.aacnnursing.org/DNP/Position-Statement

American Association of Colleges of Nursing (AACN). (2006). *The essentials of doctoral education for advanced nursing practice.* Retrieved from http://www.aacnnursing.org/Portals/42/Publications/DNPEssentials.pdf

American Organization of Nursing Executives (AONE). (2018). *Nurses again top Gallup poll of trusted professions.* Retrieved from http://www.aone.org/news/nurses-again-top-gallup-poll-of-trusted-professions

American Nurses Association (ANA). (n. d.). *Tips: Writing letters to the editor.* Practice and Policy. Retrieved from https://www.nursingworld.org/practice-policy/advocacy/federal/tips-writing-letters-to-the-editor/?letter_KEY=1602

American Nurses Association (ANA). (2001). *Code of ethics for nurses.* Silver Spring, MD: Author.

American Nurses Association (ANA). (2010). *Nursing scope and standards of practice* (2nd ed.). Silver Spring, MD: Author.

American Nurses Association (ANA). (2017a). *Hello, Congress? It's nurses. We need to talk.* Capitol Beat. Retrieved from http://anacapitolbeat.org/2017/01/19/hello-congress-its-nurses-we-need-to-talk/

American Nurses Association (ANA). (2017b). *Tips and tricks for visiting your senator's office.* Capitol Beat. Retrieved from http://anacapitolbeat.org/2017/01/05/tips-and-tricks-for-visiting-your-senators-office/

American Public Health Association (APHA). (n.d.). *Tips for speaking at a town or public meeting.* Retrieved from https://www.apha.org/-/media/files/pdf/advocacy/town_hall_or_public_meeting.ashx

American Public Health Association (APHA). (2016). *Write an op-ed.* Retrieved from https://www.apha.org/search-results?q=Write%20an%20op-ed

Bardach, E., & Patashnik, E. M. (2016). *A practical guide for policy analysis: The eightfold path to more effective problem solving.* Thousand Oaks, CA: CQ Press.

Bodenheimer, T. S., & Grumbach, K. (2016). *Understanding health policy: A clinical approach* (7th ed.). New York, NY: McGraw Hill.

Brennan, N., Cafarella, N., Kocot, S. L., McKethan, A., Morrison, M., & Nguyen, N., . . . Williams, R. D. (2009). Improving quality and value in the U.S. health care system. Brookings Institution. Retrieved from https://www.brookings.edu/research/improving-quality-and-value-in-the-u-s-health-care-system/

Bustamante, A. V., Morales, L. S., & Ortega, A. N. (2014). Racial and ethnic disparities in health care. In Kominski, G. (Ed.), *Changing the U.S. health care system: Key issues in health services policy and management.* (pp. 103–134). San Francisco, CA: Jossey-Bass.

Center on Budget and Policy Priorities (CBPP). (2016). *A quick guide to SNAP eligibility and benefits.* Washington, DC: Author. Retrieved from http://www.cbpp.org/research/a-quick-guide-to-snap-eligibility-and-benefits

Claxton, G., Rae, M., Levitt, L., & Cox, C. (2018). *How have health care prices grown in the U.S. over time?* Retrieved from https://www.healthsystemtracker.org/chart-collection/how-have-health-care-prices-grown-in-the-u s-over-time/#item-start

Cook, J. T., & Poblacion, A. P. (2016). Estimating the health-related costs of food insecurity and hunger. *2016 Hunger Report.* Washington, DC: Bread for the World Institute. Retrieved from http://www.hungerreport.org.

Davis, K., Stremikis, K., Schoen, C. & Squires, D. (2014). *Mirror, mirror on the wall, 2014 update: How the U.S. health care system compares internationally.* New York, NY: The Commonwealth Fund. Retrieved from http://www.commonwealthfund.org/publications/fund-reports/2014/jun/mirror-mirror

Evidence-based policy. (2018). In *Definitions.net*. Retrieved from https://www.definitions.net/definition/evidence-based%20policy

Feeding America. (2011). *Food banks: Hunger's new staple research brief*. Chicago, IL: Author. Retrieved from http://www.feedingamerica.org/hunger-in-america/our-research/hungers-new-staple/hungers-new-staple-full-report.pdf

Fieldhouse, A. (2014, June 26). 5 years after the great recession, our economy still far from recovered. *Huffington Post*. Retrieved from http://www.huffingtonpost.com/andrew-fieldhouse/five-years-after-the-grea_b_5530597.html

Food Bank Council of Michigan. (2015). *Myths and realities about hunger in Michigan*. Lansing, MI: Author. Retrieved from http://fbcmich.org/files/resources/64/Myths%20and%20realities%20About%20Hunger%202015.

Food Corps. (2018). *About Food Corps*. Portland, OR: Author. Retrieved from https://foodcorps.org/about/

Food Research & Action Center. (2015). *Profile of hunger, poverty, and federal nutrition programs*. Washington, DC: Author. Retrieved from http://frac.org/wp-content/uploads/2016/10/mi.pdf

Forgotten Harvest (2017). Agency information. Oak Park, MI: Author. Retrieved from http://www.forgottenharvest.org/

Ganz, P. A., Hays, R. D., Kaplan, R. M. & Litwin, M. S. (2014). Measuring health-related quality of life and other outcomes. In Kominski, G. (Ed.), *Changing the U.S. health care system: Key issues in health services policy and management*. (pp. 307–341). San Francisco: Jossey-Bass.

Gleaner's Community Food Bank. (2017). *About us*. Detroit, MI: Author. Retrieved from http://www.gcfb.org/?gclid=CIfUtZSutNMCFYK1wAodDEEA7A

Gundersen, C. A., Dewey, A., Crumbaugh, M., Kato, M., & Engelhard, E., (2016). *Map the meal gap 2016: Food insecurity and child food insecurity estimates at the county level*. Chicago, IL: Feeding America. Retrieved from www.feedingamerica.org/mapthegap.

Gundersen, C. A., & Ziliak, J. P., (2015). Food insecurity and health outcomes. *Health Affairs, 34*(11), 1830–1839. doi:10.1377/hlthaff.2015.0645

HealthCare.gov (n.d.). *Patient Protection and Affordable Care Act*. Retrieved from https://www.healthcare.gov/glossary/patient-protection-and-affordable-care-act/

Hughes, R., Serebryanikova, I., Donaldson, K., & Leveritt, M. (2011). Student food insecurity: The skeleton in the university closet. *Nutrition & Dietetics, 68*(1), 27–32.

Institute of Medicine (IOM). (1999). *To err is human: Building a safer health system*. Washington, DC: National Academies Press. Retrieved from http://www.nationalacademies.org/hmd/~/media/Files/Report%20Files/1999/To-Err-is-Human/To%20Err%20is%20Human%201999%20%20report%20brief.pdf

Institute of Medicine (IOM). (2001). *Crossing the quality chasm: A new health system for the 21st century*. Washington, DC: National Academies Press. Retrieved from www.nationalacademies.org/hmd/~/media/Files/Report%20Files/2001/Crossing-the-Quality-Chasm/Quality%20Chasm%202001%20%20report%20brief.pdf

Institute of Medicine (IOM). (2011). *Hunger and obesity: Understanding a food insecurity paradigm*. Workshop summary. Washington DC: The National Academies Press.

Johns Hopkins Bloomberg School of Public Health. (n. d.). *The art and craft of policy briefs: Translating evidence and engaging stakeholders*. Baltimore, MD: Author. Retrieved from https://www.jhsph.edu/research/centers-and-institutes/womens-and-childrens-health-policy-center/de/policy_brief/video

Jung, N. M., de Bairros, F. S., Pattussi, M. P., Pauli, S., & Neutzling, M. B. (2017). Gender differences in the prevalence of household food insecurity: A systematic review and meta-analysis. *Public Health Nutrition, 20*(5), 902–916. http://dx.doi.org.ezproxy.research.udmercy.edu:2048/10.1017/S1368980016002925

Lavarreda, S. A., & Brown, E. R. (2014). Public health insurance. In Kominski, G. (Ed.), *Changing the U.S. health care system: Key issues in health services policy and management*. (pp. 157–189). San Francisco, CA: Jossey-Bass.

Lewenson, S. B., & Nickitas, D. M. (2016). Nursing's history of advocacy and action. In D. M. Nickitas, D. J. Middaugh, & N. Aries (Eds.), *Policy and politics for nurses and other health professionals* (pp. 3–13). Burlington, MA: Jones & Bartlett Learning.

Michigan Department of Technology, Management & Budget. (2017). *Michigan and US jobless rates.* Retrieved from http://milmi.org

Miller, D. P., Larson, M. J., Byrne, T., & Devoe, E. (2016). Food insecurity in veteran households: Findings from nationally representative data. *Public Health Nutrition, 19*(10), 1731–1740. http://dx.doi.org.ezproxy.research.udmercy.edu:2048/10.1017/S1368980015003067

Murthy, V. H. (2016). Food insecurity: A public health issue. *Public Health Reports, 131*(5), 655–657. doi:10.1177/0033354916664154

National Education Policy Center. (n. d.). *Policy briefs.* Boulder, CO: Author. Retrieved from http://nepc.colorado.edu/publications/policy-briefs

Parkhurst, J. (2017). *The politics of evidence: From evidence-based policy to the good governance of evidence.* New York, NY: Taylor & Francis Group.

Ponce, N. A., & Ko, M. (2014). Multilevel social determinants of health. In Kominski, G. (Ed.), *Changing the U.S. health care system: Key issues in health services policy and management.* (pp. 135–155). San Francisco, CA: Jossey-Bass.

Porche, D. J. (2019). *Health policy: Application for nurses and other healthcare professionals.* Burlington, MA: Jones & Bartlett Learning.

Pourat, N., & Kominski, G. F. (2014). Private health insurance. In Kominski, G. (Ed.), *Changing the U.S. health care system: Key issues in health services policy and management.* (pp. 191–221). San Francisco, CA: Jossey-Bass.

Ruark, P. (2015). *Racial disparities persist in child poverty.* Lansing, MI: Michigan League for Public Policy. Retrieved from http://www.mlpp.org/racial-disparities-persist-in-child-poverty#more-31803

Schmidt, L., Shore-Sheppard, L., & Watson, T. (2015, November 30). The effect of safety net programs on food insecurity. *Journal of Human Resources, 51*(3), 589–614. doi:10.3386/w19558

Schweitzer, S. O., & Comanor, W. S. (2014). Promoting pharmaceutical access while controlling prices and expenditures. In Kominski, G. (Ed.), *Changing the U.S. health care system: Key issues in health services policy and management.* (pp. 269–304). San Francisco, CA: Jossey-Bass.

Sherman, A., & Trisi, D., (2015). *Safety net more effective against poverty than previously thought.* Washington, DC: Center on Budget and Policy Priorities. Retrieved from http://www.cbpp.org/research/poverty-and-inequality/safety-net-more-effective-against-poverty-than-previously-thought

Shi, L., & Singh, D. A. (2019). *Delivering health care in America: A systems approach.* Burlington, MA: Jones & Bartlett Learning.

Smedley, B. D., Stith, A. Y., & Nelson, A. R. (2003). *Unequal treatment: Confronting racial and ethnic disparities in health care.* Washington, DC: National Academies Press. Retrieved from https://www.nap.edu/read/12875/chapter/1#iv

Smith, A. L. (2013). *Nurses care, which is why they're advocating for Michigan Medicaid expansion.* Retrieved from http://www.eclectablog.com/2013/07/nurses-care-which-is-why-theyre-advocating-for-michigan-medicaid-expansion.html

Snyder, R., Calley, B., & Pscholka, A. (2017). *A path toward out future-state of Michigan.* FY 18 Executive Budget Presentation. Retrieved from https://www.michigan.gov/documents/budget/FY18_Executive_Budget_Presentation_550969_7.

Squires, D., & Anderson, C. (2015). *U.S. health care from a global perspective: Spending, use of services, prices, and health in 13 countries.* New York, NY: The Commonwealth Fund. Retrieved from http://www.commonwealthfund.org/publications/issue-briefs/2015/oct/us-health-care-from-a-global-perspective

Tower, M. (2016, June 12). Seniors struggle to make ends meet in wake of SNAP food assistance cuts. *Saginaw News.* Retrieved from http://www.mlive.com/news/saginaw/index.ssf/2016/02/saginaw_seniors_struggle_to_ma.html

Trump. D. (2017). *America First: A budget blueprint to make America great again.* Washington, DC: Office of Management and Budget. Retrieved from http://www.budget.gov

U.S. Department of Agriculture (USDA). (n.d.). *The benefits of increasing the Supplemental Nutrition Assistance Program (SNAP) participation in your state.* Washington, DC: Author. Retrieved from https://www.fns.usda.gov/sites/default/files/bc_facts.pdf

U.S. Department of Agriculture (USDA). (2016). *Definitions of food security.* Washington, DC: USDA Economic Research Service. Retrieved from https://www.ers.usda.gov/topics/food-nutrition-assistance/food-security-in-the-us/definitions-of-food-security/

U.S. Department of Agriculture (USDA). (2017). *National and/or state level monthly and/or annual data—Latest available month January 2017*. Washington, DC: USDA; Supplemental Nutrition Assistance Program (SNAP). Retrieved from https://www.fns.usda.gov/pd/supplemental-nutrition -assistance-program-snap

Wax, S. G., & Stankorb, S. M. (2016). Prevalence of food insecurity among military households with children 5 years of age and younger. *Public Health Nutrition, 19*(13), 2458–2466.

Wayne Metropolitan Community Action Agency (2016). *2016 Wayne County community needs assessment*. Detroit, MI: Author. Retrieved from http://www.waynemetro.org/wp-content /uploads/2016/10/2016-Community-Needs-Assessment-v082016.pdf

Whittle, H. J., Palar, K., Hufstedler, L. L., Seligman, H. K., Frongillo, E. A., & Weiser, S. D. (2015). Food insecurity, chronic illness, and gentrification in the San Francisco Bay area: An example of structural violence in United States public policy. *Social Science and Medicine, 143*, 154–161. http://dx.doi.org/10.1016/j.socscimed.2015.08.027

Wisely, J., & Tanner, K. (2015, September 17). Income rise helps poverty rate in Michigan. *Detroit Free Press*. Retrieved from http://www.freep.com/story/news/local/michigan/2015/09/16/poverty -falling-incomes-rising/32507559/

Yancey, A. K., Bastani, R. & Glenn, B. A. (2014). Racial and ethnic disparities in health status. In Kominski, G. (Ed.), *Changing the U.S. health care system: Key issues in health services policy and management.* (pp. 71–101). San Francisco, CA: Jossey-Bass.

Zimet, S. (2017). *Health budget hearing testimony*. Albany, NY: Hunger Action Network of New York State. Retrieved from http://www.nysenate.gov

Helpful Resources

American Association of Colleges of Nursing (AACN), Government Affairs http://www.aacnnursing .org/

American Association of Retired Persons (AARP) https://www.aarp.org/

American Nurses Association (ANA) https://www.nursingworld.org/

American Enterprise Institute (AEI) https://www.aei.org/

Brookings Institution https://www.brookings.edu/

Cato Institute https://www.cato.org/

Centers for Disease Control (CDC) Health Disparities & Inequalities Report https://www.cdc.gov /minorityhealth/chdireport.html

Democrats Action Center https://www.democrats.org/

Economic Policy Institute (EPI) https://www.epi.org/

Educational Policy Institute http://www.educationalpolicy.org/

Health Affairs http://content.healthaffairs.org/cgi/changeuserinfo/basic

Henry J. Kaiser Family Foundation (KFF) https://www.kff.org/health-reform/

Kettering Foundation https://www.kettering.org/

Library of Congress https://www.congress.gov/

National Academies of Sciences, Engineering, and Medicine http://www.nationalacademies.org /hmd/

National Institute for Public Policy (NIPP) http://www.nipp.org/

Office of Policy Analysis https://www.doi.gov/ppa

Organisation for Economic Co-operation and Development (OECD) http://www.oecd.org/

RAND Corporation https://www.rand.org/

Republican National Committee (GOP) Action Center https://www.gop.com/

Robert Wood Johnson Foundation (RWJF) https://www.rwjf.org/

The Commonwealth Fund http://www.commonwealthfund.org/

2016 Platform Comparison https://downloads.frcaction.org/EF/EF16I163.pdf

SECTION II

The DNP Project

CHAPTER 5

The Phenomenon of Interest

Katherine Moran and Rosanne Burson

CHAPTER OVERVIEW

Nursing practice is guided by science and theory. Nursing, as a profession, historically has been considered a practice discipline that is complex, varied, and underdetermined. There is an inherent societal obligation for the nurse to use good clinical judgment based on evidence-based practice that is informed by research. The nurse must "attend to changing relevance as well as changes in the patient's responses and nature of his clinical condition over time" (Benner, Tanner, & Chesla, 2009, p. xiv). However, because practice in the individual case is open to variations that are not necessarily accounted for by science (underdetermined), the nurse must use clinical reasoning to select and use relevant science (Benner, Tanner, & Chesla, 2009). This means that the nurse must be able to recognize important changes and/or trends in the patient's condition and use good clinical judgment when providing nursing care.

CHAPTER OBJECTIVES

After completing the chapter, the learner will be able to:

1. Understand the meaning of nursing phenomena in relation to the identification of issues that are in need of change.
2. Consider personal practice interests and expertise in contemplating phenomena.
3. Scan the literature for potential areas of interest.
4. Evaluate potential nursing theories as a framework for the nursing phenomenon.
5. Explore the phenomenon through patterns of knowing.
6. Apply the process of concept analysis to the phenomenon or a characteristic of the phenomenon.

The complex nature of nursing practice provides many opportunities to explore nursing phenomena. The focus of this chapter is to explore phenomena of interest for the doctor of nursing practice (DNP) project. Nursing theory and nursing knowledge are briefly explored to help the DNP student understand the significance of nursing phenomena. Along with the guidance received from his or her advisor, a variety of strategies are introduced to help the DNP student select a phenomenon of interest for the DNP project.

The nurse must be able to recognize important changes and/or trends in the patient's condition and use good clinical judgment when providing nursing care.

▶ The Expertise of Nursing Practice

In 2011, the Institute of Medicine (IOM) and the Robert Wood Johnson Foundation (RWJF) put forth a report that highlights the value of nursing and outlines the central role that nurses will play in the future health of our nation. In this report, *The Future of Nursing: Leading Change, Advancing Health,* nurses are called to lead and manage collaborative efforts with other healthcare practitioners to improve health care. Understanding the unique attributes of the expert nurse and expert nursing practice will help the nursing profession meet the challenges set forth by the Institute of Medicine (2011).

According to Morrison and Symes (2011), expert nursing practice includes a degree of involvement and engagement with patients that demonstrates intuitive knowledge and skilled know-how through knowing the patient, reflective practice, and risk taking. According to Benner, Tanner, & Chesla (2009),

> Expert nursing practice occurs when the nurse is able to see the situation in alternative ways, either through introspection or by consulting others; allowing the nurse to realize the true meaning of the present and past events. The nurse reflects on the goal or perspective that seems evident to them and on the action that seems appropriate to achieving their goal; referred to as deliberative rationality. (p. 16)

This unique skill set places the practicing scholar in the best position to identify those areas of clinical concern that require further research and/or improvement and

In this day of attention to patient-centered care and outcomes, the aspects of care delivery that nurses provide by their inherent understanding of phenomena require further examination, demonstration, and dissemination.

to help ensure that the healthcare needs of patients within the community, organization, or healthcare unit are being addressed.

The ability of the nurse to be tuned in to the meaning of the event *to the patient* and to choose individualized interventions that are unique for this patient at this time are the ultimate contributions that he or she offers. This *hidden work* is what influences the patient's experience and often positively affects clinical outcomes. The profession has not articulated well the skill set nurses bring to the table that enhances the work that is done. This is partly because the relationship and caring aspect of nursing has been seen as the *soft side* of nursing and historically is not valued as much as the science-based technical aspects. For example, within the advanced practice role, the perceived value from organizations and other practitioners has been the utilization of the medical model in providing care. Nursing care is not measured, although in fact that may be the very thing that assists patients in meeting outcomes. In this day of attention to patient-centered care and outcomes, the aspects of care delivery that nurses provide by their inherent understanding of phenomena require further examination, demonstration, and dissemination. These processes will serve to highlight the hidden work of nursing and to validate its importance to the patient's healthcare experience and outcome.

> *The hidden work of the nurse is what influences the patient's experience and often positively affects clinical outcomes.*

▶ Identifying the Phenomenon of Interest

What are the phenomena that are of interest to the DNP student? When asked this question individually, DNP students may have difficulty adequately articulating the details of their interest. Perhaps it is because they have not been able to get their arms around a specific area of focus, or maybe their interests are too broad and not sufficiently narrowed to begin to articulate intent. Although the student's advisor provides direction and support as the student considers a variety of phenomena, it is a question that each student must answer individually. The DNP project phenomenon of interest must center on a topic that is meaningful to the practice doctorate student and is *valued* by the practice setting. Further, as mentioned, practicing scholars are in the best position to identify those areas of clinical concern that require further research and/or improvement. Identifying the phenomenon of interest is the first step in developing the DNP project.

What Is a Phenomenon?

While some students may start the DNP program with a good understanding of the phenomenon they want to explore, as mentioned, others may not yet have a phenomenon in mind or they may not have a full understanding of what is meant by the term *nursing phenomenon*. To better understand what constitutes a phenomenon, it is important to understand the meaning of the word. According to

Merriam-Webster, *phenomenon* is defined as "a fact or event of scientific interest susceptible to scientific description and explanation; an exceptional, unusual, or abnormal person, thing, or occurrence" ("Phenomenon," 2018, para. 1). *Nursing phenomenon*, on the other hand, is described as "a type of factor influencing health status with the specific characteristics; aspect of health of relevance to nursing practice" (International Classification for Nursing Practice [ICNP], n.d., para. 1). Hence, the phenomena within the realm of nursing are complex in nature. These phenomena incorporate humans and their environment and relate to all aspects of human function as an individual, family member, or member of community—within the context of the physical or biological environment and human-made environments of norms, attitudes, and policy (ICNP, n.d.). Consequently, it is not surprising that many DNP projects deal with complex health-related issues (Christenbery, 2011).

One way to approach identifying the phenomenon of interest is to consider the areas of the DNP student's clinical expertise. Phenomenon identification derives from a practice situation that resonates. Practice experience occurs between the nurse and the patient. Further, reflecting on aspects that the student has observed within a particular patient population may give some direction. The expert nurse draws on this understanding and has developed specific interventions that align with the known phenomenon. For example, in working with patients with diabetes who are in need of insulin initiation, the nurse notes that there are often multiple barriers. Patients may experience fear of insulin related to injections or hypoglycemia. The patient may have insidious thoughts related to feelings of failure and guilt for having not been *perfect* in his or her approach to lifestyle behavior change and other recommendations from the healthcare provider. Patients may have decreased self-efficacy or empowerment issues that limit their ability to self-manage and maintain motivation. There may be family history whereby a family member started insulin, and this appeared to contribute to his or her demise. Misunderstanding the other factors related to the family member's experience can exacerbate the difficulty the patient experiences as he or she tries to overcome this new hurdle. The expert nurse has the skill set to help the patient explore the specific barriers that are contributing to his or her inability to move forward, toward better glucose control and improved health. The identified phenomenon of barriers to insulin initiation may be the beginning of an intense exploration of the topic, resulting in an intervention that improves outcomes for patients.

When considering potential topics or phenomena of interest for the DNP project, it may be helpful to begin by casting a wide net and to think about areas of interest from a broad, general perspective. Multiple methods can be used to help the student identify a pertinent topic. For example, it may be helpful to review research reports found in the Cumulative Index to Nursing and Allied Health Literature (CINAHL) database. Reviewing published reports could help the DNP student identify topics that need further exploration or studies that could be replicated on a smaller scale (to validate findings or increase generalizability). Scanning the table of contents of professional journals or even a professional organization's website may help the student identify topics of concern relevant to nursing. By way of example, a website to peruse regarding pertinent topics is the Doctors of Nursing Practice (www.doctorsofnursingpractice.ning.com/), an online community of DNP graduates and DNP students that highlights practice innovation and professional growth.

However, remember that the goal is to identify an area of interest specifically for the DNP project; therefore, the project should include subject matter in which the student has some expertise, such as his or her area of practice or specialty. The student should ask himself or herself if *there is something about this practice setting that needs further inquiry.* Perhaps a population of patients is not reaching their healthcare goals because of some common barrier, or maybe a current healthcare policy (organizational or legislative) is interfering with optimal patient care. In both of these examples, a clinical problem results in a trigger that leads to identifying a phenomenon worth exploring. This is what is meant by identifying a clinical problem in the *context of the needs of the organization or population.* Recognizing and understanding issues of concern within specific organizations is a skill set and competency that is expected from DNP students. For example, DNP *Essential* I-2 states that the DNP program prepares the graduate to ". . .determine the nature and significance of health and healthcare delivery phenomena; describe

As the student is exposed to problems and needs from a local context, he or she should consider phenomena that are contributing to the current outcomes the organization is experiencing. Often, looking at the issues from the lens of phenomena can be a driving force for innovation.

the actions and advanced strategies to enhance, alleviate, and ameliorate health and health care delivery phenomena as appropriate; and evaluate outcomes" (American Association of Colleges of Nursing [AACN], 2006, p. 9). That is why the student needs to learn how to identify, then come to understand, an issue before starting the DNP project. To better understand how to determine the needs of an organization or population see Chapter 6 for more information on conducting an organizational assessment.

At this beginning stage of discernment, a question the student should ask is, *What is interesting to me?* A student should consider not just areas of interest but include areas of passion that will take the student through the journey and energize him or her to complete the process. Another important understanding for the student is that doctoral study is transforming and takes time. The initial topics of interest will most likely *morph* as the student is exposed to new concepts in his or her educational program. The student will view the phenomenon through many new lenses, which will change the appearance of the original idea. This is a normal part of the process. The student will reflect continuously on the phenomenon, and it will gradually evolve into the DNP project.

Examples of DNP phenomena of interest are provided in **TABLE 5-1**.

Once a broad category or area of interest is identified, the next step is to drill down to a more specific focus. This is crucial. *Areas of interest* that are too broad or vague may become unmanageable, causing frustration and wasted time. Narrowing

Areas of interest that are too broad or vague may become unmanageable, causing frustration and wasted time.

TABLE 5-1 DNP Phenomenon Topics

Examples of DNP phenomena of interest

- Barriers to family presence during emergency department resuscitative efforts
- Access and barriers to utilization of palliative care
- Unreported blood and body fluid exposure
- Disruptive behavior in the emergency department
- Provider barriers to postpartum depression treatment
- Cost effectiveness of crisis stabilization unit with a psychiatric unit

Data from Vanderbilt University School of Nursing. (2017). *2017 Doctor of Nursing Practice Scholarly Projects*. Retrieved from https://nursing.vanderbilt.edu/dnp/pdf/2017_dnp_booklet.pdf

the focus gives the student the opportunity to demonstrate a comprehensive understanding of the topic. Remember, the DNP student must be able to successfully complete the project; an incomplete project does not inform nursing practice, and it does not equate to a valid program deliverable, which is required for graduation!

To effectively narrow the focus, it is helpful to start by reviewing what is already known about the topic and, conversely, what is not known about the topic. For example, perhaps the DNP student has a good understanding of the healthcare needs of the immigrant population, but now the student wants to focus on health promotion activities used by recent immigrants. This topic could be further narrowed to *health promotion strategies used by Latino women who emigrated to the United States from Latin America*. One method used to narrow a topic is to ask the following questions: Who, what, where, and when? *Who* is the population of interest? *What* is it about this population that is interesting? *Where* is the population found? *When* did the observation occur? Is it a current or historical observation or related to a specific period of life?

As the subject matter moves from a broad category to a more focused topic, multiple potential elements of interest will begin to emerge. One word of caution is needed regarding narrowing the project focus: Care should be taken to prevent the focus of the project from being narrowed too much. If the topic is narrowed to very specific criteria, there is a real risk that there will be no (or very little) information available in the literature to inform the project.

▶ Identification of a Problem or Concern

Now that a topic has been identified, it is time to think about *why* this topic is important or what is it about this topic that is a concern. Is there a need to change nursing practice to improve patient outcomes in an organization or for a specific population? Is there an unmet societal need that may benefit from a policy initiative? Does this concern occur frequently enough to warrant further exploration? What does the literature reveal about this topic?

When reviewing the literature at this point in the project development process, the goal is really only to *browse* the literature in order to gain a general understanding

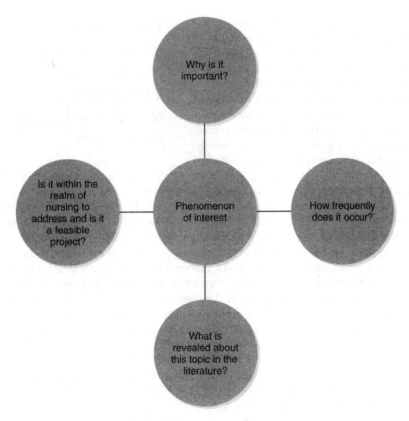

FIGURE 5-1 Process used to identify the phenomenon of interest.

of the topic, determine how much work has been done, and determine if this is indeed something worth exploring further.

If one determines that the topic is interesting, it is time to take it one step further—to begin to think about *how* to address this or *if* anything can be done about it. Finally, remember to consider the resources that will be needed to investigate this phenomenon.

Reviewing the idea with an advisor will help the student identify potential barriers and help him or her determine the feasibility of implementing the project. Remember, if the student is able to clearly articulate the value of the topic, implementing the project is feasible, and there are nursing strategies that could be explored to address the concern, the topic is worth further investigation (see **FIGURE 5-1**).

▶ Using Nursing Theory to Explore a Phenomenon

Theory provides an orderly way to view phenomena. Nursing theory was initially developed to guide practice through the clarification of the nursing domain. Theory provided a way for nurses to convey professional convictions and gave nurses a means of systematic thinking about nursing practice (McEwen & Wills, 2018).

Nursing theory is made up of concepts (words or phrases used to describe the concept) and propositions (statements that describe the relationship among the concepts) that help to explain a phenomenon of interest (Jensen, 2015). Sometimes the term *construct* is also included in the description of a theory. A construct is used to describe something that is not directly or indirectly observed, such as social support (Schmidt & Brown, 2015). Theory can be classified based on scope/level of abstractness or type/purpose, as depicted in **FIGURE 5-2**.

> **Theory *is used to guide nursing practice, and it provides an orderly way to view phenomena.***

Level of abstractness refers to the complexity of the theory and the specificity or concreteness of the concepts and proposition (McEwen & Wills, 2018). For example, grand theories are most abstract because they are used to explain the discipline of nursing and include very broadly defined concepts. The concept of *health*, for example, is broad, with potentially broad interpretation. Nursing recognizes that the concept of health encompasses more than simply the absence of disease. Health is a dynamic process that changes over time and can vary based on the individual's circumstances, experiences, and exposures to internal and external environments.

Because this concept is complex and broad in scope, it is not easily tested. A few examples of grand theories include Dorothea Orem's self-care deficit theory, Rosemarie Parse's theory of human becoming, and Imogene King's open system theory. These theories provide a philosophical umbrella under which nursing practice functions. Many of these theories were developed in the last century and serve to create paradigms that support nursing practice.

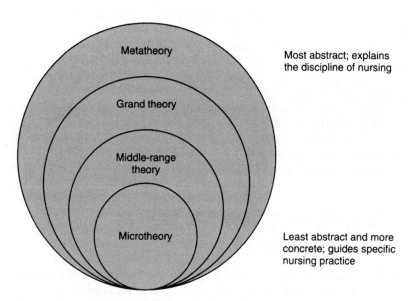

FIGURE 5-2 Levels of abstraction in nursing theory.

Data from McEwen, M., & Wills, E. M. (2019). *Theoretical basis for nursing* (5th ed.). Philadelphia, PA: Wolters Kluwer Health/Lippincott Williams & Wilkins.

Grand theories are often the theories learned at the bachelor's level of nursing. Unfortunately, the abstractness of the grand theory is often difficult for the novice nurse to integrate intentionally within his or her practice. For some nurses, the disconnect between theory and practice may start here and continue even as nurses advance in their clinical experience. Beginning DNP students often comment that they are unsure about the usefulness of theory to practice. If grand theories were presented as philosophies to novice nurses, perhaps the understanding of how practice is grounded would become clearer. Grand theories have been very important to nursing's knowledge development and will continue to form a base on which theories specific to practice can build.

The next level of abstraction in theory classification includes middle-range theories. As the name implies, these theories are found in the middle of the ladder of abstraction (between abstract and concrete) and are more limited in scope than grand theories. As a result, middle-range theories tend to be more generalizable to nursing practice and can be tested. The focus for middle-range theories is on understanding nursing-related phenomena, so they are very useful for the scholar-practitioner. Some examples of middle-range theories include Nola J. Pender's health promotion model, Merle Mishel's uncertainty in illness theory, and E. Lenz and L. Pugh's theory of unpleasant symptoms.

The final level of abstraction includes practice theories. These theories are used to guide specific areas of practice; therefore, they are very concrete and narrow in scope, and they include concepts that are measurable and easily tested (McEwen & Wills, 2018). "Situation-specific theory" is another term that highlights practice theory, which focuses on the context in which the theory is being used. This type of theory, as the name implies, is specific to the situation and encompasses the particular needs of a unique group of patients. An example of a situation-specific theory is Ramona Mercer's conceptualization of maternal role attainment/becoming a mother. Because situation-specific theory is within a local context and supports the use of evidence-based research that is appropriate to the situation at hand, DNP students find this appealing in practice.

There is a fluid relationship among theory, research, and practice that is important to understand. Each informs and impacts the other (see **FIGURE 5-3**). Theory is validated through research, which can lead to further theory development.

Both theory and research are used to inform practice. Similarly, information gleaned through theory application in practice can inform theory development and/or continued research. The symbiotic relationship among theory, research, and practice is important to recognize because of the potential opportunities for further study that can emerge when using theory to explore a phenomenon. This type of exploration is valuable to nursing because of the potential to add to nursing knowledge.

For example, complex patient care and social issues can be identified and subsequently addressed using theory. From the perspective of a scholarly project, the DNP student can use theory to recognize the antecedents to health-related events that negatively impact a population (e.g., those events that lead to colon cancer in women or to prostate cancer in men). Theory can help the DNP student recognize health and illness patterns within a population and the subsequent implications (Christenbery, 2011).

In addition to helping the DNP student recognize health patterns, theory also helps the student develop patient-centered nursing interventions to promote health

FIGURE 5-3 This figure depicts the reciprocal relationship among theory, research, and practice.

Data from McEwen, M., & Wills, E. M. (2019). *Theoretical basis for nursing* (5th ed.). Philadelphia, PA: Wolters Kluwer Health/Lippincott Williams & Wilkins.

and wellness and a framework to evaluate the effectiveness of these interventions (Christenbery, 2011).

For many DNP students, there are "a-ha!" moments related to the realization that they have been using nursing theory in their practice all along. Nursing theories have continued to evolve, and the exploration of theories that are relevant to each student's practice is an important aspect of the process of doctoral education. Connecting appropriate theory to the DNP project will offer a supporting framework and will deepen the understanding of the chosen phenomenon.

▶ Looking at a Phenomenon Through a Different Lens

Theoretical Framework

Clearly, theories can and should be used to study a phenomenon of interest. As mentioned previously, using one or even several theories to view a phenomenon is a valuable exercise because it helps the DNP student better describe or explain the phenomenon. However, sometimes just the process of identifying a theory to help inform the project can be a daunting task.

Several strategies can be used to make this process more manageable. First, it is helpful to begin by identifying the concepts (and relationships among the concepts) that describe the phenomenon of interest under consideration. This can be accomplished by reviewing the literature. Look for published articles that include the phenomenon of interest and then identify the concepts used to describe the phenomenon, as well as the theory or theories chosen to inform the work. The DNP student can then select a theory to use as a framework that best represents the concepts that describe his or her phenomenon of interest. A concept analysis can also begin to further inform the understanding of the phenomenon and will be discussed later in the chapter. In addition to reviewing the literature, there are multiple resources, both electronic and in print, that can provide the DNP student with an overview of the numerous theories available for use (see Helpful Resources). Finally, technology will be an asset as the student considers reviewing the huge amount of data involved in the exploration of various theories. A great place to start is websites where the student can begin looking at all the nursing theories available.

As the DNP student considers various theories for use, keep in mind a series of questions to evaluate each theory. These questions should reflect the student's perception of practice and include:

1. Does this theory reflect the student's personal nursing practice?
2. Does this theory help to describe, explain, and predict the phenomenon in which the student is interested?
3. Can this theory be used as a guide in the framework of the DNP project?
4. Does the theory offer a way to develop, assess, implement, and evaluate innovations that the project explores?
5. Will the use of this theory help to support excellent nursing practice?

For example, the student who is looking at phenomena focused on interpersonal relationships may consider nursing theories that give a framework to the relationship that develops between nurse and patient. The student may consider Hildegard Peplau's theory of interpersonal relations in nursing, Jean Watson's caring science, or Rosemarie Parse's human becoming theory, in which there are interpersonal effects on both the nurse and patient.

Theories outside of nursing are also worthy of consideration as the phenomenon is evaluated. Interdisciplinary aspects of DNP work encourage the review of theories specific to the phenomenon. For example, if the phenomenon is related to health behavior, an exploration of the various theories within this framework is recommended. Examples of health behavior theories from other disciplines include the health belief model, the theory of planned behavior, and the social cognitive theory. Another example is a phenomenon related to societal aspects where there may be congruence with complexity science, critical, feminist, or environmental theory. During this period of immersion, it is important for the student to develop a broad understanding of the available theories to identify links to the phenomenon of interest. A thorough and updated text will give the DNP student a starting place for this review and professional development (see Helpful Resources). Examination of the phenomenon within a specific theoretical framework will clarify aspects of the phenomenon and give direction to the DNP project. This process takes time and is often incorporated in theory coursework, which supports DNP *Essential* I: Scientific Underpinnings for Practice and DNP *Essential* III: Clinical Scholarship and Analytic Methods for Evidence-Based Practice.

Ways of Knowing

Another way to explore and understand the phenomenon of interest is to view it through the multiple lenses of the *patterns of knowing*. The fundamental patterns of knowing in nursing were initially identified by Carper in 1978 as part of her doctoral work. The patterns of knowing were developed in an attempt to help nursing as a profession better understand the characteristic ways that nurses think about phenomena that are a concern of nursing. This was done not to extend the range of knowledge but rather to understand what it means to *know* and what types of knowledge are important to nursing (Carper, 1978).

The ways of knowing are important concepts in the development and application of nursing theory. They also provide a holistic framework designed to direct practice, education, and research. The DNP student can further explore a specific phenomenon of interest by viewing it through the lens of one or several patterns of knowing. Again, this process will give the student insight, aids in informing the project, and helps the student better describe or explain the phenomenon of interest.

Carper's original four fundamental patterns of knowing are *empirical knowing*, referred to as the science of nursing; *esthetics*, referred to as the art of nursing; *personal knowledge*, allowing for a therapeutic use of self; and *ethical knowledge*, or the moral knowledge in nursing (see **FIGURE 5-4**). These patterns are separate but interdependent and interrelated; they are not mutually exclusive.

Empirical knowledge includes knowledge that is objective and quantifiable. It is tested, replicated, and proved through scientific methods.

Empirical knowledge is systematically organized into general laws and theories for the purpose of describing, explaining, and predicting phenomena of concern to nursing.

Empirical knowledge is systematically organized into general laws and theories for the purpose of describing, explaining, and predicting phenomena of concern to nursing (Cody, 2013). Evidence-based practice is just one example of empirical knowledge that informs nursing practice. The nurse using evidence to inform practice develops a skill set and knowledge base from well-documented scientific knowledge that has been rigorously tested. Chinn and Kramer (2018) clarified the

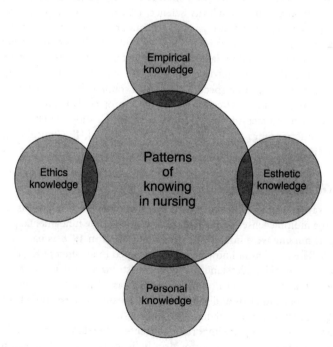

FIGURE 5-4 This figure depicts the four original fundamental patterns of knowing by Barbara A. Carper.

Data from Chinn, L. P., & Kramer, M. K. (2018). *Integrating theory and knowledge development in nursing* (10th ed.). St. Louis, MO: Mosby-Elsevier.

conceptualization of the empirical pattern by questioning what is the science and how does it work. The DNP student can apply this questioning process to determine aspects of the pattern of knowing for the phenomenon of interest. Critical questions defined by Chinn and Kramer (2018) will be asked in each subsequent pattern of knowing to substantiate the pattern in relation to the phenomenon.

Esthetic knowledge is used by nurses to better understand each patient's unique health experience; the nurse is able to sense the meaning in the moment and tailor the patient's nursing care without conscious deliberation. Esthetic knowledge encompasses the lived experience and is expressive in nature. The nurse is able to assist the patient in coping with the experience through perceived insight that is gleaned from *being in the moment* with the patient.

> *Esthetic knowledge implores the nurse to use skills of empathy, caring, and engagement to care for individual patients.*

It is important to note that the *perception* referred to in esthetic knowledge is more than simple recognition; it is the gathering of important details and nuances that together create the experience as a whole (Carper, 1978). It gives meaning to variables that cannot be quantitatively formulated (McEwen & Wills, 2018). The nurse understands what is *significant in the patient's experience* and, as a result of this perception, is able to determine what is needed to help the patient move forward. By using esthetic knowledge, the nurse is able to see the holistic needs of the patient and act appropriately. Activities that have been considered as simple or basic nursing care can have a profound effect on patient outcomes. Unfortunately, the true value of these acts is often overlooked. Esthetic critical questions ask about the meaning and significance of the experience to the patient (Chinn & Kramer, 2018).

Personal knowledge encompasses the way nurses view themselves and the patient (McEwen & Wills, 2018). Personal knowledge is largely expressed in personality; it is subjective and incorporates experience and reflection. Using personal knowledge, the nurse is able to view the patient from a holistic perspective rather than from a strictly biological or medical perspective, promoting wholeness and integrity. These interpersonal contacts and relationships with patients are examples of what is meant by *therapeutic use of self.* Through personal knowledge, the nurse may come to understand that there is something sacred in the relationship between the patient and the nurse, that what nurses do involves more than providing protection, promotion, and optimization of health and abilities; nurses facilitate healing and wellness through that human connection. The nurse questions what he or she knows about an experience through reflection to identify personal knowledge (Chinn & Kramer, 2018).

> *Using personal knowledge, the nurse is able to view the patient from a holistic perspective rather than from a strictly biological or medical perspective, promoting wholeness and integrity.*

Ethical knowledge is based on obligation to service and respect for human life. Nurses draw on ethical knowledge when moral dilemmas arise to address conflicting norms and interests and to provide insight into areas that cannot be tested (McEwen & Wills, 2018). Ethical knowledge requires rational examination and evaluation of what

> # Ethical knowledge *is based on obligation to service and respect for human life.*

is good, valuable, and desirable as it relates to the maintenance or restoration of health. Ethical issues could arise from situations involving consent, distributive justice, or personal integrity, to name a few. In these cases, the nurse may be challenged to overcome fear because of uncertainty of outcomes or have conflicting feelings resulting from personal core values or beliefs. The nurse must act with *moral courage* and address the situation with conviction and confidence, doing what is right for the patient and asking what is right and responsible (Chinn & Kramer, 2018).

Now, consider a phenomenon of interest viewed through the lens of the ways of knowing: caring for the adult patient with chronic obstructive pulmonary disease (COPD) who continues to smoke cigarettes. When viewing this phenomenon using empirical knowledge, the data are clear: smoking cigarettes is detrimental to one's health; it damages lung tissue and is certainly a concern for the patient with COPD.

Using esthetic knowledge, however, the nurse is able to recognize the forces driving a patient's decision to smoke. Perhaps through structured interviews or focus groups with patients with COPD, the nurse is able to use skills of empathy, caring, and engagement to better understand the needs of the patient with COPD who smokes. Perhaps the nurse identifies the long smoking history, extraordinary family or work stressors, and the desire to quit, but the lack of perceived coping strategies available to use to be successful in this endeavor.

The nurse reflects on what is learned and incorporates information from previous experiences or similar situations. This personal knowledge helps inform the nurse. The nurse should recognize personal biases and how personal values and beliefs can either help the patient move forward or serve as a roadblock that sabotages all efforts. In the latter case, the DNP student should carefully consider whether this is a phenomenon that he or she is comfortable pursuing. Remember, the key in all patient–nurse relationships is a *therapeutic* use of self.

Finally, using ethical knowledge, the nurse examines the situation and evaluates what is good, valuable, and desirable as it relates to the maintenance or restoration of health from the *patient's perspective*. The nurse has a moral obligation to inform the patient of the risks of smoking but also to consider quality of life and what is required to maintain or improve that quality.

It is imperative to look at your phenomena through each lens. The student may have a bias toward one lens or another. In the preceding example, a nurse who looks only through the empirical lens will not be able to incorporate the patient perspective from the esthetic and ethical lens or the impact of the nurse's personal knowing on the situation. This is known as "patterns gone wild," and the impact is a stunted view of the phenomena that does not allow the full view and experience of the phenomena (Chinn & Kramer, 2018). Patterns gone wild predictably limits the ability of the nurse to understand each unique human interaction within all patterns and may prevent the development of specific patient-centered interventions and positive outcomes that would have been attained.

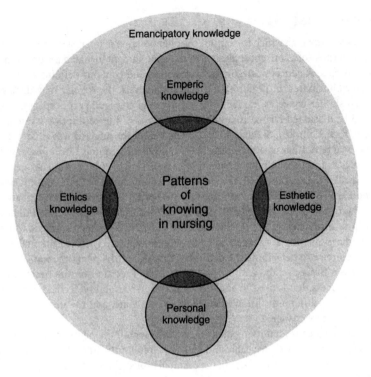

FIGURE 5-5 This figure depicts the revised fundamental patterns of knowing by Barbara A. Carper and includes Chinn and Kramer's addition of emancipatory knowing.

Data from Chinn, L. P., & Kramer, M. K. (2018). *Integrating theory and knowledge development in nursing* (10th ed.). St. Louis, MO: Mosby-Elsevier.

In 2008, Chinn and Kramer added a final pattern of knowing termed *emancipatory knowing* (see **FIGURE 5-5**). The emancipatory knowing pattern explores *what is* from a social, cultural, and political stance and envisions *what can be* (Chinn & Kramer, 2018). Equity, justice, and transformation are considered in this new vision, while surrounding and connecting with the four fundamental patterns of knowing (Chinn & Kramer, 2018). Having the ability to look at the power structures in place that contribute to social problems and being able to consider other options are at the root of this pattern—to create a new lens to view the world.

Emancipatory knowing is *expressed* in praxis, whereby the nurse reflects on issues that are not fair and initiates changes to eliminate the injustices. This is also termed *reflection in action* (Chinn & Kramer, 2018). The phenomenon of interest may be framed by emancipatory knowing, while the DNP project is also a demonstration of praxis.

> Emancipatory knowing *is expressed in praxis, whereby the nurse reflects on issues that are not fair and initiates changes to eliminate the injustices.*

Concept Analysis

Another lens through which to examine the phenomenon of interest is a concept analysis. The purpose of a concept analysis is to allow the student to match the phenomenon with concepts. A concept categorizes information and contains defining characteristics called attributes. In performing a concept analysis, the scholar may distinguish between similar concepts, explain a term, or refine ambiguous concepts. An example will be discussed related to a published analysis of the concept of "overcoming" (Brush, Kirk, Gultekin, & Baiardi, 2011). The aim of the analysis was to "develop an operational definition of overcoming and explicate its meaning, attributes, and characteristics as it relates to homeless families" (Brush et al., 2011, p. 160). As described in the article, the process used is based on Walker and Avant's (2011) concept analysis method, which is an excellent resource to review prior to initiating a concept analysis.

The result of the concept analysis will provide a precise operational definition or help to more clearly define the problem. Concept analysis also helps to define standardized nursing language and to develop new tools. The concept analysis is a formal exercise to determine the defining attributes of the phenomenon. Although the analysis is precise, the end product is variable. Precision occurs because of the specific process that is used to analyze the concept. Variability occurs because people see things differently, knowledge changes over time, and the understanding of the concept may change.

The first step is identifying a critical concept within the phenomenon. This step will keep the analysis manageable and will be helpful in the overall understanding of the phenomenon, which will benefit the eventual project. Frame the concept of interest within an introduction that describes the concept of interest and provides definition. Avoid umbrella terms; the more specific the definition of your concept is, the more manageable it becomes. For example, in the article reviewed, the authors noted that in a previous qualitative study of homeless mothers, *overcoming* their situation was frequently mentioned as a desired outcome. Through concept analysis, the authors were able to explore definitions of overcoming in dictionaries and the literature. Using all sources of definition, from dictionaries and colleagues to ordinary and scientific sources, gives a broad view of the concept. This process is important because identifying the uses of the concept from practice and literature further defines the concept.

Defining attributes of the concept is the primary work of concept analysis. The student should look at characteristics that appear consistently. In the previous example, three key attributes were identified from the literature that allowed for the development of a clear definition. "Overcoming is thus defined as a deliberate and thoughtful process of changing or conquering a self-perceived problematic circumstance, challenge or adversity in order to live a healthier and happier future existence" (Brush et al., 2011, p. 162).

The authors then identified antecedents to and consequences of the concept overcoming. Antecedents are events that must occur prior to the concept, whereas consequences are outcomes of the concept. This process allows for a deeper and more specific understanding of the concept. Antecedents in the example of overcoming include recognition of the need to change, demonstrated readiness to change, and determination to change. Possible consequences of overcoming include a return to a more stable, better quality of life (Brush et al., 2011).

Once the antecedents and consequences are recognized, the empirical referents are identified that allow for measurement of the concept and demonstrate that it has occurred. The authors in this example mentioned that there are no direct measurements but suggested using measures of related constructs such as resilience, hope, optimism, self-efficacy, and perceived support (Brush et al., 2011).

Finally, a model, a borderline, and a contrary case are discussed. This allows one to clearly define what the concept *is* (model), to recognize a case that has *some* of the characteristics of the concept (borderline), and to clearly recognize what the concept *is not* (contrary). Each type of case study serves to highlight and clarify characteristics. In the continuing example of overcoming, each case compared the characteristics of the person with the previously discussed antecedents and the resultant consequences.

A concept analysis of a phenomenon or a characteristic of a phenomenon can assist the scholar in defining a problem or distinguishing between similar concepts. This is a creative process. Having just considered the process of concept analysis, what concepts of interest come to mind in relation to practice and phenomena of interest?

Foundational Tenets of Nursing Knowledge

One part of the scholarly process involves considering personal and professional philosophies that are a framework for one's practice. The scholar will likely identify a framework that has been in place in the background, but perhaps not with full awareness. Bunkers (2000) described 16 foundational tenets that are grounded in nursing theory and conceptual frameworks. Examples of the foundational tenets include appreciating the meaning of lived experiences of health and cultivating an attitude of openness to uncertainty and difference (Bunkers, 2000). Reflecting on foundational tenets that have grounded the student's practice can lead to appropriate theories and frameworks to support the work.

As one ponders phenomena of interest, consider the aspects of practice that impact both the nurse and the patient in the delivery of care. **TABLE 5-2** is a worksheet for the student to use when contemplating a phenomenon of interest.

TABLE 5-2 Phenomenon Assessment Worksheet	
Aspects of the Phenomenon	**Phenomenon of Interest**
Personal Interest Expertise	What is my phenomenon of interest? What is my interest level in relation to this phenomenon? What is my level of expertise in relation to this topic?
Literature	What does the literature document regarding this phenomenon? Are there gaps in the literature related to this topic?

(continues)

TABLE 5-2 Phenomenon Assessment Worksheet	*(continued)*

Patterns of knowing
  Empirical
  Esthetic
  Personal
  Ethical
  Emancipatory
	What knowledge do I have of the phenomenon looking through each pattern?

Applicable theories Nursing theories Non-nursing theories	What theories may support the structure of a project utilizing this phenomenon?
Related concepts/concept analysis	What concepts are part of the phenomenon that need further definition?
Foundational tenets	Which of the foundational tenets are important aspects of this phenomenon? How important are the identified tenets to my professional practice?
Peer contributions	What do my peers think about my thoughts about this phenomenon?
Faculty consultation	What input has faculty provided regarding the phenomenon?

▶ Keeping Your Options Open

Selecting a phenomenon of interest for the DNP project is a fluid process, informed by the literature and flexible to change. The scholar will spend considerable time mulling over the potential ideas. Conversations with fellow students and faculty will also add to the richness of the experience. Having said that, certainly time constraints will play an important part in the decision-making process, such as the timeline to graduation! Therefore, it is important to carefully consider the options and discuss them with an advisor; however, remember that the ultimate decision should be made by the DNP student. When the student is passionate about the topic, and the topic is personally meaningful, the time and work involved in completing the project successfully become a labor of love.

> Selecting a phenomenon of interest *is a fluid process, informed by the literature and flexible to change.*

Once the DNP student has considered the phenomenon of interest, ideas will evolve and may develop into potential scholarly projects. Review Chapter 3, Scholarship in Practice, to consider types of scholarship that can develop the project. To illustrate an in-depth exploration of a phenomenon of interest, the following excerpt is presented by Dr. Katherine A. Marshall (see **EXEMPLAR 5-1**). Note the impact and sustainability of identifying a phenomenon that is important to the practitioner and to the organization. Phenomenon identification that drives innovation can result in continued organizational improvements that support patient, population and system outcomes.

EXEMPLAR 5-1 Identifying the Project Topic

Katherine A. Marshall, DNP, RN, PMHCNS-BC

My clinical practice involves the assessment, treatment, and planning of care for community-bound psychiatric and dementia patients for a Metro-Detroit home healthcare agency. This terminal and vulnerable population has challenged the healthcare system with unique needs and rapidly growing costs for care. Hospitalizations are frequent, futile, and often conclude with decreased functional ability and poor quality of life. My expertise in this arena fueled my passion to address the need for clinical staff to identify impending dehydration and malnutrition and impact futile hospital admissions. The agency, like many other healthcare facilities, has felt the impact of the growing dementia population and identified an interest in making changes related to the care of this population. A match between my interests and that of the organization became evident.

A review of the agency's hospital admission records for dementia patients revealed that these patients had higher rates of admission for dehydration and malnutrition than other admission diagnoses. The data were alarming and trending toward increased hospital admissions, increased costs, and undesirable outcomes for dementia patients. In addition, patients and families were impacted negatively with each and subsequent admissions. Upon hospital discharge, patients were physically weaker from being bedbound and presented with greater confusion; all of this ultimately decreased the patients' quality of life.

Identifying clinical phenomena and characteristics that place this population at risk for hospitalization would provide possible opportunities to decrease hospitalization rates and improve quality of life by developing best practice guidelines and system improvements related to preventive interventions, care, and treatment of the dementia patient in home health care. A literature review identified a gap in standards of care related to this population. After realizing this gap, the first step was to explore and describe retrospectively the incidence and correlations of variables or factors that predict or precede dehydration and malnutrition in the home care agency's dementia patients hospitalized for dehydration and malnutrition—in order to give attention to opportunities for improvement related to the care of this population.

The Outcome and Assessment Information Set (OASIS) Start of Care document, a comprehensive assessment tool completed at the start of care, provided the data on the identified variables. Through the literature review, variables were identified that have a potential influence on the condition of dehydration and malnutrition. Potential

(continues)

variables of influence that were identified and extracted from the OASIS were primary residence and degree of support, comorbidities, basal metabolic rate, incidence of urinary tract infections (UTIs), and nutrition score. Demographic data included gender, ethnicity, and age. Forty-four subjects with dementia had been admitted to the hospital with an admission diagnosis of dehydration and malnutrition over a 2-year period. While a single variable or collection of variables were not identified that would predict risk for hospitalization for dehydration and malnutrition, there were areas identified that would benefit from increased clinical attention and process improvement.

This first step prompted an early intervention by a multidisciplinary team within the agency to assess and educate the patient and family on dementia progression, including the signs and symptoms of dehydration and malnutrition. Further, clinicians now have an increased awareness that dehydration and malnutrition are likely and common events in the dementia patient. A high priority is placed on education, prevention, and early intervention to avoid the unnecessary and taxing hospitalization of the dementia patient. Patients and families are introduced to and provided with palliative care and hospice resources earlier in their home care experience, thus avoiding unnecessary hospitalizations and invasive futile treatments.

It is critical to identify a phenomenon of interest where the student has expertise and knowledge and then to match this to an organization's need to move the topic from an area of interest to an identified area of improvement. Using the literature helped me develop an understanding of the current state of the art, while the data from my organization framed the topic within the local context. These first steps set the stage for a project that is both evidence based and effective within the specific organization. Continued and increased attention and improvement has been realized in the dementia population served by the home care agency since the inception of the DNP project. In addition, the project has acted as a springboard for addressing other system and clinical issues that confront the dementia population and their caregivers.

To date, the project has been published in a peer-reviewed journal and several presentations and posters have been delivered. I was also asked to sit as a commissioner on my community's Commission on Aging as an expert in dementia and aging. As the population ages, the incidence of individuals with cognitive impairment in the community treated by the agency has increased and created unique issues in all areas of care. This has prompted the agency to support more clinicians in obtaining their American Nurses Association (ANA) Certification in Mental Health. The agency has also asked that I develop a module on dementia that all clinicians can view to increase their knowledge level and receive continuing education credit.

The agency created easy hold tumblers fitted with a straw that hold 16 ounces of fluids and can be kept at the bed or chair side as a reminder to drink. Clinicians are encouraged to provide the tumblers to patients and provide specific education on the use of the tumbler to increase hydration.

In addition, interactions with caregivers in facilities have helped to elucidate the need for literacy-sensitive education and educational materials, so that education provided by clinicians can be more effectively implemented by the caregiver in the living environment.

This DNP project led to multiple changes and improvements regarding the day-to-day practice of nursing and collaboration with other disciplines in the care of this special population and their caregivers striving to provide the best quality of life.

Impact

- Determining the phenomenon of interest in the context of the organizational need can ultimately impact the success of the project as well as sustainability.
- Including a theoretical framework to describe and explore a phenomenon of interest reflects a scholarly approach to exploring all aspects of a practice problem, contributing to a successful project outcome (See Chapter 15 for a published article that includes a theoretical framework).

Key Messages

- Nursing practice is guided by science and theory, and conversely practice ultimately informs science and theory.
- The complex nature of nursing practice provides many opportunities to explore nursing phenomena.
- The *hidden work* of the nurse is what influences the patient's experience and often positively affects clinical outcomes.
- The DNP project phenomenon of interest must center on a topic that is meaningful to the practice doctorate student and is *valued* by the practice setting.
- A *nursing phenomenon* is "a type of factor influencing health status with the specific characteristics; aspect of health of relevance to nursing practice" (ICNP, n.d., para. 1).
- As the scholar ponders phenomena of interest, he or she should consider the aspects of practice that impact both the nurse and the patient in the delivery of care.
- When the value of the phenomenon of interest can be clearly articulated, there is an identifiable need within society, implementing the project is feasible, and nursing strategies could be explored to address the concern, the topic is worth further investigation.
- Examining a phenomenon within a specific theoretical framework will clarify aspects of the phenomenon and give direction to the DNP project.
- The DNP student can examine a phenomenon of interest by viewing it through the lens of one or several patterns of knowing, which will help the student describe or explain the phenomenon of interest and give the student deeper insight.
- Conducting a concept analysis may help the DNP student to match the phenomenon with concepts, distinguish between similar concepts, explain a term, or refine ambiguous concepts.
- After the DNP student thoughtfully reflects on the phenomenon of interest, the phenomenon will gradually evolve into the DNP project.

Action Plan—Next Steps

1. Identify your areas of clinical expertise, patient populations, and interests.
2. Consider phenomena that you have noted in patient experiences.
3. Become immersed in the literature related to the phenomenon.
4. Observe the phenomenon through multiple lenses, such as the patterns of knowing.

5. Contemplate your nursing framework as evidenced by the foundational tenets.
6. Review potential applicable theories within and outside nursing.
7. Discuss your ideas with your advisor, faculty, peers, and colleagues.
8. Allow your ideas to develop and gel.
9. Identify potential organizations/arenas that could support your area of interest.
10. Enjoy the creativity and the potential of the DNP project.
11. Begin to think about a plan for the project in relation to the phenomenon.
12. Begin to consider the resources you will need to develop your project.

References

American Association of Colleges of Nursing (AACN). (2006). *The essentials of doctoral education for advanced nursing practice.* Retrieved from http://www.aacnnursing.org/Portals/42/Publications/DNPEssentials.pdf

Benner, P., Tanner, C. A., & Chesla, C. A. (2009). *Expertise in nursing practice: Caring, clinical judgment and ethics.* New York, NY: Springer Publishing Company.

Brush, B., Kirk, K., Gultekin, L., & Baiardi, J. (2011). Overcoming: A concept analysis. *Nursing Forum, 46,* 160–168.

Bunkers, S. S. (2000). The nurse scholar of the 21st century. *Nursing Science Quarterly, 13*(2), 116–123.

Carper, B. A. (1978). Fundamental patterns of knowing in nursing. *Advances in Nursing Science, 1*(1), 13–24.

Chinn, L. P., & Kramer, M. K. (2018). *Integrating theory and knowledge development in nursing* (10th ed.). St. Louis, MO: Mosby-Elsevier.

Christenbery, T. L. (2011). Building a schematic model: A blueprint for DNP students. *Nurse Educator, 36*(6), 250–255.

Cody, W. K. (Ed.). (2013). *Philosophical and theoretical perspectives for advanced nursing practice* (5th ed.). Burlington, MA: Jones & Bartlett Learning.

Institute of Medicine (IOM). (2011). *The future of nursing: Leading change, advancing health.* Washington, DC: National Academies Press. Retrieved from http://www.nap.edu/catalog/12956.html

International Classification for Nursing Practice. (n.d.). *Nursing phenomena classification.* Retrieved from http://www.omv.lu.se/icnpbeta/dbrun/hierarchies/1A_Nursing_Phenomena.htm

Jensen, E. (2015). Linking theory, research, and practice. In N. A. Schmidt & J. M. Brown (Eds.), *Evidence-based practice for nurses: Appraisal and application of research* (pp. 133–149). Burlington, MA: Jones & Bartlett Learning.

McEwen, M., & Wills, E. M. (2019). *Theoretical basis for nursing* (5th ed.). Philadelphia, PA: Wolters Kluwer Health/Lippincott Williams & Wilkins.

Morrison, S. M., & Symes, L. (2011). An integrative review of expert nursing practice. *Journal of Nursing Scholarship, 43*(2), 163–170.

Phenomenon. (2018). *Merriam-Webster.* Retrieved from https://www.merriam-webster.com/dictionary/phenomenon

Schmidt, N. A., & Brown, J. M. (2015). *Evidence-based practice for nurses: Appraisal and application of research.* Burlington, MA: Jones & Bartlett Learning.

Walker, K. C., & Avant, L. O. (2011). *Strategies for theory construction in nursing* (5th ed.). Upper Saddle River, NJ: Prentice Hall.

Helpful Resources

Butts, J. B., & Rich, K. L. (2018). *Philosophies and theories for advanced nursing practice.* Burlington, MA: Jones & Bartlett Learning.

McEwen, M. & Wills, E. M. (2019). *Theoretical basis for nursing* (5th ed.). Philadelphia, PA: Wolters Kluwer Health/Lippincott Williams & Wilkins.

Meleis, A. I. (2010). *Transitions theory: Middle range and situation specific theories in nursing research and practice.* New York, NY: Springer Publishing Company.

nurses.info. (2010). *Theories: Middle-range nursing theories.* Retrieved from http://www.nurses.info /nursing_theory_midrange_theories.htm

Nursing Theories. (2012, January 31). *Introduction to nursing theories.* Retrieved from http:// currentnursing.com/nursing_theory/introduction.html

Nursing Theory. (2018). *Nursing theories and models.* Retrieved from http://www.nursing-theory .org/theories-and-models/

Parker, M. E., & Smith, M. C. (2010). *Nursing theory and nursing practice.* Philadelphia, PA: F.A. Davis.

Peterson, S. J., & Bredow, T. S. (2012). *Middle range theories: Application to nursing research.* Philadelphia, PA: Wolters Kluwer Health/Lippincott Williams & Wilkins.

CHAPTER 6

Developing the DNP Project

Katherine Moran

CHAPTER OVERVIEW

Melnyk (2013) purports that DNP programs should prepare nurses as "expert clinicians to generate internal evidence (i.e., evidence generated through outcomes management, quality improvement, and evidence-based practice [EBP] projects) and to translate evidence produced through rigorous research into practice to improve healthcare quality, patient outcomes, and organizational or health policy" (p. 443). Therefore, the DNP project should involve rigorous scholarly inquiry with a focus on advancing nursing knowledge by identifying issues related to clinical practice, helping influence change that will lead to an improvement in clinical practice, and/or contributing to solutions. As one can imagine, developing the DNP project requires considerable thought and planning. The experience can easily become overwhelming without some direction to guide the DNP student who is beginning the process. The goal of this chapter is to introduce the DNP student to elements of a scholarly project that need to be considered early in the development phase.

CHAPTER OBJECTIVES

After completing the chapter, the learner will be able to:

1. Conduct a literature search.
2. Write a literature review.
3. Conduct an organizational assessment.
4. Formulate a problem statement.

(continues)

▶ Developing the DNP Project

In preparation for the development of the DNP project, the student should spend time exploring phenomena that he or she finds interesting. In Chapter 5, The Phenomenon of Interest, the doctor of nursing practice (DNP) student learned the definition of *nursing phenomenon*, explored a variety of strategies to use to identify a phenomenon of interest for the DNP project, and undoubtedly recognized the value of utilizing multiple methods to explore the phenomenon comprehensively. It is important that the DNP student allows enough time to go through this process because it helps him or her gain deeper insight into the phenomenon of interest and identify a direction for the DNP project.

Once the student identifies a phenomenon of interest for the DNP project, he or she is ready to begin the DNP project development process.

Conducting a Literature Search and Writing the Literature Review

As mentioned in Chapter 5, a literature review is conducted to sum up what is known and what is not known about the topic of interest, but it can also help illuminate the value of the phenomenon of interest and identify the appropriate methods to use to examine the phenomenon (Polit & Beck, 2018). However, at this point in the process, instead of browsing the literature to better understand or describe a phenomenon, it is time to carefully review the literature to support the value and/or the need to study the phenomenon of interest and to answer the clinical question. The literature review should summarize the current evidence on the topic; in this way, it helps identify a void in knowledge or a gap between the current state of the phenomenon of interest and the desired state.

> *The literature review is a method used to support the value and/or the need to study the phenomenon of interest.*

The ability to perform a comprehensive literature review and articulate the findings effectively is essential. Today, technology has made it possible to access information quickly and efficiently using a computer and the internet. However, there is more to a literature review than the process involved in performing a search; therefore, it is beneficial to learn key strategies for conducting a literature review as well as interpreting the results.

According to Timmins and McCabe (2005), an effective literature search is a "crucial stage in the process of writing a literature review, the significance of which is often overlooked" (p. 41). Certainly, the process can be very labor intensive, especially if time has not been taken to develop an organized search strategy. To ensure a successful outcome, a literature search should be based on a systematic, thorough, and rigorous approach that is unbiased, up to date (within the last 5 years is ideal), and reproducible (Polit & Beck, 2018; Timmins & McCabe, 2005).

McGrath, Brown, and Samra (2012) propose using the following six steps to systematically search the literature: (1) identify the problem and construct the question, (2) choose the appropriate databases, (3) formulate the search strategy, (4) conduct the search, (5) evaluate the results, and (6) if the results answer the clinical question, then use the results; however, if the results do not answer the clinical question, then refine the search strategy.

To begin, write out the clinical question to help define the focus (key words) for the search. For example, for an evidence-based focus this often includes writing the question using a PICO approach, which stands for *Population* (describes the patient population, i.e., age, gender, etc.); *Intervention, influence, or exposure* (names the clinical intervention or therapies of interest, or identifies the potentially harmful influences or exposures of concern); *Comparison* (identifies a comparison intervention or the intervention is compared with usual care); and *Outcomes* (describes the outcome or consequences). With some clinical questions it may also be helpful to use a PICOT question, which includes the *Time frame* (describes the timing in relation to the intervention and/or duration for data collection). While not all projects will require a PICOT question, all will require an understanding of the purpose of the project, the age and race (if appropriate) of the population, and perhaps disease condition (McGrath, Brown, & Samra, 2012).

There are several effective approaches to reviewing the literature. One method includes looking through databases, journals, and books to develop a list of relevant material. Another useful method involves identifying a relevant article and using the reference list to identify other potentially useful articles, books, or sources of pertinent data (Timmins & McCabe, 2005). Both methods provide a means to begin gathering relevant information and set the parameters for the search.

When using a database to begin a search, it is important to identify a database that contains information relevant to the phenomenon of interest, and to formulate a search strategy that includes the proper key words and subject headings in order to assure a good outcome (McGrath, Brown, & Samra, 2012). A database is a large collection of information organized to allow users rapid search and retrieval (Database, 2018). The information contained in a database or repository is stored in a form that is quickly searchable and readily retrievable, based on the words used in the query. A variety of databases exist; some require a subscription to access, and some are freely available to all. Databases may contain general information, cross-disciplinary topics, or subject-specific citations. Even databases that contain the same subjects may be different from one another. For example, PubMed is a comprehensive resource for biomedical literature, and the Cumulative Index to Nursing and Allied Health Literature (CINAHL) is a comprehensive resource for nursing and allied health literature. See **BOX 6-1** for a list of common databases.

BOX 6-1 Examples of Databases Used when Conducting a Literature Search

- *Business Source Premier* is a business research database. This is the industry's most popular business research database and features the full text for more than 2100 journals. Full-text versions are provided back to 1965, and searchable cited references are provided back to 1998 (EBSCO Industries, Inc., 2012, para. 1).
- *Cochrane Collaboration/Cochrane Nursing Care Network* develops and distributes systematic reviews of interventions for many healthcare professionals.
- *CINAHL*, the Cumulative Index to Nursing and Allied Health Literature, is a comprehensive resource for nursing and allied health literature. CINAHL has expanded to offer four databases, including two full-text versions. The CINAHL databases are available on EBSCO Health (EBSCO Industries, Inc. 2018, para 1).
- *Emerald Fulltext* is a collection of business, management, and social science journals. The database covers all major management disciplines.
- *Joanna Briggs Institute* provides the best available evidence to inform clinical decision-making at the point of care.
- *National Guideline Clearinghouse* is a useful resource to identify summaries of evidence-based clinical practice guidelines.
- *PubMed/MEDLINE*, established by the National Library of Medicine, indexes biomedical literature to help provide health professionals access to information necessary for research, health care, and education. PubMed comprises more than 28 million citations for biomedical literature from MEDLINE, life science journals, and online books. Citations may include links to full-text content from PubMed Central and publisher websites (PubMed, n.d., para 1).

Next, it is important to develop a thorough yet logical search strategy. Taking time to choose appropriate search terms, whether keywords or subject headings, will help to organize the inquiry and defend the interpretation of the results once the review is complete. It is helpful to consult a librarian at this stage in the process. Librarians can help identify the appropriate keywords, subject headings, and limits for the search so that the information received is not overwhelming and is relevant to the topic.

Consider, for example, the following keywords: *asthma* and *children*. A search of the CINAHL database (2013 to present) identified 2274 references. It is clear that the keywords are too broad to identify any specific, relevant information regarding this population. In this case, the librarian can help identify a more appropriate search strategy to use, along with the proper Boolean (or logical) operators and limits to further narrow the search.

The method used to organize the literature should be logical to the user and allow for easy retrieval. A variety of methods can be used to achieve the same outcome. Some individuals find it helpful to use index cards to capture pertinent information about an article, and others rely on electronic reference or citation management software to record and organize references, such as EndNote, ProCite, or RefWorks; one of these products may be available for use through the university at no cost to the student (see Helpful Resources). Because most people have a personal computer today, more and more people are managing the data electronically in files created on the computer. The information can be categorized under major headings and then further categorized in subfolders within the major headings. Consider, for example, a diabetes management case scenario. A major heading for a literature review category could be *diabetes management*, and within that folder could be sub-folders for *fasting blood glucose* or *cholesterol*. To further organize the information captured in the electronic folders, some individuals develop a literature summary table. A summary table is used to organize the literature based on information that is important to the user, that is, the year of publication, author, name and type of the work, sample size, methods, and results (if the work is research). See **TABLE 6-1** for an example of a literature summary table.

Irrespective of the method used, the value here is to capture the search process used, the reference information, the key ideas, and/or a brief summary of the literary work to refer to when writing the literature review.

When conducting the literature search, it is important to keep in mind the need to attain primary source material whenever possible. Primary sources are original materials that have not been filtered through interpretation or evaluation from another author (secondary source). Primary sources present "original thinking, report on new discoveries, or share fresh information" (University of Minnesota Crookston, 2018, para. 2). The problem associated with secondary sources relates to the interpretation of the intent of the original author. Therefore, when information is found through a secondary source, it is important to take the time to search for the primary work. Generally, reference information regarding the primary source can easily be obtained from the secondary source reference list.

In addition to commercially published research, the student may need to search for grey literature. According to GreyNet International (2018),

> Grey literature is a field in library and information science that deals with the production, distribution, and access to multiple document types produced on all levels of government, academics, business, and organization in electronic and print formats not controlled by commercial publishing, i.e., where publishing is not the primary activity of the producing body. (para. 2)

Grey literature can be helpful because it often includes timely information that can be used to minimize publication bias and provide a more thorough view of the evidence. Examples of organizations that may provide useful grey literature include the World Health Organization and the National Institutes for Health and Care Excellence (McGrath, Brown, & Samra, 2012).

Once the literature is compiled, the information gathered must be interpreted, critiqued, and synthesized. This is a very important step in the process. It involves selecting information that is most applicable to the phenomenon of interest that is of the highest quality. Determining the level of evidence is needed to assure the information included in the review is credible and appropriate for inclusion in practice. This can be done by rating the evidence based on methodological rigor (precision of the design) and research design. For example, the American Association of Critical Care Nurses (AACN) levels of evidence considers meta-analysis and meta-synthesis of controlled trials as the highest level of evidence (level A) because, theoretically, they have less potential for bias. These are followed by well-designed controlled studies (level B); studies from a variety of designs (level C); peer-reviewed professional organizational standards based on clinical studies (level D); theory, expert opinion, and case reports (level E); and finally, anything produced by industry (level M) is considered the lowest level of evidence (Peterson et al., 2014).

TABLE 6-1 Example of a Literature Summary Table

Year	Author, Title, Journal	Purpose	Design (descriptive, systematic review, observational etc.)	Sample	Result
2008	Kelleher and Andrews. An observational study on the open-system endotracheal suctioning practices of critical care nurses. *Journal of Clinical Nursing*	Compare endotracheal suction (ETS) practices of critical care nurses with recent research recommendation.	Nonparticipant structured observational design	45	Participants varied in their ETS practices. They did not follow best practice recommendations, resulting in lower quality ETS treatment.
2008	Evangelista, Moser, Westlake, Pike, Ter-Galstanyan, and Dracup. Correlates of fatigue in patients with heart failure. *Progress in Cardiovascular Nursing*	1. To determine how prevalent fatigue is in patients with systolic heart failure (HF). 2. To identify clinical and psychological states associated with HF.	A cross-sectional, correlational design	150	Fatigue levels were moderately intense and highly prevalent in the sample population. Fatigue had predictable clinical dimensions and psychosocial correlates. Fatigue may influence patients' adherence to their medical regimen, social relationships, and quality of life.

| 2008 | Jacobson, Myerscough, De-Lambo, Fleming, Huddleston, Bright, and Varley. Patients' perspectives on total knee replacement. *American Journal of Nursing* | To describe patients' pre- and postoperative experiences with total knee replacement (TKR). | Qualitative descriptive design | 27 | Four overarching themes: 1. Many patients delayed having surgery for months to years, even though they had pain. 2. Once they decided to have surgery, they spent time waiting and worrying about the outcome. 3. Patients struggled with the need for independence and to accept the new knee. 4. Postoperatively, patients experienced pain after surgery and with rehabilitation but were hopeful they would regain function. |

Reproduced from Brown, S. J. (2018). *Evidence-based nursing: The research-practice connection* (3rd ed.). Burlington, MA: Jones & Bartlett Learning.

When describing the literature, the student should form logical conclusions that justify the problem statement and (when applicable) answer the research question (Machi & McEvoy, 2016). The student should consider the following questions when evaluating his or her conclusions:

1. What is the stated conclusion?
2. What are the reasons that support the conclusion?
3. Do the reasons stated have convincing data to support them?
4. Does the conclusion logically follow from those reasons? (Machi & McEvoy, 2016, p. 41)

Sometimes knowledge about a subject may be incomplete, or there may even be opposing views expressed in the literature. Therefore, interpreting and synthesizing the literature can be a difficult process. The reality is, there may not be one single truth about a phenomenon because a multitude of individuals are contributing to the knowledge base. Further, each contributor has a specific purpose in mind for that contribution, which adds in some way to the value of the overall knowledge base. The task at hand, then, is to articulate where the literature is congruent, where and how it differs, and the overall message based on the review. The review should offer a summary of knowledge currently available. Price (2009) stated, "Even where more is debated than agreed it is possible to point to the richness and the complexity of the literature available" (p. 49).

Remember, from the perspective of the phenomenon of interest, the interpretation and summary of the literature review offers an opportunity to substantiate the need for the original inquiry by identifying the void in knowledge or a gap between the current state of the phenomenon of interest and the desired state. Further, it offers a lead-in to why the phenomenon is important, or it describes the benefits of investigating the phenomenon.

Therefore, it is essential that the concluding points of the review refer back to the purpose and focus of the literature review (Price, 2009). Reviewing examples of a literature review published in a peer-reviewed professional journal may help the student understand how the evidence is synthesized to support the project. An example is provided in Chapter 15 of a quality improvement project by Duffy, Rodgers, Shever, and Hockenberry (2015) that focused on preventing central line–associated bloodstream infections in pediatric oncology patients.

Organizational Assessment

As mentioned in Chapter 5, practicing scholars are in the best position to identify those areas of clinical concern that require further research and/or improvement, which allows them to develop the clinical question in the context of the needs of an organization or population. When the DNP student is considering a quality improvement project, this is of critical importance to the success of the project because the project must be *valued* by the practice setting. In other words, the student should avoid identifying a project *then* looking for an organization to welcome a change initiative. The DNP student should first take the time to complete an assessment at the organization of interest to enhance project implementation, organizational change, and determine the potential for sustainability.

An organizational assessment (OA) is a systematic process that is used to gain information about the organization's performance and factors that impact performance. This process is critical for the DNP student to engage in to determine areas within the organization that need improvement, but also to help gain support for the project need. For example, as part of the organizational assessment the student will review the organization's strategic plan to determine if the project is in line with the goals of the organization. It would be difficult to gain support for a project that does not align with an organization's strategic goals. Further, the results of the organizational assessment not only provide information in regards to planning and decision making, but also can provide meaningful feedback that can be shared with stakeholders about the organization's performance and make it easier to identify resources that can help move a change initiative forward (Reflect & Learn, n.d.).

Conducting an organizational assessment requires a systematic approach that encompasses the review of the organizational motivation, such as the mission and vision, strategic plan, history, and culture. The OA also includes the operational framework that identifies the effectiveness of the organization, the efficiencies, and financial stability. In addition, the assessment should capture the organizational capacity, such as strategic leadership and management, the organization's infrastructure (technology, program and process management, etc.), as well as linkages to other organizations. Finally, a review of the external environment should be assessed to identify factors that impact the well-being of the organization, such as the political, sociocultural, and economic environment (Canadian International Development Agency, 2006; Reflect & Learn, n.d.). There are many tools available to guide the student in conducting an organizational assessment. See Chapter 13, The DNP Project Toolbox, for more information on organizational assessment tools.

To *assess* involves estimating or determining the importance, value, or significance of the object of interest. In this context, performing an assessment in relation to a phenomenon of interest involves a comprehensive analysis that could be used to highlight the variance from what is found in the *current state of being* to what could be found in a *future or desired state of being*. In some situations, an organization may have a desired state in mind and may enlist the DNP student to assist the organization to achieve the desired state. Even in this scenario, it is important to begin with an assessment to confirm the organization's prediction. Once the assessment is complete, the difference between the current and desired state is then *measured* to determine if there is an actual need. In other words, an *assessment* of the organization, department, or unit of practice conducted by the DNP student will (1) help identify the gap between the current and desired state of being but also will (2) provide data that support the need for change. Using data to drive change is essential in the current healthcare arena. This process can also make it easier to secure project funding; because financial resources are often limited, projects are often prioritized within the system and implemented only when there is compelling evidence that supports the need for change. The assessment can also help identify what resources are currently being used and what resources exist to address the current needs. Simply stated, a comprehensive assessment provides a means to easily identify where opportunities exist. This process serves a significant purpose when conducting a scholarly project.

SWOT Analysis

An assessment can be used to evaluate the strengths and weaknesses of a variety of phenomena, such as the strengths and weaknesses of a community, organization, program, project, or even a process. One tool used to perform an assessment is called a strengths, weaknesses, opportunities, and threats (SWOT) analysis. The SWOT analysis is an assessment of both internal and external attributes and threats to the phenomenon of interest. For example, perhaps the focus of the assessment is on evaluating a diabetes education program. The *internal* attributes of the program are those traits that are helpful to the program. They may include efficient processes, experienced staff, or an aesthetically appealing environment. These intrinsic factors have a positive influence on the program outcome. On the other hand, weaknesses of the program include any *internal* traits that could be harmful to the program. Perhaps there is underlying tension between key stakeholders (registered nurses, dietitians, social workers, psychologist, exercise physiologist, etc.), ineffective communication, or gaps in critical knowledge. These intrinsic factors can disrupt the program and potentially interfere with the ability of the program to meet its objectives. Together, these two evaluations provide a general perspective of the current situation.

The extrinsic factors are then examined to identify any potential *external* opportunities that could help the program. Perhaps there are opportunities to collaborate with other community members, or maybe key stakeholders are willing to provide additional support in an area identified as a program weakness. Finally, those external factors that may threaten or potentially harm the program, or interfere with the program's ability to achieve objectives are also examined. Extrinsic threats may include significant external competition (that is changing the marketplace), or perhaps there is a very real threat that the primary program funding source will be withdrawn. Either of these external factors, or others like these, could have a catastrophic effect on program outcomes if left unaddressed.

Once this process is complete, a determination can be made regarding how to proceed. This could include using the identified strengths to take advantage of the identified opportunities, or, in contrast, it may include using the identified strengths to minimize internal weaknesses or even overcome identified external threats.

The evaluation of the internal strengths and weaknesses, in conjunction with the evaluation of the external opportunities and threats, provides a broad view of the current situation. However, remember that the SWOT analysis is just one of many assessment tools that can be used to assess the phenomenon of interest. Chapter 13, The DNP Project Toolbox, includes examples of additional assessment tools the student may find helpful. See **FIGURE 6-1** for an illustration of the SWOT analysis model.

Conducting a Needs Assessment

Once the broad-view or "macro-level" assessment is complete, the DNP student can drill down to the "micro level" to determine the most important or immediate needs of the organization. Conducting a *needs assessment* is fairly straightforward. First, determine what it is that you want to know (which may have been identified through the SWOT analysis), who the best person(s) is to answer the question(s), and how the data will be gathered; then, outline the data analysis plan and determine how you will share the findings with the organization.

The assessment ... can lead to the identification of a gap in the current state of a phenomenon or help validate current perceptions.

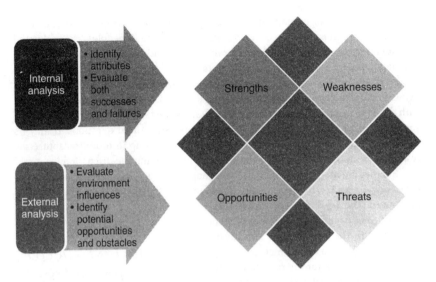

FIGURE 6-1 An example of a SWOT analysis chart.

One very important first step in performing a needs assessment is to create an assessment plan. To begin the process, have a clear objective in mind. As mentioned, think about what needs to be determined. The answer to this question establishes the direction the assessment will take and the questions that need to be asked to obtain the pertinent information. Finally, it also helps narrow the target audience. The next step involves identifying who would be best prepared to answer the assessment questions. Is it an individual or a group of individuals? If several individuals need to provide input, how will those individuals be chosen? Choosing the appropriate individuals is important because a representative sample of the population is necessary to ensure that the data captured are valid. A more detailed discussion related to identifying key stakeholders follows this section.

Finally, once the DNP student identifies who is best equipped to answer the assessment questions, a decision will need to be made regarding how the data will be collected, such as via interviews, focus groups, or surveys, and how the results will be evaluated.

Interviews can be conducted in person, over the telephone, or through an internet resource, such as Skype. The advantages of interviews are that (1) the response rates tend to be higher compared to surveys, (2) respondents have an opportunity to ask questions to gain clarity on a question that they may have otherwise left blank, and (3) additional information is gained by observing the respondent, which can help in interpreting responses (Polit & Beck, 2018). Regardless of the technique used, the student will want to have a structured set of questions prepared that may include both closed- and/or open-ended questions. The key is to carefully construct the questions so that they are clear to the respondent; are sensitive to the psychological state of the respondent; and, when using questionnaires or surveys, are the appropriate grade level and are presented in a meaningful order that encourages cooperation (Polit & Beck, 2018). Developing appropriate questions can be a labor-intensive process. Therefore, the DNP student should allow time in the project schedule for survey development and testing to assure the best outcomes are achieved.

A focus group or community forum serves the same purpose as an individual interview, except it is conducted with a small group of 5 to 10 people. When selecting individuals to participate in the focus group, care should be taken to attract a diverse population with a broad view of the phenomenon of interest. The DNP student can choose to send an invitation to potential participants or may choose to invite participants in person; however, he or she should also send a reminder prior to the event with the date, time, and location identified. During the focus group the DNP student should guide or facilitate the discussion using the structured questions. It may be useful to solicit additional help to conduct the focus group in order to capture the responses from the participants and/or assist in facilitating the discussion.

Surveys are used to gain quantitative data that are primarily closed ended, such as yes-or-no answers, but may include a few open-ended questions to add clarity. As mentioned, the DNP student should allocate sufficient time for survey development and testing in the project plan. The advantages of using a survey format are that it provides anonymity for the respondent and can easily be dispersed via the postal service or electronically via email. Another advantage is that respondents can then answer the survey at their convenience; but the downside is the response rates tend to be low.

Once the information is obtained, the data are analyzed. The data analysis method used will be dependent on the types of questions that are asked, such as quantitative (closed-ended) or qualitative (open-ended) questions. The DNP student will want to consult with his or her advisor to determine the best method to use for data analysis. See Chapter 7 for more detailed information on this topic. Once complete, the results of the analysis should be shared with the organization. Communicating the assessment results can be accomplished using a formal (presentation or white paper) or informal process (verbal communication), depending on the student's relationship with the organization and the preference of the organization's key stakeholders (see Chapter 15, Disseminating the Results).

The process of conducting a needs assessment is fairly straightforward. First, determine what it is that you want to know, who the best person(s) is to answer the question(s), and how the data will be gathered; then outline the data analysis plan and determine how you will share the findings with the organization.

Keep in mind that when the purpose of the assessment is simply to verify that the phenomenon of interest is worth exploring or to identify the perceived state of the phenomenon, a DNP scholar–created questionnaire will suffice. As mentioned, this type of assessment could be accomplished fairly quickly by conducting a small focus group or community forum or by surveying a convenience sample of the target population. When the results of the assessment are the central purpose for the project, measures need to be taken to ensure that a valid and reliable tool is used to conduct the assessment and that appropriate statistical methods are used to analyze the data. This type of assessment takes a considerable amount of time and resources to complete and may require institutional review board (IRB) approval (discussed later in this chapter). However, a comprehensive assessment, such as a community or organizational *needs assessment*, provides valuable data that describe the current state of the phenomenon of interest, how the proposed project could address the findings, knowledge of approaches that could be most effective, as well as the potential project impact (McCawley, 2009).

Developing the Problem Statement

The definition of a *problem*, according to Merriam-Webster, is "a question raised for inquiry, consideration or solution . . . [or] an intricate unsettled question" ("Problem," 2018, para. 1). Both definitions are fairly straightforward; they indicate that a question is involved. However, defining a *problem statement* has not been quite as forthcoming. In fact, it has not been consistently described in the literature. Some consider the purpose of the project and problem statement as one in the same, whereas others lump together the objective, hypothesis, or summary of the content as the problem statement (Hemon & Schwartz, 2007). In an attempt to bridge this gap, for the purposes of this discussion and in the context of the DNP project, a problem statement will encompass a *phenomenon in need of inquiry that is examined in order to develop a potential solution.*

The problem statement is an introduction to the intent of the project. It should include enough information for the reader to gain an understanding of the issues surrounding the phenomenon of interest and the reason the project was selected as an area of focus. The problem statement provides the background to the problem and justification for investigating the phenomenon of interest, as demonstrated through the literature review.

Hemon and Schwartz (2007) indicated that a problem statement should include four components:

1. Lead-in
2. Declaration of originality
3. Explanation
4. Indication of the central focus (p. 308)

Using this definition as a guide to formulate a problem statement, the *lead-in* should include information that helps to set the stage; it is the first introduction to the problem. To illustrate this concept, consider the following lead-in: *Successful diabetes management in the primary care setting is a difficult, costly, and labor-intensive process*

> *The problem statement encompasses a phenomenon in need of inquiry that is examined in order to develop a potential solution.*

> *Articulating the problem statement . . . The goal is to identify an issue, describe it clearly but succinctly, and adequately articulate why it is important that the problem be addressed.*

that requires proven skills in lifestyle counseling (Moran, Burson, Critchett, & Olla, 2011). The information provided in this lead-in introduces the audience to the phenomenon of interest: diabetes management in primary care. It also highlights the area of concern: multiple factors that make it difficult to provide successful diabetes management in this care setting.

The lead-in statement is then followed by the *declaration of originality*, supported by information from the literature review. The intent here is to substantiate the need for the inquiry by identifying the void in knowledge or the gap between the current state of the phenomenon and the desired state. Continuing with the previous case example, consider the following: *Although many studies have proved the value of addressing the needs of people with diabetes in this care setting, there is a paucity of studies that look at clinically effective interventions or strategies in relation to cost* (Moran et al., 2011). In this case, the need for the investigation or declaration of originality is substantiated by the paucity, or scarcity, of studies available that look at interventions or strategies in relation to cost in this care setting.

Next, the *explanation* of the phenomenon should highlight the value of the project and/or the benefits of investigating the phenomenon. The explanation of the purpose in the example centered on the need to improve diabetes clinical and cost outcomes in the primary care setting. Finally, the *indication of central focus* should tie all the previously mentioned components together to form a complete package, which is accomplished by articulating and/or defining what the project will accomplish. To clearly communicate the central focus, consider beginning this concluding statement by simply proclaiming the purpose of the project or study: "The purpose of this study was to implement and evaluate a care delivery model integrating the Registered Nurse-Certified Diabetes Educator in the Patient Centered Medical Home to assist in achieving positive clinical and cost outcomes in diabetes care" (Moran et al., 2011, p. 783).

Another approach that may be used to facilitate writing the problem statement is to begin by defining *who, what, where, when,* and *why*. In other words, *who* the problem involves, *what* the issue is, *when* and *where* the problem is occurring, and *why* it is important to investigate.

It is important to clearly define *who* is affected by the problem; this information will be included in the lead-in. Using the previous example, the specific group identified in the problem statement is primary care providers and their patients. The *what* and the *where* in this statement involve providing successful diabetes management for patients with diabetes within the primary care setting. This defines the boundaries of the problem. One can conclude that providing diabetes management for patients with diabetes in this specific care setting is difficult and possibly not effective. Discussing the impact of the issue or why this problem is important would also be appropriate here. For example, one could link the phenomenon of interest with patient outcomes. In this case, including information in the literature regarding less-than-optimal overall glucose control in this care setting could be considered. This introduces the reader to the potential negative impact on the stakeholders, that is, patients with diabetes and their healthcare providers. One could even link the less-than-optimal clinical outcomes in this setting to the current cost of care of patients with diabetes. Regardless of the approach used, the goal is to identify an issue, describe it clearly but succinctly, and adequately articulate why it is important that the problem be addressed. Remember, a well-written problem statement will engage the audience and leave them with a desire to read more.

Identifying Key Stakeholders

Once the problem statement for the potential project is developed, it is critical to identify and reach out to the key stakeholders. Stakeholders are those individuals or groups who touch the project in some way or have an interest in the project outcome. These individuals can affect or could be affected by the outcome of the project. The student should consider those individuals or groups who are invested from the micro and macro level because they can provide informed and unique perspectives on issues that may have otherwise been overlooked.

Key stakeholders . . . are those individuals or groups who touch the project in some way or have an interest in the project outcome.

To begin, list all the individuals or groups who may be interested in the project. Who the potential stakeholders are depends on the project, of course, but a few examples may include service users, mentors, colleagues, organizational leaders, and community organizations. In the diabetes management example, the key stakeholders could include patients, families, healthcare providers, healthcare staff, healthcare institutions, payers, and even the community. Think about stakeholders who could benefit from the project, those who may have to make changes to current processes as a result of the project, and those who have something to lose. Determining the type of influence a stakeholder may have on the project's success is critical. Positive influence stakeholders may be willing to champion the project or support the project in some way, whereas negative influence stakeholders may be a restraining force.

Once all stakeholders are identified, consider which stakeholders are vital to the success of the project. These are the key stakeholders. The task at hand now is to determine what can be done to get stakeholder support or to reduce stakeholder resistance. This may include identifying the potential benefits of the project for certain stakeholders, such as outlining the project costs and benefits and developing strategies to minimize any perceived negative impact by other stakeholders.

This process may seem cumbersome and time consuming, but it is a valuable use of time because it helps to garner support for the project and minimize potential roadblocks. Consider Pareto's principle, or the 80–20 rule. It is very applicable to planning the DNP project: 20% of the work consumes 80% of the needed time. Furthermore, identifying and engaging key stakeholders is a good use of time because stakeholders can provide objective guidance on project implementation, identify options and/or solutions to address identified issues, provide input in areas in which there is an information gap, or help identify specific resources that are available to support the project.

Determining Project Goals

Project goals describe what the student intends on delivering within the context of the project.

A goal is "the end toward which effort is directed" ("Goal," 2018, para. 1). In the case of the DNP project, it is what the student strives to achieve. Project goals describe what the student intends on delivering within the context of the project. Generally, a project's overall goal is relatively high level, though it should provide enough information to define when the project is complete. The project goal is the underpinning for decision-making.

When considering potential project goals, think visionary! Perhaps the goal is to achieve a specific milestone, to test a hypothesis, to share insights or discoveries learned through the process, or to improve a process or outcome within an organization. For example, perhaps after conducting an organizational needs assessment the student identifies that there has been a steady increase in the number of medication administration errors occurring in the medical intensive care unit (MICU) over the past 9 months. After sharing this information with the organization, a decision is made to investigate the cause, determine the best course of action, and finally implement a quality improvement project with the aim of reducing the medication error rate in the MICU. The possibilities are limited only by imagination and available resources, including time. To this last point, it is crucial that the chosen project goal be achievable within the prescribed DNP program time frame; otherwise, there is a very real risk of not meeting program deadlines, which could result in failure to progress.

Once the goal has been identified, the next step is to define it. When articulating the goal of the project, clarity is the key. It is vital that the goal be clearly identified to ensure that everyone knows what event will mark the completion of the project. From here, the student can work backward to identify the interim goals (or objectives) that must be met in order to achieve the final desired outcome.

Defining the Project Scope

The project scope includes all the work that needs to be accomplished in order to fulfill the project goals. It helps to define when the project begins and when the project ends. To define the project scope, the student will need to consider the boundaries of the project. This includes identifying what will and will not be included (features and functions), along with identifying the deliverables. Defining the project scope early on in the process helps the student during the implementation process. It is much easier to determine what is relevant to the project and what is not when clear boundaries have been identified up front. In the medication administration error scenario, the scope is defined by unit (MICU) and only includes medication errors. In this case, the scope may also include all three shifts, and it may include parenteral and oral medications, etc. To this last point, it may be easier for the student to understand all the dimensions of the project if the various components are diagrammed or graphed; this gives a visual representation of the project scope.

The project scope includes all the work that needs to be accomplished in order to fulfill the project goals.

When defining the project scope, consider the following: What will make this project personally meaningful? Certainly, the ultimate goal of the DNP project is to provide a medium for the student to demonstrate achievement of the DNP *Essentials*, which translates to an outcome that directly or indirectly benefits society. This is of great significance, and as such, what is and is not included in the project should be determined by the student after assessing what he or she believes is of most value.

This process fosters personal investment in the outcome and makes the entire project more meaningful to the student. After all is said and done, the student owns the project and is responsible for achieving the deliverables.

Once the scope of the project is clear, the objectives of the project should be defined. This will help keep the project on track, clarify any assumptions, and avoid any unintended surprises. Objectives should describe what will be done (a measurable component) and when it will be completed. There may be a wide variety of types of objectives, depending on the type of DNP project. For example, in the medication administration error scenario the DNP student conducts a root cause analysis and determines that there is a system issue that is contributing to the increase in medication administration errors in the MICU. As a result of these findings a plan is developed, based on best practice, to address the problem. An example objective for this quality improvement project could be: *Amend the current medication administration policy and procedure to include safety checks and medication administration safe zones to decrease medication administration errors within 3 months after the new policy has been implemented.* An objective could include cost metrics, technical processes, or other measurable success criteria as indicated by the project. The key is to be as specific as possible. The student must accurately capture the conditions that are necessary to achieve the project's overall goal. One final point, the student will want to carefully consider the DNP program deliverables in the project goals and objectives. See Chapter 15, Disseminating the Results, for more information on program deliverables.

Determining the Theory and Framework

The next step in the process is to articulate the necessary features or functions that are required to meet the objectives. To begin, the student will need to outline the implementation process. Using a conceptual framework may be helpful in this phase of project development because it assists in identifying and categorizing the various components of the project. A conceptual framework is a "group of concepts that are broadly defined and systematically organized to provide a focus, a rationale, and a tool for the integration and interpretation of information" ("Conceptual framework," 2018, para. 1). The Donabedian model is an example of a conceptual framework that focuses on three main categories: structure, process, and outcome (Donabedian, 1988). Using this framework, the student is able to identify all the concepts that affect the project structure (the setting in which the project will be implemented and who will be involved in the project), the process (what will be done and how it will be delivered), and, finally, the outcome (what will be measured, reviewed, or assessed).

The Donabedian model is just one example of a conceptual framework; there are many to choose from. Vogel, Appel, and Winker (2018) describe how they used the health belief model (HBM) as a framework to guide a quality improvement project to improve human papillomavirus (HPV) vaccination among young males. For example, they capitalized on the parents'/guardians' desires to avoid adverse outcomes for their children by offering HPV education, which then increased their perceived seriousness of this condition. Since the likelihood of increased vaccine uptake was dependent on the parents'/guardians' overall perceived benefits outweighing the perceived barriers, education proved to be helpful. In this example, each of the HBM core components was considered in relation to HPV vaccination uptake among males in their target population.

In addition to a conceptual framework, the student will also need to consider a theoretical framework to help inform and/or guide the project. As indicated in Chapter 5, a theoretical framework is used to guide the student's perspective by further defining the project variables, identifying the known relationships among variables, and providing a framework for examining outcomes. Theory helps to explain or predict the relationships around the phenomenon of interest. If this is the case, the student and the student advisor need to determine the framework(s) that best capture the components of the student's scholarly project. More detailed information regarding the implementation process is covered in Chapter 14, Project Implementation.

Quality Improvement

Since many DNP projects are focused on improving processes and outcomes in practice, it is important to understand what is meant by quality improvement and how implementation science may be used to impact these outcomes. The Health Resources and Services Administration (HRSA) (2011) defines quality improvement as a systematic and continuous process that leads to measurable improvement in healthcare services and the health status of targeted groups. Further, because a health organization's quality is linked to the organization's service delivery approach or underlying systems of care, the principles of quality improvement should focus on the systems/processes of care, the patients, the care team, and the use of data to drive change (p. 1).

Using the prior discussion of Donabedian's (1988) framework to address the medication errors in the MICU, the key components of the organization's systems, processes, and outcomes of care can be depicted. For example, the organization's *system or structure* would include resources (infrastructure, people, materials, technology), the *process* would include what is done and how it is done, and the *outcome* would include the results of the care provided (patient satisfaction, change in health behavior and health status). The organization's resources and processes need to be evaluated together in order to improve the end result.

While the structure and resources for an organization are generally easy to recognize, it may be difficult for some organizations to identify their processes because of the complex nature of health care. To better understand the processes used within an organization and the subsequent impact on outcomes, a process map can be used to diagram the events that lead to an outcome. A process map typically includes identifying and mapping the sequence of activities involved in a particular outcome (which includes identifying what is performed, who performs it, when it is performed, etc.). Following this process allows one to visualize opportunities for improvement (see Chapter 13 for an example of a process map).

When evaluating outcomes, one measure of quality that is of particular importance in health care is the degree to which the patient's needs are met, such as access to care, culturally sensitive care, and patient safety. It should be no surprise that in order to meet the patient's needs effectively and to continue to improve quality, it takes an interprofessional team. According to HRSA (2011), the healthcare team has the knowledge, skills, and experience to make needed and long-lasting improvements. It is because of the unique perspectives from each team member that creativity and innovation evolve. The DNP student engaged in this process will have an opportunity to demonstrate his or her leadership competencies in facilitating the work of the interprofessional team. The importance of this role cannot be understated, because behind every effective team is an equally effective leader who is able to organize and facilitate the work of the team.

Finally, the team will need to use data to drive the change. This will include quantitative data (frequencies) for measurement of change but also qualitative data to provide context for the needed improvements (HRSA, 2011). Determining what is most important to measure can be difficult. For this reason, HRSA (2011) recommends beginning with standardized performance measures, which are derived from practice guidelines that are designed to measure systems of care (see Agency for Healthcare Research and Quality [AHRQ] Clinical Guidelines and Recommendations, www.ahrq.gov/professionals/clinicians-providers/guidelines-recommendations/). Good performance measures should be relevant, measurable, accurate, and feasible. The data should be collected at established intervals and then analyzed to determine opportunities for change.

Implementation Science

A new and developing interprofessional research field in health care is *implementation science research*, also known as dissemination science or health services research. The focus of implementation science research is identifying and implementing best-practice approaches to health care in a variety of healthcare settings with an ultimate goal of improving outcomes. According to the Fogarty International Center (2018), implementation science is:

> . . . the study of methods to promote the adoption and integration of evidence-based practices, interventions, and policies into routine healthcare and public health settings. Implementation research plays an important role in identifying barriers to, and enablers of, effective global health programming and policymaking, and leveraging that knowledge to develop evidence-based innovations in effective delivery approaches. (para. 1)

There is an increasing need for this type of research in health care to improve outcomes. It is well-known that there is a gap that exists between research and practice, which has resulted in a delay in adopting evidence-based approaches that have been proved to positively impact healthcare outcomes. Implementation science research holds promise for bridging this gap. This can be accomplished in a variety of ways, such as by using scientific methods to compare evidence-based interventions, develop new approaches to improve healthcare delivery, evaluate a population-based intervention, improve program quality and performance, or identify strategies that promote the integration of evidence into practice. An example of a model that addresses integration is Rogers's diffusion of innovation theory. Rogers (2003) explains that diffusion, which is "the process by which an innovation is communicated through certain channels over time among the members of a social system" (p. 5), occurs when there are key characteristics present in an innovation. These include (1) *relative advantage,* which is the degree that an innovation appears better than the alternatives (measured in terms of economics, social prestige, convenience, and satisfaction); (2) *compatibility*, which is the degree the innovation is seen as consistent with existing values, previous experiences, and needs of those who would adopt it; (3) *complexity*, which is the degree in which the innovation is seen as difficult to use or even understand; (4) *trialability*, which is the degree that an innovation could be experienced or experimented with on a limited basis; and 5) *observability*, which refers to how visible the results of the innovation are to those likely to adopt it (Rogers, 2003).

However, because this field is still evolving, there is a need to recognize how implementation science research differs from other forms of research. Scientific rigor must be balanced with the need to conduct research in real-world settings. It is important to keep in mind that implementation science research may not produce results with the same precision as other forms of research; however, that does not mean that implementation science research is not of high quality. Therefore, implementation science should include the elements of good science, such as data collection and analysis methods that are replicable and available for public review, propositions that are logical and lead to falsifiable hypotheses, and methods that are evaluated by subject matter experts (Quality Enhancement Research Initiative [QUERI], 2014a).

The DNP student embarking on a project focusing on implementation of evidence into the clinical setting and/or evaluation of the implementation process should consider an implementation framework to help guide them. For example, the Iowa model of evidence-based practice to promote quality care is useful because it includes steps to accomplishing a change in practice (Titler et al., 2001). The model incorporates the patient, the provider, and the social system. Through a series of steps, the practitioner identifies either a problem-focused trigger or knowledge-focused trigger that indicates the need for change.

Another example of a model that may be useful for implementing evidence into practice is the QUERI (Quality Enhancement Research Initiative) (2014b). This six-step model includes (1) selecting conditions based on patient populations that are at high risk of disease and/or disability; (2) identifying evidence-based guidelines and/or best practices; (3) measuring existing practice patterns and outcomes; (4) implementing improvement programs; (5) assessing feasibility, implementation, and impacts of the program on the patient, family, and system; and (6) evaluating the impact of the program on health-related quality of life.

Finally, formative or process evaluation is a component of implementation science that focuses on the process of implementation, rather than the outcomes of implementation. The information gleaned through formative evaluation also contributes to the overall understanding of project outcomes. Through formative evaluation, an understanding of the context (where the project is implemented) can help mitigate barriers to implementation and provide insight to factors that will assure sustainability. Data collection methodologies used in formative evaluation include both quantitative measures (e.g., a scale to assess readiness to change) and qualitative measures (e.g., open-ended questions used to gain insight to project facilitators and barriers) (QUERI, 2014c).

These examples illustrate how DNP-prepared nurses as well as DNP students may use implementation science methods to explore a clinical concern and be included as part of implementation science research teams, as the DNP competencies (which are rooted in quality improvement) are in perfect alignment with the requirements for implementation science research.

▶ Defining the Project Type

The DNP project can take many forms (see **BOX 6-2**). The boundaries for the project are determined by the DNP program requirements. While all projects will exemplify some of the DNP *Essentials*, such as interprofessional collaboration or use of data and informatics, they may not exemplify all of the *Essentials*.

Quality Improvement

The definition of *quality* as it relates to health care is subjective; it differs based on who is defining it. For the patient, quality may include accurate, skillful, and compassionate care. Healthcare providers, on the other hand, may define quality as achievement of the desired health outcome, whereas healthcare payers (health insurance companies) are likely to include some aspect of cost effectiveness. Quality improvement projects in health care encompass those efforts that seek to improve services for the future. According to the Institute of Medicine (IOM), *healthcare quality* is defined as "the extent to which health services provided to individuals and patient populations improve desired health outcomes. The care should be based on the strongest clinical evidence and provided in a technically and culturally competent manner with good communication and shared decision making" (Peerpoint, 2012, para. 1).

The IOM (2001) summary report *Crossing the Quality Chasm* outlines six aims for improvement that are built on the need for health care to be:

1. *Safe*: avoiding injuries to patients from the care that is intended to help them
2. *Effective*: providing services based on scientific knowledge to all who could benefit, and refraining from providing services to those not likely to benefit
3. *Patient-centered*: providing care that is respectful of and responsive to individual patient preferences, needs, and values, and ensuring that patient values guide all clinical decisions
4. *Timely*: reducing waits and sometimes harmful delays for both those who receive and those who give care
5. *Efficient*: avoiding waste, including waste of equipment, supplies, ideas, and energy
6. *Equitable*: providing care that does not vary in quality because of personal characteristics such as gender, ethnicity, geographic location, and socioeconomic status (p. 3)

BOX 6-2 Examples of DNP Projects

- Quality improvement
- Translating evidence into practice
- Clinical or practice-based inquiry
- Healthcare delivery innovation
- Program development and evaluation
- Demonstration project
- Healthcare policy
- Generating new evidence or knowledge

Quality Improvement Focus

As mentioned, healthcare quality improvement projects generally focus on analyzing elements of specific areas of performance in order to gain some measure of improvement. Given the current focus on healthcare quality by the IOM, the DNP scholar is well positioned to influence healthcare quality at the micro level (reducing medical errors on a specific care delivery unit) and/or macro level (leading efforts to reduce infant morbidity and mortality at the state level).

Quality Improvement Methods

Several different quality improvement methods have been used effectively in the healthcare arena. A few of the most common tools used in quality improvement projects are presented in Chapter 13. The following are a few examples of the quality improvement methods used by DNP scholars:

- FADE model: *Focus* (define the process that needs improvement), *Analyze* (collect the data and analyze), *Develop* (determine the plan of action), *Execute* (implement the plan), and *Evaluate* (measure the change and continue to monitor).
- Model for Improvement: A framework developed by Associates in Process Improvement (Langley et al., 2009) that is used by the Institute for Healthcare Improvement (IHI) to guide improvement work. The model includes three focus questions:
  1. What are we trying to accomplish?
  2. How will we know that a change is an improvement?
  3. What changes can we make that will result in improvement?

  By asking these questions, the organization is actually setting aims, establishing measures, and selecting changes. The changes are then tested using several PDSA cycles (see below). After refining the change using the PDSA cycle, the change is then implemented on a broader scale and is eventually spread through other parts of the organization.

- Shewhart Cycle: Uses rapid cycles of improvement until an optimal process is reached. This model uses the PDSA cycle to test change—*Plan* (plan a change), *Do* (implement the plan), *Study* (analyze the results), and *Act* (take action based on the results).
- Six Sigma: Focuses on identifying and eliminating defects in a process in order to reduce variability and improve outcomes. This model uses the DMAIC strategy—*Define* (define the opportunity for improvement, the project goals, and the key stakeholders), *Measure* (determine what to measure and collect the data), *Analyze* (analyze the data to determine the root cause), *Improve* (implement a solution and continue to collect data to evaluate the outcome), and *Control* (develop and initiate a monitoring plan).

Other Quality Improvement Considerations

The goal of this chapter is to provide a broad overview of the types of DNP projects currently being developed, not to provide specific instruction on how to conduct these types of projects. Students who choose to complete a quality improvement project as evidence of their scholarly work need to be aware of quality improvement requirements. For example, the Standards for Quality Improvement Reporting Excellence (SQUIRE) 2.0 guidelines (2015) focus on the "use of formal and informal theory in planning, implementing, and evaluating improvement work; the context in which the work is done; and the study of the intervention(s)" (Ogrinc et al., 2015, p. 501). Selecting a mentor with expertise in quality improvement is desirable.

Nursing Research

While it is recognized that DNP students will primarily be focused on projects that improve practice and will therefore be using quality improvement frameworks, there is also a recognition that some students will choose to engage in *implementation science research* or other forms of research to improve practice. For this reason, information that is important for the DNP student to consider related to research is included. *Research*, in general, is defined as an "investigation or experimentation aimed at the discovery and interpretation of facts, revision of accepted theories or laws in the light of new facts, or practical application of such new or revised theories or laws" ("Research," 2018, para. 1). When considering the more specific nature of *nursing research*, Houser (2018) defined it as a "systematic process of inquiry that uses rigorous guidelines to produce unbiased, trustworthy answers to questions about nursing practice" (p. 5).

Research Focus

The National Institute of Nursing Research (NINR), an organization dedicated to improving the health and health care of Americans through funding of nursing research, "supports and conducts clinical and basic research and research training on health and illness, research that spans and integrates the behavioral and biological sciences, and that develops the scientific basis for clinical practice" (NINR, 2016, p. 6). This could be accomplished through clinical problem analysis, knowledge generation (especially when collaborating with PhD colleagues), or translating evidence into practice.

Research Question

As mentioned at the beginning of this chapter, a method often used to develop a good clinical and/or research question is the PICOT approach. For example, a clinical question using the PICOT format could be: Do patients with type 2 diabetes who attend a 6-week diabetes management program experience lower HbA_{1c} results than those patients who do not attend the program? In this case, the P indicates patients with type 2 diabetes, the I is a diabetes management program, the C represents patients who do not attend the program, the O is the HbA_{1c} results, and the T is 6 weeks. This format helps the scholar focus on elements of the question that are of interest (Brown, 2018; Polit & Beck, 2018).

Research Method

The research methods may be qualitative (when the goal is to understand the lived experience around the phenomenon of interest), quantitative (when the goal is to test a hypothesis, measure a phenomenon, or examine how the phenomenon of interest works), or a mixed method (both quantitative and qualitative).

Research Design

The research design may be nonexperimental (descriptive, correlational, predictive, or quasi-experimental design) or experimental (used to test cause and effect) in nature. The design is determined based on the research question or purpose, the availability of subjects and time frame, the skills of the researcher, ethical factors, amount of control required, the resources available to conduct the study, and expectations of the audience for research (Houser, 2018). The overall study plan—the details of how the study will be conducted—will be determined by the research design.

Other Research Considerations

1. *The institutional review board (IRB).* Before beginning a research project, approval is required from the university's IRB and/or from the review board where the study is conducted. The IRB, an independent ethics committee, comprises a group of individuals who "oversee all research involving human subjects and ensures studies meet all federal regulation criteria, including ethical standards" (Houser, 2018, p. 482). Applying for and receiving IRB approval can be a labor-intensive and time-consuming process. Once the application for IRB approval is submitted, it can take anywhere from several weeks to several months to receive approval, depending on the type of review (expedited or full review). See Chapter 10, Creating and Developing the Project Plan, for more information regarding submitting for IRB approval.

   > *The institutional review board . . . oversees all research involving human subjects and ensures that studies meet all federal regulation criteria and ethical standards.*

2. *Time and resources.* Because of the short time frame associated with the typical DNP program, the student will need to choose a project with a fairly well-defined scope to complete the DNP program requirements on time. Not only does the actual study need to be completed on schedule, but the analysis and interpretation of the results need to be conducted and the final documentation (i.e., a research report) produced. In cases in which the project is large or complex, some DNP programs have allowed DNP students to complete the project together, with each student being responsible for specific elements of the project.

3. *Expertise.* If research is the focus of the DNP scholarly work, the student should work with a study team and/or individual researcher with expertise in conducting research. See Chapter 7, Aligning Design, Method, and Evaluation with the Clinical Question, for information on collecting and mining the data.

Pilot Study

A pilot study, also known as a feasibility study, is a smaller study that is done to determine if a larger study is practical and/or achievable. A pilot study could be done to ensure validity and reliability of instruments and data collection procedures, or to assess costs, efficiency, and/or accuracy (Houser, 2018). A pilot study conducted to determine feasibility should replicate the larger study as close as possible (i.e., setting, intervention, data collection, and analysis).

Pilot Study Focus

A pilot study is useful because it can identify areas of concern around a study design that can then be fixed before implementing the study on a larger scale. For instance, there may be issues with the randomization process of participants or with the data collection procedure. A pilot study can also be used to determine if the level of intervention is appropriate (for example, length of the intervention) or to see if the intervention causes adverse effects. Using the case example presented earlier, a pilot study was used to determine if providing diabetes education, management, and support using a registered nurse–certified diabetes educator would be cost effective and improve clinical outcomes.

Pilot Study Methods and Design

The methods and design used in a pilot study are analogous with those of a larger research study.

Other Pilot Study Considerations

A pilot study can be especially helpful for a student because it gives him or her some experience. It also allows for preliminary testing of a hypothesis and, as mentioned previously, it can help reduce unanticipated problems in the main study; this may save time and/or money if procedural issues inherent in the study design are discovered before it is implemented on a larger scale.

1. *The institutional review board.* If the pilot study involves human subjects, approval from the university and study setting IRB may be required. Remember that it may take anywhere from several weeks to several months to receive IRB approval (depending on the type of review), so careful planning is essential.

2. *Time and resources.* Although a pilot study can be completed in significantly less time than a large study, a fair amount of time is still required to complete the study in its entirety, including the analysis and interpretation of the results and final documentation. Again, careful planning is essential.

3. *Expertise.* As mentioned, if research is the focus of the DNP scholarly work, the student should work with a study team and/or individual researcher with expertise in conducting research.

Healthcare Delivery Innovation

The current U.S. healthcare system is at a crossroads. New methods for care delivery and approaches to disease management are being evaluated to determine if there is a more cost-effective means to meet the healthcare needs of the population. The focus is shifting from acute, episodic care to prevention. Clinical teams are exploring the benefits of redefining care around medical conditions. For these and other reasons, DNP healthcare delivery projects are also popular choices for scholarly work. These projects often include an intervention or innovative approach to healthcare delivery that has an ultimate goal of positively affecting outcomes.

Healthcare Delivery Innovation Focus

The focus may include designing and evaluating new models of care, implementing and evaluating evidence-based practice guidelines, integrating telehealth into chronic disease management, or even redesigning care delivery systems in resource-poor settings. The potential projects in this category are extensive. The DNP student may consider using an implementation science or quality improvement approach when addressing these types of practice projects.

Healthcare Delivery Innovation Methods

The method used to deliver the project is dependent on the focus. For example, a DNP student embarking on a quality improvement project may use quantitative methods to answer the clinical question but may also want to consider qualitative methods to provide additional clarity. Projects that organize care using a team approach are gaining momentum because payers are looking for ways to improve clinical outcomes and efficiency. For example, the DNP student could choose to partner with a hospital- or community-based organization to coordinate delivery of care. Certainly, collaborating with other healthcare providers in the area or even health payers can be an effective approach when implementing a scholarly project.

Other Healthcare Delivery Innovation Considerations

When considering implementation of a healthcare delivery innovation, regardless of the specific type of project or methods used to implement the project, there should be a focus on the cost effectiveness of the innovation as well as the clinical effectiveness. For instance, in the case study that was used to illustrate how to write a problem statement, the focus of the study was on implementing clinically effective interventions or strategies in the primary care setting to address the needs of a diabetes population. However, the authors chose to also include the cost associated with implementing this type of intervention. The results were that the model was both clinically and cost effective in the population studied (Moran et al., 2011). In the end, the authors were able to make a business case for implementing the registered nurse–certified diabetes educator in the patient-centered medical home.

Healthcare Policy Analysis

Healthcare policies must be evaluated frequently to ensure that they are still relevant to society, that is, they continue to meet societal needs. Policy analysis helps with this process. The DNP student who engages in healthcare policy analysis within a scholarly project works to evaluate the historical evolution of the policy and determines if there is still congruence within the current social context. If there is incongruence, the results of the analysis may be used for policy modification recommendations (Porche, 2019). The policy analysis may be the first step in formulating a project plan to address the healthcare needs identified. The DNP project should include planning, implementation, and evaluation components to address policy needs identified in the analysis to impact healthcare outcomes (AACN, 2015).

Healthcare Policy Analysis Focus

The intent of the analysis may be descriptive, to describe how and why the policy came to be and to describe the current state of a policy, or it may be prescriptive, to consider what could occur if a proposed policy is implemented.

Healthcare Policy Analysis Methods

Multiple approaches can be used in policy analysis depending on the impetus for conducting the analysis (i.e., qualitative or quantitative). The DNP student may decide to use one of the following models, as outlined by Porche (2019); however, keep in mind there are other models that are not described here:

- *Eightfold path* uses a problem-solving process to clarify the problem and identify solutions. See Chapter 4 for an example of a policy analysis using the eightfold path model.
- *Participatory policy analysis (PPA)* is used to ensure that the ideals of democracy are included in policy alternatives.
- *Logical-positivist model* uses a deductive reasoning approach to analyze a policy (hypothesis testing).
- *Forecasting model* focuses on the assessment of technology adoption.
- *Political feasibility model* focuses on the fit of the policy with the values/interests of stakeholders.
- *Economic viability model* involves analyzing policies from an economic and financial perspective.
- *Value analysis model* looks at the values that are important in policy (e.g., access, efficiency, privacy, consent, etc.).
- *Five "E" model* uses five variables to analyze a policy: (1) effectiveness, (2) efficiency, (3) ethical considerations, (4) evaluating alternative options, and (5) positive and feasible recommendations for change.

Other Healthcare Policy Analysis Considerations

Policy analysis can focus on micro-level issues (efficient allocation of resources) or macro-level issues (structural focus, sociocultural issues). The policy analysis process can use a variety of methods to obtain relevant data. However, conducting the analysis is only one part of the picture. Disseminating the results of the analysis to the appropriate stakeholders is a critical component of policy analysis; it is a part of the implementation and evaluation portion of the DNP project.

Program Development and Evaluation

Programs that are developed to address health and healthcare needs are of critical importance and essential to the health of our nation. Gaps in healthcare access or delivery across the nation have been addressed through implementation of a variety of healthcare programs. They can be complex and multifaceted or relatively simple, such as providing health education to a community.

Program Development and Evaluation Focus

The types of programs that DNP scholars could potentially develop are vast and wide reaching. A DNP program development and evaluation project may include an intervention that involves planning and implementing activities that will ultimately improve the health of a specific group or decrease known health problems within a community ("Program development," 2018). The process involves identifying a gap in care, developing a program to address the need, and finally evaluating the outcome.

Program Development and Evaluation Focus Methods

Methods used for program planning and evaluation are variable but may include items such as surveys, individual interviews, and, more recently, focus groups. As mentioned, focus groups comprise individuals who represent a defined target population. These and other methods are used to gather information to determine the program needs, participant satisfaction, policy making, organizational development, and outcome evaluation. Irrespective of the method used to glean the desired information, it is imperative that the expectations are clear to the participants and the purpose well-articulated.

Other Program Development and Evaluation Focus Considerations

The DNP student embarking on a program development and evaluation project may benefit from the guidance of an expert in program development, implementation, and evaluation, especially as it relates to his or her area of interest. It may be helpful to include such an individual on the DNP project team (if applicable). It is also recommended by the AACN (2015) Implementation of the DNP Task Force to include an organizational mentor as part of the project team to be a liaison within the organization. Acting in this capacity, the mentor could open doors to key personnel and inform the project from the organizational perspective.

Clearly, the potential project options for the DNP scholar are boundless. In fact, there are many more options than are listed within this chapter. When considering the options, the key is to focus on a phenomenon that meets the needs of society and/or organization, is interesting, and in which the DNP scholar has sufficient expertise; to choose a project that will result in a personally meaningful outcome (because the time commitment to complete scholarly work is significant); and to develop a network of support in areas in which the DNP scholar has limited knowledge. There are many outstanding exemplars of DNP scholarly work. Consider the work by Dr. Rachel Cardoza, which involved a practice innovation that focused on vulnerable underserved palliative populations and a funding plan for expansion of services into the community (see **EXEMPLAR 6-1**).

EXEMPLAR 6-1 A Standardized Palliative Care Referral Workflow and Educational In-Service at an Outpatient Congestive Heart Failure Clinic

Rachel Cardoza, DNP, RN, AGNP-C

The DNP project starts with trying to change the world and ends with what will be meaningful and sustainable work. As a DNP student, choosing an organization for project work is key to the success and sustainability of scholarly work. Entering into my project, I knew I had interdisciplinary DNP project champions that included nursing, social work, and physicians who would support and adapt to the scholarly needs and help me identify areas for change, growth, and improvement. As a DNP student, the academic practice partnership in palliative care highlighted not only an emerging specialty but also the product that a DNP-prepared nurse practitioner can provide. Palliative Care, as a specialty, is less than 10 years old in this organization. Palliative Care is supportive, person-centered care for those with life-limiting illnesses and incorporates care aligned with patient preference and also comfort management. It is not hospice care, but the specialties often align closely due to many of the interdisciplinary certifications. My project allowed me to establish a foundational relationship to work towards innovative practice change improving palliative care practice at the individual and system level. My DNP project work included a focus on vulnerable, underserved, palliative populations and a funding plan for expansion of services into the community.

Fast forward 3 years, my DNP student project blossomed into a new position as a palliative care nurse practitioner. The position involved patient care, building on DNP scholarly work, but also continuing to change practice, mentor future DNP students, and demonstrate the added value of a DNP-prepared nurse. As a DNP-prepared nurse, I understand the importance of measuring process and outcomes to easily demonstrate the benefits of change. A key strategy that I used, and now all DNP students within this organization use, involved identifying key stakeholders and leaders within the organization. Once those key personnel were identified, it was important to understand what they valued in terms of data, finances, and outcomes, so that I could build a business case for expansion and improvement of palliative care services and develop a plan for a successful project within the organization.

I became employed as the first DNP-prepared nurse in palliative care shortly after completion of my DNP project work. My new DNP position included program development, which led to an opportunity to secure $400,000 in philanthropy funding from the organization's foundation to support practice change. The need for a *DNP Project succession process* (to continue the work I had started) was identified after reviewing referral patterns and issues in a small population. A second DNP student was able to expand on my work in a more profound way because of the relationships and value that had already been established. The job description grew over time based on the work of the DNP students that followed and came to fruition within two successive years of my original DNP scholarly work. This DNP Project succession process continues today. Two successive years of students have started their DNP scholarly experience in this setting, and former DNP students are seeking employment opportunities as a result of their project work.

The more the organization understood the role of the DNP-prepared nurse, the more impact was realized as these nurses worked to improve practice within the organization. The DNP students were deliberate in measuring quality with each successive project; these measures included decrease in hospital utilization and increase in median hospice length of stay.

(continues)

EXEMPLAR 6-1 A Standardized Palliative Care Referral Workflow and Educational In-Service at an Outpatient Congestive Heart Failure Clinic *(continued)*

Next, came the dissemination of the results of DNP work as both a student and employee at National Home-Based Services and Hospice and Palliative Conferences, which was enhanced because of the skills attained as a doctoral-prepared nurse and the focus on interdisciplinary project team partnership. Ultimately, this DNP work aligns with the Institute of Healthcare Improvement's (2018) "triple aim" and with what some organizations have adopted as the "quadruple aim," which includes improving quality, controlling costs, enhancing patient and family experience, while supporting clinical staff satisfaction (Bodenheimer & Sinsky, 2014).

Impact

- Project planning leads to a successful DNP project. This process requires careful alignment with the needs of the organization, appropriate identification of priority practice concerns, assessment of the barriers and facilitators to implementation and factors that will assure sustainability, and careful selection of the best method and/or approach to use to both address the practice concern and to evaluate the outcome.

Key Messages

- The literature review is a method used to support the value of and/or the need to study the phenomenon of interest.
- The assessment can lead to the identification of a gap in the current state of a phenomenon or help validate current perceptions.
- The problem statement encompasses a phenomenon in need of inquiry that is examined to better understand the phenomenon in order to develop a potential solution.
- When articulating the problem statement, the goal is to identify an issue, describe it clearly but succinctly, and adequately articulate why it is important that the problem be addressed.
- Key stakeholders are those individuals or groups who touch the project in some way or have an interest in the project outcome.
- Project goals describe what the student intends on delivering within the context of the project.
- The project scope includes all the work that needs to be accomplished in order to fulfill the project goals.
- The IRB oversees all research involving human subjects and ensures that studies meet all federal regulation criteria and ethical standards.

Action Plan—Next Steps

1. Conduct a literature review.
2. Conduct an organizational assessment.
3. Write the problem statement.

4. Identify key stakeholders.
5. Define the project goals and scope.
6. Select a project theory and framework.
7. Determine the project type.
8. Submit for IRB review (if required).

References

Agency for Healthcare Research and Quality (AHRQ). (2018). *Guidelines and measures.* Retrieved from https://www.guidelines.gov/

American Association of Colleges of Nursing (AACN). (2015). *Implementation of the DNP Task Force.* Retrieved from http://www.aacn.nche.edu/news/articles/2015/dnp-white-paper

Brown, S. J. (2018). *Evidence-based nursing: The research-practice connection* (3rd ed.). Burlington, MA: Jones & Bartlett Learning.

Bodenheimer, T. & Sinsky, C. (2014). From triple to quadruple aim: Care of the patient requires care of the provider. *Annals of Family Medicine, 12*(6), 573–576.

Canadian International Development Agency. (2006). *Organizational assessment guide.* Retrieved from http://documents.reflectlearn.org/Offline%20Docs%20for%20Your%20Introductory%20Guide%20to%20OA/OA%20Guide-E.pdf

Cochrane Nursing Care. (2018). Retrieved from http://nursingcare.cochrane.org/

Conceptual framework. (2018). *The Free Dictionary.* Retrieved from http://medical-dictionary.thefreedictionary.com/conceptual+framework

Database. (2018). *Merriam-Webster.* Retrieved from http://www.merriam-webster.com/dictionary/database

Donabedian, A. (1988). The quality of care: How can it be assessed? *Journal of the American Medical Association, 260,* 1743–1748.

Duffy, E. A., Rodgers, C. C., Shever, L. L., & Hockenberry, M. J. (2015). Implementing a daily maintenance care bundle to prevent central line–associated bloodstream infections in pediatric oncology patients. *Journal of Pediatric Oncology Nursing, 32*(6), 394–400.

EBSCO Industries, Inc. (2012). *Business Source Premier.* (2012). Retrieved from http://www.ebscohost.com/academic/business-source-premier

EBSCO Industries, Inc. (2018). *CINAHL databases.* Retrieved from https://www.ebscohost.com/nursing/products/cinahl-databases

Emerald Publishing. (2018). *About Emerald Publishing.* Retrieved from http://www.emeraldgrouppublishing.com/about/index.htm

Fogarty International Center. (2018). *Implementation science information and resources.* Retrieved from http://www.fic.nih.gov/News/Events/implementation-science/Pages/faqs.aspx

GreyNet International. (2018). Retrieved from http://www.greynet.org/home/aboutgreynet.html

Goal. (2018). *Merriam-Webster.* Retrieved from https://www.merriam-webster.com/dictionary/goal

Health Resources and Services Administration (HRSA). (2011). *Quality improvement.* Retrieved from http://www.hrsa.gov/quality/toolbox/508pdfs/qualityimprovement.pdf

Hemon, P., & Schwartz, C. (2007). What is a problem statement? *Library and Information Science Research, 29,* 307–309.

Houser, J. (2018). *Nursing research: Reading, using, and creating evidence.* Burlington, MA: Jones & Bartlett Learning.

Institute of Medicine (IOM). (2001). *Crossing the quality chasm: A new health system for the 21st century.* Washington, DC: National Academies Press. Retrieved from http://www.nationalacademies.org/hmd/~/media/Files/Report%20Files/2001/Crossing-the-Quality-Chasm/Quality%20Chasm%202001%20%20report%20brief.pdf

Joanna Briggs Institute. (2018). Retrieved from joannabriggs.org/

Langley, G. L., Moen, R. D., Nolan, K. M., Nolan, T. W., Norman, C. L., & Provost, L. P. (2009). *The improvement guide: A practical approach to enhancing organizational performance* (2nd ed.). San Francisco, CA: Jossey-Bass Publishers.

Machi, L. A., & McEvoy, B. T. (2016). *The literature review: Six steps to success.* (3rd ed.). London, UK: Sage Publications.

McCawley, P. F. (2009). *Methods for conducting educational needs assessment: Guidelines for cooperative extension system professionals*. University of Idaho Extension. Retrieved from https://www.cals .uidaho.edu/edcomm/pdf/bul/bul0870.pdf

McGrath, J. M., Brown, R. E., & Samra, H. A. (2012). Before you search the literature: How to prepare and get the most out of citation databases. *Newborn & Infant Nursing Reviews, 12*(3), 162–170.

Melnyk, B. M. (2013). Distinguishing the preparation and roles of doctor of philosophy and doctor of nursing practice graduates: National implications for academic curricula and health care systems. *Journal of Nursing Education, 52*(8), 442–448.

Moran, K., Burson, R., Critchett, J., & Olla, P. (2011). Exploring the cost and clinical outcomes of integrating the registered nurse–certified diabetes educator in the patient-centered medical home. *The Diabetes Educator, 37*(6), 780–793.

National Institute of Nursing Research (NINR). (2016). *The NINR strategic plan: Advancing science, improving lives*. Retrieved from https://www.ninr.nih.gov/sites/www.ninr.nih.gov/files /NINR_StratPlan2016_reduced.pdf

Ogrinc, G., Davies, L., Goodman, D., Batalden, P., Davidoff, F., & Stevens, D. (2015). SQUIRE 2.0 (Standards for Quality Improvement Reporting Excellence): Revised publication guidelines from a detailed consensus process. *The Journal of Continuing Education in Nursing, 46*(11), 501–507.

Peerpoint. (2012). *The definition of healthcare quality and the Institute of Medicine*. Retrieved from http://www.peerpt.com/performancequality-improvement/ the-definition-of-healthcare -quality-and-the-institute-of-medicine/

Peterson, M. H., Barnason, S., Donnelly, B., Hill, K., Miley, H., Riggs, L. & Whiteman, K. (2014). Choosing the best evidence to guide clinical practice: Application of AACN levels of evidence. *Critical Care Nurse, 34*(2), 58–68.

Polit, D. F., & Beck, C. T. (2018). *Essentials of nursing research: Appraising evidence for nursing practice*. Philadelphia, PA: Wolters Kluwer/Lippincott Williams & Wilkins.

Porche, D. J. (2019). *Health policy: Application for nurses and other healthcare professionals*. Burlington, MA: Jones & Bartlett Learning.

Price, B. (2009). Guidance on conducting a literature search and reviewing mixed literature. *Nursing Standard, 23*(24), 43–49.

Problem. (2018). *Merriam-Webster*. Retrieved from http://www.merriam-webster.com/dictionary /problem

Program development. (2018). *The Free Dictionary*. Retrieved from http:// medical-dictionary.the freedictionary.com/program + development

PubMed. (n.d.). Retrieved from http://www.ncbi.nlm.nih.gov/pubmed/

Quality Enhancement Research Initiative (QUERI), (2014a). *Applying theories, frameworks, and models*. Retrieved from https://www.queri.research.va.gov/implementation/ImplementationGuide _1.pdf

Quality Enhancement Research Initiative (QUERI), (2014b). *Methods used in implementing research into practice*. Retrieved from https://www.queri.research.va.gov/implementation/Implementation Guide_3.pdf

Quality Enhancement Research Initiative (QUERI), (2014c). *Formative evaluation*. Retrieved from https://www.queri.research.va.gov/implementation/ImplementationGuide_4.pdf

Reflect & Learn (n.d.). Your introductory guide to OA. Retrieved from http://www.reflectlearn.org /discover/your-introductory-guide-to-oa#_What_is_an

Research. (2018). *Merriam-Webster*. Retrieved from http://www.merriam-webster.com/dictionary /research

Rogers, E. M. (2003). *Diffusion of innovations*. New York, NY: Simon & Schuster, Inc.

Standards for Quality Improvement Reporting Excellence (SQUIRE) 2.0 (2015). *Revised standards for quality improvement reporting excellence*. Retrieved from http://squire-statement.org/index .cfm?fuseaction=document.viewDocument&documentid=1&documentFormatId=1&vDoc LinkOrigin=1&CFID=33187921&CFTOKEN=601f5bf702fd3c6d-A613A60E-1C23-C8EB -801327165B903DC1

Timmins, F., & McCabe, C. (2005). How to conduct an effective literature search. *Nursing Standard, 20*(11), 41–47.

Titler, M. G., Kleiber, C., Steelman, V. J., Rakel, B. A., Budreau, G., & Everett, L. Q. . . . Goode, C. J. (2001). The Iowa model of evidence-based practice to promote quality care. *Critical Care Nursing Clinics North America, 13*, 497–509.

University of Minnesota Crookston. (2018). *Primary, secondary, and tertiary sources.* Retrieved from https://www.crk.umn.edu/library/primary-secondary-and-tertiary-sources

Vogel, N. P., Appel, S. J., & Winker, G. (2018). Improving HPV vaccination rates among young males in rural areas of the United States. *The Nurse Practitioner, 43*(1), 1–6.

Helpful Resources
Citation Management Resources

EndNote, https://endnote.com/product-details/basic/
EQUATOR Network, https://www.equator-network.org/
RefWorks, http://www.refworks.com/

Data Resources

Agency for Healthcare Research and Quality (AHRQ). *Clinical guidelines and recommendations.* http://www.ahrq.gov/professionals/clinicians-providers/guidelines-recommendations/
Agency for Healthcare Research and Quality (AHRQ). Quality indicators. http://www.qualityindicators.ahrq.gov/
American Nurses Association (ANA). http://www.nursingworld.org
Business Source Premier. http://www.ebscohost.com/academic/business-source-premier
CINAHL Plus with Full Text. https://www.ebscohost.com/nursing/products/cinahl-databases
Cochrane Collaboration. http://www.cochrane.org/
Joanna Briggs Institute. http://joannabriggs.org/
National Guidelines Clearinghouse. https://www.guidelines.gov/
PsycINFO. http://www.apa.org/pubs/databases/psycinfo/index.aspx
PubMed. http://www.ncbi.nlm.nih.gov/pubmed/

Quality Improvement Resources

Agency for Healthcare Research and Quality (AHRQ). http://www.ahrq.gov
American Health Quality Association (AHQA). http://www.ahqa.org
Fogarty International Center. https://www.fic.nih.gov/Pages/Default.aspx
Institute for Healthcare Improvement (IHI). http://www.ihi.org
National Association for Healthcare Quality (NAHQ). http://www.nahq.org
National Quality Forum. http://www.qualityforum.org
Six Sigma. http://www.isixsigma.com/new-to-six-sigma/getting-started/what-six-sigma/

CHAPTER 7

Aligning Design, Method, and Evaluation with the Clinical Question

Patricia Rouen

CHAPTER OVERVIEW

The doctor of nursing practice (DNP) project process is an exciting and rich experience that sets the stage for future scholarship and contributions to nursing practice. Just as DNP projects vary in their designs and methods, implementation processes and evaluation are also diverse. The importance of a tight project that aligns the scientific approach with the appropriate design, methodology, and evaluation cannot be understated. The goal of this chapter is to introduce the DNP student to the general processes and most common components of project design, data collection, and evaluation. Resources that support DNP project work are identified, with an emphasis on interprofessional collaboration.

CHAPTER OBJECTIVES

After completing this chapter, the learner will be able to:

1. Select a design for the DNP project that is congruent with the project aim.
2. Propose methods and outcome measures for the DNP project.
3. Identify and describe the analytical approach for data evaluation in the DNP project.
4. Describe the elements of interprofessional collaboration that contribute to DNP project implementation.

▶ It Starts with Design

Design is a plan for arranging elements in such a way as best to accomplish a purpose.

— **Charles Eames**

The holistic nature of nursing practice invites DNP students to explore a wide variety of phenomena that eventually guide the DNP project. As such, DNP projects are diverse and may take on many forms, requiring different methodological approaches. In these situations, the DNP project team and student work together to determine the best design to guide the project and to ensure rigor and measure success. Just as DNP projects are diverse in scope and design, data collection methods and processes are also quite varied. A critical component of the DNP project is the congruence between the project aim(s) and study design, and the data collection and analysis plan. This congruence is a key factor in ensuring the veracity and accuracy of the DNP project outcome(s). The congruence among the design, methods, and analysis plan is discussed and evaluated by the doctoral project team as part of the project approval process. See Chapter 9, The DNP Project Team, for more information about DNP team functions.

> *The designs and methods of the DNP project should be congruent with the purpose and goals.*

DNP projects use a variety of approaches including quality improvement, program and policy evaluation, evidence-based practice (EBP) initiatives, and components of quantitative and qualitative research methodologies to evaluate, innovate, or improve practice (**TABLE 7-1**). The design choice for the project is always driven by the clinical question or issue. For example, clinical inquiry to evaluate a population health outcome, risk factor prevalence in a community, or needs of a client group, or to determine the priority health issue of a community or organization, may use a research approach. Common designs for these clinical questions are exploratory, descriptive, or correlational. These designs are considered observational and non-experimental (LoBiondo-Wood & Haber, 2018), but are valuable in determining the characteristics or needs of a unique population. Descriptive and correlational projects can also be used to assess behaviors of healthcare professionals, patients, communities, and systems or to provide baseline data that can be used to drive practice improvements.

Examples of exploratory DNP projects include:

- Perceived barriers to pain management among nursing staff in a long-term care facility
- Factors that facilitate hypertensive management in young to middle-aged African American women
- Environmental and situational factors related to job stress and turnover in staff nurses in critical care

When the DNP project aim is to initiate change via an intervention, practice improvement, or implementation of an innovative new model of care delivery, the design choice includes a research or a quality improvement (QI) approach. Experimental designs range from the randomized controlled trial to a quasi-experimental

TABLE 7-1 DNP Project Approaches

Category	Research/Practice-Based Inquiry	Quality Improvement (QI)	Evidence-Based Practice (EBP)	Program Evaluation (PE)
Definition	Systematic investigation including development, testing, and evaluation designed to develop or contribute to generalizable knowledge (U.S. Department of Health and Human Services [DHHS], 2009)	Systematic data-guided activities to monitor, evaluate, and improve quality and safety outcomes of health services and care processes (Adapted from Cronenwett et al., 2007; DHHS, 2011)	A systematic approach that integrates the review and appraisal of the best available scientific evidence combined with clinical expertise and patient/population circumstances to guide care delivery (Adapted from Melynk & Fineout-Overhold, 2015, Sackett, Rosenberg, Gray, Haynes, & Richardson, 2000)	A systematic assessment of the processes and/or outcomes of a program, guided by standards, to make judgments regarding the program, improve its effectiveness, and guide further development (Centers for Disease Control and Prevention [CDC], 2013)
Purpose	Investigate or answer a research question relevant to nursing practice	Improvement or innovation in healthcare outcomes or workflow processes	Integration of evidence into practice (Shirey et al., 2011)	Evaluation of a program's achievements and effectiveness

(continues)

TABLE 7-1 DNP Project Approaches (continued)

Category	Research/Practice-Based Inquiry	Quality Improvement (QI)	Evidence-Based Practice (EBP)	Program Evaluation (PE)
Methods	Scientific method, clinical question, or hypothesis Quantitative, qualitative, or mixed methods approaches	Plan-Do-Study-Act (PDSA) cycle Six Sigma Lean methodology failure mode effect analysis (FMEA) Root cause analysis (RCA) Structure process outcome (Donabedian, 2005)	IOWA model (Titler et al., 2001) Advancing Research & Clinical Practice through Close Collaboration (ARCC) (Melynk, Fineout-Overholt, Giggleman, & Choy, 2017) Academic Center for Evidence-based Practice (ACE) (Stevens, 2004) PARiHS (Promoting Action on Research Implementation) (Rycroft-Malone, 2004) Stetler model (Stetler, 2001) Johns Hopkins Hospital nursing evidence-based practice model (Newhouse, Dearholt, Poe, Pugh, & White, 2007) JBI model of evidence-based health care: A model reconsidered (Jordan, Lockwood, Aromataris, & Munn, 2016) Rosswurm & Larrabee model (1999)	CDC Framework (1999) Logic model (Millar, Simeone, & Carnevale, 2001) Balanced Scorecard (Kaplan & Norton, 1992) CIPP (Context, Input, Process, and Product) (Stufflebeam, 1983)

Data Collection	Multiple options Surveys, standardized instruments, physiologic measures, registries or database extraction, interviews, observations, focus groups	Multiple options Surveys, check sheets, process flow diagrams, cause-and-effect diagrams, clinical record reviews or data extraction, interviews, observations, focus groups, key informants, system/stakeholder assessment	Literature search Literature review System/stakeholder assessment Baseline and/or post-implementation measures of outcomes relevant to the practice guideline integration	Multiple options to measure the program's execution, outcomes, and impact System/ stakeholder assessment, resource review, surveys, interviews, focus groups, program costs and measures for the specific program goals
Data Analytics	Specific to the clinical question or hypothesis Emphasis on quantitative and qualitative techniques; fiscal analyses Process and outcome evaluation for intervention and implementation projects	Specific to the quality issue Quantitative and qualitative techniques Run charts Pareto charts Statistical process control Fiscal analyses	**Practice Guideline Development** Evaluation of evidence strength: *Quantitative Data* Levels of evidence: I–VII (Melnyk & Fineout-Overholt, 2015) Levels of evidence (Johanna Briggs Institute [JBI], 2014a) Grades of recommendations (JBI, 2014b)	Diverse approaches to measure processes and outcomes that can include quantitative and qualitative techniques and financial analyses

(continues)

TABLE 7-1 DNP Project Approaches   *(continued)*

			Qualitative Data CERQual (Confidence in Evidence from Reviews of Qualitative Research; www.cerqual.org). *Guideline Assessment* AGREE-II (www.agree.trust.org) **Practice Integration Evaluation** Analysis of achievement of designated outcomes with quantitative, qualitative, and fiscal techniques	PE informs and identifies opportunities for research, EBP, and QI. Interprofessional collaboration.
Intersections	Research informs QI, EBP, and program evaluation. New research can be initiated from gaps in EBP reviews. Interprofessional collaboration.	QI informs EBP. QI can identify needs for research and program development. QI can generate new knowledge. Interprofessional collaboration.	EBP informs QI. EBP evaluation identifies need for additional research. EBP can guide program development and evaluation. Interprofessional collaboration.	

Data from Centers for Disease Control and Prevention (CDC), 2013; Newhouse, 2007; Shirey et al., 2013; Schaffer, Sandau, & Diedrick, 2012.

study. In practice settings, the quasi-experimental approach is helpful because it does not require randomization or a control group (LoBiondo-Wood & Haber, 2018). This design is practical and capable of measuring change in health-related outcomes after treatment or intervention when it is not feasible to use a true experiment (Polit & Beck, 2017). Other research designs such as observational and longitudinal studies, and randomized controlled trials may be considered for QI projects in practice settings (Brown et al., 2017; Portela, Pronovost, Woodcock, Carter, & Dixon-Woods, 2015). Examples of DNP projects using this approach include:

- Improving pre-procedure and post-procedure colonoscopy processes
- Implementation of group medical visits to improve glucose control in persons with diabetes
- Implementation of a team approach to post-anesthesia care unit (PACU) handoffs

Practice improvements guided by QI models are an important source of DNP project opportunities. QI uses data-based methods to improve clinical or healthcare systems processes and outcomes (Batalden & Davidoff, 2007). There are several QI approaches that may guide the DNP project: the well-known Plan-Do-Study-Act (PDSA) cycle, Lean methodology, and the Six Sigma process (see Chapter 13, The DNP Project Toolbox). These methods focus on process refinements to control variation and ultimately improve the designated outcome. QI involves the systematic collection and analysis of data to measure change, with growing emphasis on rapid cycle change. QI methodologies such as root cause analysis (RCA) and failure mode effect analysis (FMEA) are feasible choices to guide a QI-focused DNP project. RCA uses a retrospective approach to identify root causes of an adverse event. A team approach is used to identify system process breakdowns that impacted the undesired outcome. Improvement opportunities are identified with subsequent implementation of planned changes. FMEA is a proactive prevention approach to assess a new program, procedure, or policy to anticipate possible consequences of the innovation. This QI method emphasizes prospective assessment to mitigate identified risks prior to implementation of new processes, drugs, or procedures in healthcare settings to prevent untoward outcomes. It is recommended that the QI model approach aligns with the purpose and aims of the DNP project. Competence in QI is an expectation in today's healthcare environment, and DNP projects using this approach make important data-driven contributions to practice. **TABLE 7-2** presents journal article citations representing health care and nursing QI project exemplars.

Examples of DNP projects using a QI approach include:

- A process improvement in a primary care office to reduce wait times and improve patient and provider satisfaction
- Improving medication management and reconciliation in elders in primary care
- Implementation of a discharge readiness assessment in bladder cancer patients post-cystectomy

> *Quality improvement uses data-based methods to improve clinical or healthcare systems outcomes (Batalden & Davidoff, 2007).*

TABLE 7-2 Improvement Projects Featuring Different QI Models

QI Model	Citation
PDSA	Sundberg, M. J., Parver, S., Morin, M., & Stack, A. M. (2017, May/June). An intervention to improve caregiver adherence to oral rehydration therapy. *Pediatric Quality & Safety, 2*(3), e020. doi:10.1097/pq9.0000000000000020
Lean/Six Sigma	Gavriloff, C., Ostrowski-Delahanty, S., & Oldfield, K. (2017). The impact of Lean Six Sigma methodology on patient scheduling. *Nursing Economics, 35*(4), 189–193.
RCA	Gertler, S. A., Coralic, Z., Lopez, A., Stein, J., & Sarkar, U. (2016). Root cause analysis of ambulatory adverse drug events that present to the emergency department. *Journal of Patient Safety, 12*(3), 119–124. doi: 10.1097/PTS.0000000000000072
FMEA	Alamry, A., Al Owais, S. M., Marini, A. M., Al-Dorzi, H., Alsolamy, S., & Arabi, Y. (2017). Application of failure mode effect analysis to improve the care of septic patients admitted through the emergency department. *Journal of Patient Safety, 13*(2), 76–81. doi:10.1097/PTS.0000000000000118

PDSA: Plan-Do-Study-Act cycle; FMEA: failure mode effect analysis; RCA: root cause analysis.

Qualitative inquiry is another perspective that contributes to a DNP project. These types of designs provide evidence for practice when little is known about the phenomenon of interest (Toles & Barroso, 2018). At other times, the phenomenon of interest may have been described in a population or social setting, but there is a gap in practice knowledge with a new group of clients or a new setting. Qualitative data provide a holistic understanding of phenomena, capture the real-world context, and generate evidence for practice, congruent with the nursing paradigm (Leeman & Sandelowski, 2012). The qualitative approach is flexible and feasible for use in practice. There are several different types of qualitative inquiry, such as ethnography, grounded theory, phenomenology, and case study (Toles & Barroso, 2018). If qualitative data collection is being considered for a DNP project, consultation with a researcher skilled in these methods is highly recommended.

Some DNP projects will include both quantitative and qualitative data collection with a mixed methods approach. Focus groups and interviews are the most common tool to garner data from key stakeholders to

Competence in QI is an expectation in today's healthcare environment, and DNP projects using this approach make important data-driven contributions to practice.

inform, develop, improve, or evaluate programs or services. Data garnered from focus groups or interviews include people's opinions, ideas, and beliefs on a certain topics or products that can inform and enrich a DNP project. DNP projects such as program development, quality improvement initiatives, and program evaluation often include qualitative data collection to guide the project activities.

Program evaluation (PE) is another option for the DNP project. PE is a systematic process to gather evidence that a project, program, or policy is effective and efficient. Guided by standards, program evaluation examines the processes, outcomes, and impact of the project and includes the key stakeholders or systems that participate in or are affected by the project. There are several models for program evaluation, and the selected approach should be congruent with the type of program that will be evaluated. Common models used in health care include, but are not limited to: the Logic model (Millar, Simeone, & Carnevale, 2001), the Centers for Disease Control and Prevention framework for public health programs (CDC, 1999), the Balanced Scorecard (Kaplan & Norton, 1992), and the Context-Input-Process-Product (CIPP) model (Stufflebeam, 1983).

Parameters of program evaluation differ slightly among the models, but most address stakeholder engagement, available resources, planned activities, outputs, and outcomes with an assessment of the impact of the program. Outcomes can be varied and should align with selected framework and the purpose of the project. Some processes of program evaluation are similar to intervention research or QI, including the data collected (quantitative, qualitative, and fiscal) and the options for data analysis. In their recent review of evaluation designs, Brown and colleagues (2017) advised that evidence-based interventions and quality improvement designs consider an evaluation component. An important distinction of program evaluation is the pivotal role of collaboration with key stakeholders in the development and evaluation process and the use of formative and summative evaluation during program implementation (CDC, 2013). Examples of DNP projects that address program evaluation include:

- Evaluation of a nurse practitioner–led smoking cessation program for rural adolescents
- Evaluation of a patient navigation program for colorectal cancer
- Evaluation of an army regulation electronic contingency notebook as a process improvement tool during the soldier readiness process

DNP projects also enhance evidence-based practice (EBP). EBP is a decision-making approach that incorporates clinical expertise and patient preferences with the best scientific evidence to guide healthcare interventions (Melynk & Fineout-Overholt, 2015; Sackett, Rosenberg, Gray, Haynes, & Richardson, 2000). EBP emphasizes the integration of existing knowledge (evidence) into contemporary healthcare practice (Iowa Model Collaborative, 2017), often in the form of protocols or practice guidelines. Evidence-based DNP projects are developed using a systematic process, which includes a critical appraisal of the literature to determine the best available evidence along with knowledge of the organizational culture and resources needs of the practice environment, to implement a planned change. These rigorous

Program evaluation is a systematic process to gather evidence that a project, program, or policy is effective and efficient.

methods produce a summative synthesis of the evidence with a valid practice recommendation. The evidence-based practice process quality assessment (EPQA) (Lee, Johnson, Newhouse, & Warren, 2013) should be used to evaluate the proposed EBP practice recommendation and confirm the quality of the proposed recommendation. As with other DNP projects, EBP initiatives are evaluated post implementation to measure outcome attainment and opportunities for guideline revision.

There are several models for EBP (Table 7-1) that can guide the DNP project.

> *EBP emphasizes the integration of existing knowledge (evidence) into contemporary healthcare practice (Iowa Model Collaborative, 2017).*

The six major models have several common elements and some differences. In their overview of the major models, Schaffer, Sandau, and Diedrick (2012) noted that most models are applicable to organizational settings, while others address building capacity for EBP among clinicians. In planning the DNP project, it would be important to consider the model features to select a "best-fit" approach that addresses the practice issue. Examples of DNP projects that use an EBP approach include:

- Development of a practice guideline for the prevention of sexual assault on a college campus
- Implementation of an evidence-based nutrition management protocol in adults in the neurology critical care unit
- Evidence-based care of homeless veterans: a protocol for depression

Policy analysis or evaluation is another domain for the DNP project. Health policy analysis projects address outcomes related to healthcare quality, cost, and access in the context of a specific topic or population group. Policy may be examined at the macro- or microsystem level and from different theoretical perspectives (epidemiology, sociology, etc.). Data are used to guide policy analysis via metrics that document the specific concerns with the policy's achievement of its intended actions. The methods for health policy analysis are varied but consistently require a systematic assessment (Weimer & Vining, 2016) that weighs the benefits and liabilities associated with the policy, and provides evidence related to cost and quality of the expected outcomes. Bardach and Patashnik's (2016) model recommends a summary of the policy issues, evaluation of supporting and opposing arguments, analysis of stakeholders, and anticipated impact on sentinel outcomes including population health benefits, costs, equity, and administrative feasibility (see Chapter 4, Health Care Policy and Advocacy, for an example of a policy analysis using this model). A student considering a health policy analysis for a DNP project should work with the project team to determine the most appropriate method. Examples of DNP projects that employ policy analysis include:

- Policy analysis: community-based services programs and implications for rural elder care
- Contraception and unintended pregnancy in adolescents: policy analysis of regional school-based teen programs
- Measuring advanced practice nurses understanding of reimbursement and full practice authority to support a strategic plan

▶ Diversity in DNP Projects

DNP projects are diverse and use different methodologies that address the broad perspective of nursing practice. Yet, while differences among the approaches exist, all employ interprofessional collaboration (see Chapter 8, Interprofessional and Intraprofessional Collaboration in the DNP Project) and use a systematic process that is data driven, evaluates outcomes, and provides evidence for nursing practice. **TABLE 7-3** presents an overview of the DNP project processes that may assist the DNP student in his or her project choice.

The first step is to identify the impetus for the project design. For example, in a QI project there is a gap in care or outcome issue, while an EBP project is initiated when there is a gap in evidence that impacts a clinical issue. Program development occurs in response to a needs assessment to identify and prioritize the need for a new program; research projects are initiated when there is a practice-based question that needs to be answered or a hypothesis that needs to be tested. Models that guide DNP project development are varied across all project approaches (see Table 7-1 for DNP project approaches).

All projects proceed in an orderly fashion that varies among the project options. Common elements across all of the project options include a systematic literature review and the critical appraisal of the quality of the evidence to support the DNP project idea. As the nature of the literature review differs by project type, so do the standards for appraising the evidence base for the project type. Several tools are available to guide the appraisal of the diverse forms of evidence, including randomized controlled trials, systematic reviews, cohort studies, case-control studies, cross-sectional studies, qualitative studies, evidence-based projects, qualitative research, and quality improvement initiatives (see *Helpful Resources* at the end of the chapter). Most projects collect and analyze data; all projects engage in systems and stakeholder engagement, use implementation competencies, and evaluate projects for effectiveness and sustainability.

The last step for each project type is different. For example, new research data are applied to practice and can support EBP if the topic is similar. EBP outcomes include sustained practice change. QI is an ongoing improvement approach that, once controlled, continues to be monitored with screening for the need of iterative improvements. Program evaluation may include data-driven improvements, along with plans for program sustainability and fidelity. Additional points to consider with DNP projects are that research and program implementation and evaluation can conclude with the activities that are completed and may be considered static; whereas a quality improvement initiative and implementation of EBP are dynamic, as the improvement and the standardization of process and outcome continue (Portela et al., 2015).

The rich diversity of DNP project work also generates opportunities for future work among the different approaches. For example, EBP projects have the potential to identify other QI opportunities (Newhouse, 2007; Shirey et al., 2011) and provide data that can guide program development and evaluation. Further, gaps in the evidence can prompt new research studies. QI provides contextual data that can inform EBP initiatives as well as uncover needs for research (Shirey et al., 2011) and program development. QI can also generate new knowledge. Program evaluation can identify other opportunities for QI, EBP, and research projects. Data from clinical

TABLE 7-3 At a Glance: DNP Project Processes

Research	Evidence-Based Practice	Quality Improvement	Program Development and Evaluation
Propose a hypothesis or practice-based question.	Identify a practice problem with a PICOT question.	Identify a care process or outcome issue.	Conduct a needs assessment to identify and prioritize needs.
Perform a literature review.	Conduct a relevant literature search.	Select a QI model to guide the improvement plan.	Assess literature and stakeholder priorities to develop program.
Select a study design and a sample population.	Do a critical appraisal of the evidence.	Establish goals and benchmarks. Implement the change process.	Select the evaluation framework.
Collect the data.	Synthesize the evidence.	Collect the data.	Implement the program.
Analyze the data.	Propose an evidence-based recommendation using EPQA guidelines.	Analyze the data.	Evaluate process, outcome, and fiscal data.
Disseminate findings.	Integrate the evidence into practice.	Evaluate the outcomes.	Disseminate findings.
Apply the new knowledge into practice.	Evaluate the implementation process; sustain the practice change.	Monitor data for control or set new benchmarks for continued iterative improvements.	Ongoing data-driven improvements; program sustainability and fidelity.

 Systems and Stakeholder Engagement
Implementation Competencies
Effectiveness and Sustainability

Data from Centers for Disease Control and Prevention (1999), Iowa Model Collaborative (2017), Agency for Healthcare Research and Quality (2017), Institute for Healthcare Improvement (2017), Issel & Wells (2018), Jordan, Lockwood, Aromataris, & Munn (2016), Lobiondo-Wood & Haber (2018), Melynk & Fineout-Overholt (2015), Polit & Beck (2017).

research can suggest the need for QI (Newhouse, 2007; Shirey et al., 2011) or new program development, as well as contribute to the pool of evidence-based data for practice. Policy analysis can suggest the need for QI actions to improve policy outcomes, provide data to support EBP, identify gaps in the literature that requires more research, or suggest the need for new program development and evaluation.

> *All DNP projects use a systematic process that is data driven, evaluates outcomes, and provides evidence for nursing practice.*

▶ Driven by Design: Data Collection Methods

Once the design and the specific aim(s) for the DNP project are determined, the next step is to select the data collection method. DNP projects can involve the collection of new data via surveys and interviews or evaluation of stored data from repositories such as electronic health records (EHRs) and national registries. It is critical that the data collection method is congruent with the study design and the project purpose (**TABLE 7-4**). Data collection methods should be broad enough to encompass measurement of the outcome or dependent variable, as well as the relevant independent and confounding factors thought to be related to the outcome variable.

The major data collection methods used in research and QI projects include self-report via survey or structured interviews, direct observation, and physiological measures (Polit & Beck, 2017). QI projects may also use prospective logs or tracking sheets to collect real-time data. In addition, QI initiatives include process flow diagrams and cause-and-effect diagrams to guide the data collection process. Extraction of data from EHRs or registries can be used to evaluate clinical outcomes such as disease prevalence rates or immunization compliance, costs, or patterns in service usage to identify opportunities for QI, EBP, and research projects, or the need for new programs.

> *It is critical that the data collection method is congruent with the study design and the project purpose.*

The most common qualitative data collection methods are focus groups or individual interviews, in which participants respond to open-ended questions, and investigators observe responses. These data are important for QI, EBP, and program evaluation projects as they provide insight into the organizational stakeholder's perspectives regarding the practice issue. Storytelling and written narratives are other choices for collecting qualitative data.

It is important to select the data collection method that is best suited for the DNP project goals. The data collection method should be feasible, practical, and amenable for use in the clinical setting or with the population of interest. For example, an online survey would be a method of choice if working with young adults or collecting input from stakeholders regarding a QI opportunity, while an elderly population might require survey questions to be asked aloud as part of a structured interview.

TABLE 7-4 Practice Projects: Sample Outcome Evaluation Plans

Approach	Design	Purpose	Intervention/Action/Process	Outcome Measures	Analysis
Research	Intervention	Improve health outcomes in a rural community: 1. Increase knowledge of nutrition and physical activity. 2. Improve weight and BMI (Spurrier, Suttle, Matheson, & Baker-Watson, 2018).	12-week program in a faith-based setting using 10 wellness modules related to obesity, weight, nutrition, and exercise facilitated by a nurse	Pre/post measures Weight, BMI, food logs, exercise logs Surveys: Patient-centered Assessment and Counseling for Exercise, Godin Leisure Time Exercise questionnaire 1-month post-program measures: BMI, weight	Descriptive statistics Paired *t*-tests Repeated measures ANOVA
Quality Improvement	PDSA	Improve medication management and reconciliation rates for elders in a geriatric primary care practice (Vejar, Makic, & Kotthoff-Burrell, 2015)	Goals: ↑ medication reconciliation rates; implement process for patients to bring in meds; ↓ use of dangerous OTC drugs; ↓ use of duplicate medications. Team included GNP, PA, physicians, MAs, RN, social worker, pharmacist.	Pre/post measures Medication reconciliation rates Number of patients bringing in their medications Use of high-risk medications Duplicate medication therapy Staff perception of feasibility of change	Descriptive statistics Frequencies Chi square analysis

Evidence-Based Practice	Evidence-based protocol Implementation	Education sessions to train staff and to engage patients. Several PDSA cycles over 9 months with monthly meetings.	Number of babies	Descriptive statistics t-tests
	Implement and evaluate the adoption the AAP Clinical Practice Guideline for hyperbilirubinemia in a newborn nursery (Flynn, 2017) Goals: ↑ the number of TSB tests and ↑ the appropriate use of phototherapy	Concerns regarding newborns needing screening and the preferred treatment resulted in unneeded heels sticks for the newborns. The AAP guidelines were implemented and addressed the early identification of hyperbilirubinemia with the correct testing and the suggested indications for phototherapy. Guideline implemented with a presentation and a protocol, a risk factor assessment tool, and the indications for phototherapy to support success.	Number of TSB tests per newborn decreased. Newborns' appropriate treatment with phototherapy increased.	t-tests

(continues)

TABLE 7-4 Practice Projects: Sample Outcome Evaluation Plans   *(continued)*

Approach	Design	Purpose	Intervention/Action/Process	Outcome Measures	Analysis
Program Evaluation	Program implementation and evaluation	Design, implement, and evaluate outcomes of a video monitoring program (Purvis, Kaun, McKenna, Viste, & Federov, 2018)	CNS-led program to implement and evaluate video monitoring, in lieu of a sitter, for patients in need of constant observation. The process involved forming an interdisciplinary steering committee; engaging staff, patients, and families; delivering education to all team members; training VMTs; implementation of a daily huddle; and ongoing process improvements to ensure fidelity of the program on six nursing units.	Demographic data Type of CO patient: sitter vs. video monitoring Amount of CO time in minutes: sitter vs. video monitoring Patient fall data Fiscal data	Aggregate descriptive statistics Frequencies Compared means Frequencies FTEs used

| Health Policy | Stakeholder analysis to inform policy | Descriptive qualitative study using purposive sampling to identify key stakeholders involved in HPV vaccination from public and private institutions (Carhart, Schminkey, Mitchell, & Keim-Malpass, 2018) | Phone interviews with key informants using semi-structured questions that were recorded. Stakeholders included care providers (physicians, nurses, nurse practitioners), pharmacists, industry, health department, community programs, and health researchers. Qualitative analysis was used to develop themes. | <u>Barriers</u>
Parent–child:
Interpersonal:
Organization/community
Policy level
<u>Facilitators</u>
Parent–child:
Interpersonal:
Organization/community
Policy level | Qualitative method
Themes:
■ Knowledge gap
■ Sexuality concerns
■ Time; Inconsistent recommendations
■ Lack of leadership and information
■ Ineffective mandate
Themes:
■ Realistic attitude
■ Strong support
■ Team approach
■ Outreach
■ Support from federal and health professionals |

AAP: American Academy of Pediatrics; ANOVA: analysis of variance; BMI: body mass index; CNS: clinical nurse specialist; CO: constant observation; FTE: full-time equivalent; GNP: geriatric nurse practitioner; MA: medical assistant; OTC: over the counter; PA: physician assistant; PDSA: Plan-Do-Study-Act cycle; PSA: patient safety attendant; RN: registered nurse; TSB: total serum bilirubin; VMT: video monitor technician.

All methods have strengths and limitations, and these are carefully considered during DNP project planning (see Chapter 10, Creating and Developing the Project Plan). For example, while surveys are direct measures that are versatile, they are prone to bias when respondents provide the socially acceptable answer rather than their true opinion. Direct observation is a more objective approach than self-reported survey data, but this method is vulnerable to bias from the observer's personal interests in conducting the study. Extraction of data from EHRs is economical and efficient but may be limited by the missing data points in the records. In focus groups, the dialogue permits clarification of participant responses, but the presence of others and the risk for a breach in confidentiality may limit disclosure.

When selecting measures to gather quantitative data, it is important to choose tools that have documented reliability, validity, sensitivity, and precision so that they best approximate the true meaning of the concept or parameter being measured (Polit & Beck, 2017). It is also helpful if the instruments have previously been used with the population of interest in the DNP project. Measurement of theoretical concepts, such as self-efficacy, evidence of reliability, and validity, should be documented in the project proposal (see Chapter 12, The Proposal). When biophysiological parameters are used, such as glucose, the precision (coefficient of variation) and sensitivity (lowest limit of detection) of the measure are usually reported.

In research, QI projects, EBP initiatives, and program evaluation, multiple measurement methods may be required to capture the relevant data that measure the expected outcomes of a QI or an EBP initiative, each objective of a program evaluation plan, or data that appropriately answer each clinical question of a research-oriented project. For QI, EBP, and program evaluation projects, economic measures of costs savings or burden may be included. DNP projects may also include a process and impact evaluation component that examines the actual development and implementation of a new program, quality improvement, or EBP initiative. While outcome evaluation measures the changes that occurred with the project, process evaluation assesses whether the program met its target goals for enrollment, or that the interventions were implemented as planned; impact evaluation assesses the longer-term benefits of the project's intended goals (Perrin, 2015). For example, outcome measures in an improvement project to reduce infection rates in postoperative hip replacement patients may include direct observation of the surgeon's handwashing technique, direct measure of the temperature in the operating room, checklists recording the surgical process (time under anesthesia, dose of antibiotic medication, etc.), or extraction of relevant patient-related variables, such as body mass index and glucose levels, from the electronic health record that categorize the patient's risk status. Process measures in this project would include disruptions in the system or organization that compromised the project implementation, such as switching vendors for the handwashing product. Impact evaluation may show that after 3 years, the infection rates remain lower than the expected goal or were the lowest rates in the local community.

With EBP initiatives, a major data-driven component of the project is the evidence-based guideline development that requires a systematic process to search for relevant literature and evaluate the evidence. Criteria for rigor in the development of practice guidelines are described in the AGREE II instrument and may be used to guide this type of DNP project (Brouwers et al., 2010; Brouwers, Kerkvliet, Spithoff, & AGREE Next Steps Consortium, 2016). The AGREE II criteria include the use of a systematic search strategy with inclusion and exclusion criteria, an assessment of the strengths and limitations of the evidence, and the process used to determine the recommendation decisions (Brouwers et al., 2010). The process of appraising evidence includes determination of the level and grade of evidence to determine the essential guideline components for the selected practice outcome, population group, and system setting (Johanna Briggs Institute, 2014a; Melynk & Fineout-Overholt, 2015). In addition, an assessment of the benefits and risks of the recommendations; a process for expert review; and the feasibility, appropriateness, and meaningfulness of the guideline (Johanna Briggs Institute, 2014b) is also required. **TABLE 7-5** provides more exemplars of DNP projects by project design.

TABLE 7-5 Exemplars of Completed DNP Projects

Project Domain	Diabetes Mellitus Type 2 DNP Project Exemplars	Other DNP Project Exemplars
QI	Sutton, M. D. (2015). A quality improvement project to increase diabetes self-efficacy in a rural primary care clinic through patient utilization of a diabetic logbook. *Doctor of Nursing Practice (DNP) Projects, 56.* Retrieved from https://repository.usfca.edu/dnp/56	Nardi, C. (2016). Using multi-modal education in a public health system to increase rates of cervical cancer screening. *Doctor of Nursing Practice (DNP) Projects, 80.* Retrieved from https://repository.usfca.edu/dnp/80
EBP	Garza, L. (2016). An initiative to improve primary prevention of heart disease in adults with type II diabetes based on the ACC/AHA (2013) and ADA (2016) guidelines. *Doctor of Nursing Practice, 8.* Retrieved from https://athenaeum.uiw.edu/uiw_dnp/8/	Paulson, S. S. (2017). Implementation of an innovative early warning system: Evidence-based strategies for ensuring system-wide nursing adoption. *Doctor of Nursing Practice (DNP) Projects. 105.* Retrieved from https://repository.usfca.edu/dnp/105
Program Implementation and Evaluation	Bela, C. (2017). Motivational interviewing, and healthy eating intervention with low income diabetic patients. *Doctor of Nursing Practice Capstone, 108.* Retrieved from https://scholarworks.umass.edu/nursing_dnp_capstone/108	Kaur, L. (2016). The development, implementation, and evaluation of a transgender health resource bundle. *Doctor of Nursing Practice (DNP) Projects, 84.* Retrieved from https://repository.usfca.edu/dnp/84

(continues)

		(continued)
TABLE 7-5 Exemplars of Completed DNP Projects		
Project Domain	**Diabetes Mellitus Type 2 DNP Project Exemplars**	**Other DNP Project Exemplars**
Research/ Practice Inquiry	Baker, B. (2016). Higher fat low carbohydrate diet to improve health related quality of life for overweight or obese diabetics in a primary care clinic. *Doctor of Nursing Practice Capstone, 79.* Retrieved from https:// scholarworks.umass.edu /nursing_dnp_capstone/79	Devers, G. (2018). On-line simulation in clinical end user training. *Doctor of Nursing Practice (DNP) Projects, 126.* Retrieved from https:// repository.usfca.edu/dnp/126
Policy/Social Change	Udo, I. G. (2016). Promoting diabetes self-management education and training in out-patient clinics. *Doctor of Nursing Practice Capstone.* Retrieved from https:// scholarworks.waldenu. edu/cgi/viewcontent. cgi?article=4050& context=dissertations	Zeigler, A. (2018). Development of an advanced practice provider onboarding structure. *Doctor of Nursing Practice (DNP) Projects, 119.* Retrieved from https:// repository.usfca.edu/dnp/119/

DNP Scholarly Repository Sources

- The University of San Francisco Scholarship Repository is open access: https://repository.usfca.edu/about.html.
- The University of Massachusetts, Amherst repository is open access. The DNP projects are licensed under a Creative Commons Attribution-Noncommercial-No Derivative Works 3.0 License.
- The Athenaeum, a service provided by the University of the Incarnate Word (UIW) Libraries, is an open access repository for research, scholarship, and creative works by the UIW community in all formats and media.
- Walden University: Dissertations are brought to you for free and open access by the Walden Dissertations and Doctoral Studies Collection at ScholarWorks. Follow at: http://scholarworks.waldenu.edu/dissertations.

▶ Resources for Data Collection: Registries and Surveys

When developing the DNP project, it can be helpful to search for reliable and valid surveys and tools that may be adapted for use. There are several online public resources that house well-written, previously tested survey questions from large multicenter observational studies. In addition, several national registries that can be mined for data to support a DNP project are available. A list of these resources for registries and surveys is included at the end of the chapter (see *Helpful Resources*).

▶ It Takes a Team: Data Collection

The data collection phase of the DNP project is action oriented and involves collaborators to assist with participant recruitment, instrument development, and data collection. Depending on the project design, data collection may occur in different settings and require permission from organizational leadership and the engagement of staff at each location. Consultation with PhD-prepared researchers or statisticians may be needed for instrument construction, complicated analyses such as statistical process control, or strategies to mine data from data repositories. Information technology experts are another group of professionals that contribute to data retrieval and DNP project work.

There are several administrative dimensions to the data collection process (Polit & Beck, 2017). Procedures and forms for data collection need to be developed and may include surveys, chart abstraction tools, checklists, tracking sheets, or scripted interview guides. See Chapter 13, The DNP Project Toolbox, for information on tools to support the scholarly project. If direct assessments are used, forms to record the observations will be needed. Newly developed instruments should be attractive, legible, and formatted in a logical structure to facilitate use. An assessment of the literacy level of the tool may be needed. It is helpful to pilot test instruments before implementation to evaluate the ease of use, the clarity of the items, and the amount of time needed for completion.

Procedures to recruit, screen, and obtain consent from participants, if indicated, need to be established along with the protocol for data collection. It is helpful to produce project protocol books and Gantt charts for all personnel assisting with the study. As mentioned in Chapter 10, Creating and Developing the Project Plan, a project meeting is also highly recommended to review all procedures prior to the study start. If an intervention, QI improvement, or EBP guideline implementation is planned, training sessions for the project team members (investigators, project assistants, and system staff) are needed. In more complex or lengthy projects, periodic evaluation of the project team members is indicated to ensure fidelity of the intervention or the innovation.

QI projects may involve large groups of staff, rather than individual subjects, who participate in the data collection process. A series of meetings to review the project processes and engage staff may be needed. Periodic visits to the project site encourage collaboration and provide personnel with the opportunity to ask questions or alert the DNP student to issues as they arise. These actions contribute to a successful project outcome. See Chapter 10 for a discussion on forming and training the project team.

Qualitative data collection uses smaller groups of subjects, and often only a single investigator and one assistant are needed for data collection. Subject recruitment is purposive to engage the specific types of participants required (Miller, 2010). Informed consent is needed; if the study uses focus groups, a group commitment to confidentiality is required. Open-ended questions or interviews are commonly used as the primary data collection method, with responses recorded by audiotapes. The role of the investigator is to facilitate the discussion. The study assistant observes nonverbal behaviors, taking field notes as needed.

Not everything that can be counted counts, and not everything that counts can be counted.

— William Bruce Cameron

▶ Data Management

Data security is an important issue to consider in any clinical inquiry project and requires a protocol to protect participants. In projects that collect personal health information and require human subject review, participants are assigned an identification (ID) number, and a master list of participants with their study IDs is created. This master list is stored in a secure location, with access granted only to the primary investigator and trained study staff. When possible, data collection tools should be devoid of identifying information and stored in a different secure location away from the master list. QI, EBP, and program evaluation projects often collect data in aggregate form that may or may not include protected health information.

There are several strategies used during the data collection period to facilitate efficiency and accuracy. A process for tracking responses from participants should be developed and monitored. Maintaining a project log is recommended to document issues that arise and decisions that are made as the project progresses. A data codebook is created and includes the name or label for each data item, its level of measurement, and its numeric coding scheme. For example, if gender is the variable, the codebook

Data security is an important issue to consider in any clinical inquiry project and requires a protocol to protect participants.

would indicate this is a nominal-level variable, where a value of 1 indicates female and a value of 2 indicates male. A code for missing data is also commonly created for each item.

As they are received, data collection forms should be examined for completeness and legibility. Steps to retrieve pieces of missing data may need to be implemented. If this is not possible, decisions regarding the amount of missing data that warrants exclusion of the record from the study need to be considered. Sometimes participants creatively complete data collection forms. For example, they may write in an answer rather than selecting from the ones provided. At other times, they may change their answer several times, making it difficult to determine which answer they intended to select. The DNP student will need to make decisions about the interpretation of these items. One solution is to create a new code for these variant items that is labeled "other" to distinguish these data. These concerns would invite collaboration with a PhD-prepared researcher or statistician. Decisions made should be entered into the project log to ensure consistency in the evaluation of all data forms.

When dealing with numerical data, approximately right is better than precisely wrong.

— Carl G. Tor

▶ Data Entry

When all data collection forms have been reviewed, verified, and cleaned, they are coded using the schema established in the codebook. Coded data are then entered into the selected statistical program. There are several statistical software programs available, including the Statistical Package for the Social Sciences (SPSS), the Statistical Analysis System (SAS), and Stata. Microsoft Excel is also capable of descriptive data analysis and graphics. With additional software, Excel can perform inferential statistics and produce QI metrics. The choice of statistical software should be driven by the analyses needed to accurately measure the DNP project outcome.

Data entry is a tedious, time-intensive process, and errors are common. Consequently, it is necessary to verify or check the entries to correct mistakes prior to data analysis. One option for data verification is to print all data set values and compare the numbers visually to each original data record (e.g., survey). Another option is double data entry. In this case, the data are entered twice and the two data sets compared for errors. The comparison can be done visually or, if available, the statistical computer program can compare both data sets.

Qualitative data include audiotapes from interviews and focus groups, field notes with observations of nonverbal behaviors, or written narratives. Verification of data often occurs during the data collection process, in which the researcher checks with the participant to affirm the interpretations. Management of qualitative data includes the transcription of audiotaped interviews into text for analysis. Computerized software products (e.g., NVivo, Atlas) are also available to manage verbal and written narrative data.

Data entry is a tedious, time-intensive process, and errors are common. Therefore, it is important that the student verify the entries to correct mistakes prior to data analysis.

The processes of both data management and analysis are complex and challenging. This is another dimension of the DNP project where interprofessional collaboration is paramount. Consultation with expert researchers and statisticians experienced in quantitative and qualitative inquiry is highly recommended when selecting analytical software or making decisions that affect data veracity.

However exhausted I might be, the sight of long columns of numbers was perfectly reviving to me.

— Florence Nightingale

▶ Data Analysis

Data analysis is an exciting phase of the DNP project! Statistical analyses organize and transform the numbers that represent the project outcome data into meaningful information that can be interpreted. As with the other components of the DNP project, there is a systematic process to evaluate and interpret data. The data analysis plan will differ based on the DNP project approach and can be diverse, including a broad array of outcome measures.

The first step in data analysis is to evaluate the distributions of the dependent/outcome and independent variables for normality using histograms and frequency distributions (See Chapter 13, The DNP Project Toolbox). If the distributions are normal, parametric analyses can be used. If distributions are not normal, variables can be transformed to try to achieve normality. If this is not successful, nonparametric analyses are used. The next wave of data analysis includes descriptive analysis with measures of central tendency (mean, median, and mode) and variation (range and standard deviation). These data provide an overall picture of the participants' characteristics and measures of the independent, confounding, and outcome variables.

Statistical analyses organize and transform the numbers that represent the project outcome data into meaningful information that can be interpreted.

The second set of analyses examines the relationships between the variables. These analyses usually include scatter plots, chi-square tests (crosstabs), and bivariate Pearson or Spearman rank-order correlations, depending on the measurement level of the variables. Additional analyses may include regression or the assessment of differences between groups using parametric tests (independent or pair t-tests, ANOVA) or nonparametric tests (Mann–Whitney U test, Wilcoxon signed-rank test, Kruskal–Wallis test) if congruent with the project aim and type of data that were collected. Additional statistical tests may be conducted to answer questions related to the DNP project outcome.

QI data can be analyzed using histograms, scatter plots, pie charts, line graphs, frequencies, and descriptive statistics using the same analytical programs. Change in the dependent variable from an innovation can also be measured with traditional statistical analyses. Additional QI analyses such as control and run charts, Pareto charts, or value stream maps can be created using Excel with QI macros if congruent with the DNP project plan. For well-developed QI processes, statistical process control is the sentinel analytic technique. See Chapter 13, The DNP Project Toolbox, for examples created using QI macros.

Qualitative data analysis involves thoughtful review of transcribed audiotaped data or written narratives to identify themes or patterns in the data. Statistical programs such as NVivo or Atlas can be used to corroborate and support the investigator's suppositions. Data are analyzed inductively via specific, rigorous techniques to organize answers around the clinical inquiry question (Miller, 2010). Qualitative analysis seeks understanding about a phenomenon rather than a specific answer.

When analyses are complete, the challenge is to interpret the findings and apply them in the context of the clinical question as outcomes. What is the meaning in the

The data analysis plan will differ based on the DNP project approach and can be diverse including a broad array of outcome measures.

data? How does it inform the clinical phenomenon? What are some of the possible explanations for the findings? What are the implications of the findings? Are there opportunities for systems improvements? How might these data be used to change practice? How does this work contribute to nursing practice?

At the same time, the limitations of the data are evaluated. Where is the bias or error in the study? How does this impact the conclusions? If the study were repeated, what improvements could be made? This phase of data analysis requires dedicated thinking time to reach thoughtful conclusions. It is also another time in the scholarly process where consultation with the DNP team and collaboration with other researchers and statistical or QI specialists can be helpful.

In God we trust, all others bring data.

— W. Edwards Deming

▶ Telling the Story

The last part of the project is the dissemination of findings. Dissemination can include an article for publication, or presentations at professional or community meetings (see Chapter 15, Disseminating the Results). If the project was conducted in a specific setting or with a special population, the findings should be shared with those groups. If the data inform policy, they should be shared with the relevant stakeholders. The diffusion of the project outcome is just as important, if not more important, than the actual work itself.

When preparing papers or presentations to share the project data, a structured format is helpful (Oermann, Turner, & Carman, 2014). There are specific guidelines for the reports of experimental and observational research, program evaluation (CDC, 2013), as well as for QI reports and EBP initiatives. The recommended formats are included in the *Helpful Resources* section at the end of this chapter.

As is mentioned in Chapter 15, Disseminating the Results, in general, most papers and presentations begin with an introduction and background to establish the need for the project and its significance to nursing practice or healthcare delivery. This is followed by the methods section, which describes the project design, the sample or population studied, institutional review board or quality council approval, and the protocols for data collection and measurements.

The project findings are also reported in a systematic fashion, starting with the participant response, if indicated, and a description of the sample characteristics or the clinical setting for a QI or an EBP project report. This is followed by the data outcomes organized around the clinical issue, program goals, or the improvement process. It is important to focus on the major points in this section. It is not necessary to provide

There are specific guidelines for the reports of research, program evaluation, QI reports, and EBP initiatives.

every piece of data; the main outcomes are sufficient. If there were unanticipated findings that are relevant, they should be noted.

The last part of the paper or presentation is the discussion. This is the opportunity to give meaning to the findings for the audience or reader. The discussion should include the implication of the data for practice and opportunities for future change or improvement. The major findings and their implications should be discussed first, followed by other results considered important. The data are often compared to other studies in the literature or other improvement processes. The limitations of the data are summarized and the next steps for future innovation are presented.

The doctoral project is the summative scholarly product in DNP programs, and it demonstrates the synthesis of the student's academic work and achievement of the essential DNP competencies. The project, when viewed as a program outcome, should make a substantive contribution to nursing practice. DNP projects are diverse and address relevant patient, systems, or population issues with an emphasis on improving health- and healthcare-related outcomes. The project deliverables are disseminated professionally and provide a foundation for continued practice scholarship.

Impact

The alignment of the clinical question with methods and appropriate evaluation assures rigor of DNP projects to produce outcomes with impact.

Key Messages

- The DNP project design drives the selection of methods, measures, and the data evaluation plan.
- DNP projects are diverse and encompass multiple different perspectives.
- Interprofessional collaboration is essential for a successful DNP project.
- The DNP project is the work of many, not the work of one—it takes a team!

Action Plan—Next Steps

1. Ensure that all appropriate team members have been brought to the table.
2. Verify that there is congruence between the clinical issue, selected design, and methods.
3. Choose a statistical software program to use for data analysis.
4. Consult with a PhD colleague or statistician when analyzing the data and interpreting the results.

References

Agency for Healthcare Research and Quality (AHRQ). (2017). *Patient centered outcomes research.* Retrieved from https://www.ahrq.gov/pcor/index.html

Alamry, A., Al Owais, S. M., Marini, A. M., Al-Dorzi, H., Alsolamy, S., & Arabi, Y. (2017). Application of Failure Mode Effects Analysis to improve the care of septic patients admitted through the Emergency Department. *Journal of Patient Safety, 13(2),* 76–81. doi:10.1097/PTS.0000000000000118.

American Association of Colleges of Nursing (AACN). (2015). *The doctor of nursing practice: Current issues and clarifying recommendations. Report from the task force on the implementation of the DNP*. Retrieved from http://www.aacnnursing.org/Portals/42/DNP/DNP-Implementation.pdf

American Association of Colleges of Nursing (AACN). (2017). Fact sheet: *The doctor of nursing practice (DNP)*. Retrieved from https://www.aacnnursing.org/News-Information/Fact-Sheets/DNP-Fact-Sheet

Bardach, E., & Patashnik, E. M. (2016). *A practical guide for policy analysis: The eightfold path to more effective problem solving* (5th ed.). Thousand Oaks, CA: CQ Press.

Batalden, P. B., & Davidoff, F. (2007). What is quality improvement and how can it transform health care? *Quality and Safety in Health Care, 16*, 2–3. doi:10.1136/qshc.2006.022046

Bauer, M. S., Damschroder, L., Hagedorn, H., Smith, J., & Kilbourne, A. (2015). An introduction to implementation science for the non-specialist. *BMC Psychology 3*, 32. doi: 10.1186/s40359-0089-9.

Beyea, C., & Slattery, M. (2013). Historical perspectives on evidence-based nursing. *Nursing Science Quarterly, 26*(2), 152-155. doi: 10.1177/0894318413477140.

Brouwers, M., Kho, M. E., Browman, G. P., Burgers, J. S., Cluzeau, F., Feder, G., & Zitzelsberger, L. for the AGREE Next Steps Consortium. (2016). AGREE II: Advancing guideline development, reporting and evaluation in healthcare. *Canadian Medical Association Journal, 82*, E839–E842. doi:10.1503/090449.

Brown, C. H., Curran, G., Palinkas, L. A., Aarons, G. A., Wells, K. B., Jones, L., . . . Cruden, G. (2017). An overview of research and evaluation designs for dissemination and implementation. *Annual Reviews of Public Health, 38*, 1–22. Retrieved from publhealth.annualreviews.org, https://doi.org/10.1146/annurev-publhealth-031816-044215

Carhart, M. Y., Schminkey, D. L., Mitchell, E. M., & Keim-Malpass, J. (2018). Barriers and facilitators to improving Virginia's HPV vaccination rate: A stakeholder analysis with implications for pediatric nurses. *Journal of Pediatric Nursing, 42*, 1–8. doi:10.1016/j.pedn.2018.05.008

Carter, E. J., Mastro, K., Vose, C., Rivera, R., & Larson, E. L. (2017). Clarifying the conundrum: Evidence-based practice, quality improvement or research? The clinical scholarship continuum. *Journal of Nursing Administration, 47*(5), 266–270. doi:10.1097/NNA.0000000000000477

Centers for Disease Control and Prevention (CDC). (1999). A framework for program evaluation. Retrieved from https://www.cdc.gov/mmwr/PDF/rr/rr4811.pdf

Centers for Disease Control and Prevention (CDC). (2013). *Developing an effective evaluation report: Setting the course for effective program evaluation*. Atlanta, GA: Centers for Disease Control and Prevention, National Center for Chronic Disease Prevention and Health Promotion, Office on Smoking and Health, Division of Nutrition, Physical Activity and Obesity. Retrieved from http://www.cdc.gov/eval/materials/developing-an-effective-evaluation-report_tag508.pdf

Cronenwett, L., Sherwood, G., Barnsteiner, J., Disch, J., Johnson, J., Mitchell, P., . . . Warren, J. (2007). Quality and safety education for nurses. *Nursing Outlook, 55*(3), 122–131.

Damschroder, L. J., Aron, D. C., Keith, R. A., Kirsh, S. R., Alexander, J. A., & Lowery, J. (2009). Fostering implementation of health services research findings into practice: A consolidated framework for advancing implementation science. *Implementation Science, 4*, 50. Retrieved from http://www.implementationscience.com/content/4/1/50.

Donabedian, A. (2005). Evaluating the quality of medical care. *Milbank Quarterly, 83*, 691–729. doi:10.1111/j.1468-0009.2005.00397.x

Flynn, M. E. (2017). A quality improvement project to decrease serum bilirubins and increase appropriate phototherapy use by following the AAP guidelines in the well nursery. *Pediatric Nursing, 43*(3), 143–148.

Gavriloff, C., Ostrowski-Delahanty, S., & Oldfield, K. (2017). The impact of Lean Six Sigma methodology on patient scheduling. *Nursing Economics, 35*(4), 189–193.

Gertler, S. A., Coralic, Z., Lopez, A., Stein, J., & Sarkar, U. (2016). Root cause analysis of ambulatory adverse drug events that present to the emergency department. *Journal of Patient Safety, 12*(3), 119–124. doi: 10.1097/PTS.0000000000000072

Institute for Healthcare Improvement. (2017). *Quality improvement essentials toolkit*. Retrieved from www.ihi.org/resources/pages/tools/Quality-Improvement-Essentials-Toolkit.aspx

Iowa Model Collaborative. (2017). Iowa model of evidence-based practice: Revisions and validation. *Worldviews on Evidence-Based Nursing, 14*(3), 175–182. doi:10.1111/wvn.12223.

Issel, L. M., & Wells, R. (2018). *Health program planning and evaluation: A practical systematic approach for community health* (4th ed.). Burlington, MA: Jones & Bartlett Learning.

Johanna Briggs Institute. (2018). *Critical appraisal tools.* Retrieved from http://joannabriggs.org /research/critical-appraisal-tools.html

Jordan, Z., Lockwood, C., Aromataris, E. C., & Munn, Z. (2016). *The updated JBI model for evidence-based healthcare.* The Joanna Briggs Institute. Retrieved from http://joannabriggs.org /assets/docs/approach/The_JBI_Model_of_Evidence_-_Healthcare-A_Model_Reconsidered.pdf

Kaplan, R. S., & Norton, D. P. (1992). The balanced scorecard – measures that drive performance. *Harvard Business Review, 70*(1), 71–79.

Lee, M. C., Johnson, K., Newhouse, R. P., & Warren, J. I. (2013). Evidence-based practice process quality assessment: EPQA guidelines. *Worldviews on Evidence-Based Nursing, 10*(3), 140–149. doi: 10.1111/j.1741-6787.2012.00264.x

Leeman, J., & Sandelowski, M. (2012). Practice-based evidence and qualitative inquiry. *Journal of Nursing Scholarship, 44*(2), 171–179.

Lobiondo-Wood, G., & Haber, J. (2018). *Nursing research: Methods and critical appraisal for evidence-based practice* (9th ed.). St Louis, MO: Elsevier.

Melnyk, B. M., & Fineout-Overholt, E. (2015). *Evidence-based practice in nursing and healthcare: A guide to best practice* (3rd ed.). Philadelphia, PA: Wolters Kluwer Health.

Melynk, B. M., Fineout-Overholt, E., Giggleman, G., & Choy, K. (2017). A test of the ARCC model improves implementation of evidence-based practice, healthcare culture and patient outcomes. *Worldviews on Evidence-Based Nursing, 14*(1), 5–9. doi:10/1111/wvn.12188.

Millar, A., Simeone, R. S., & Carnevale, J. T. (2001). Logic models: A systems tool for performance management. *Evaluation and Program Planning, 24*, 73–81.

Miller, W. R. (2010). Qualitative research as evidence: Utility in nursing practice. *Clinical Nurse Specialist, 24*(4), 191–193.

Newhouse, R. (2007). Diffusing confusion among evidenced-based practice, quality improvement and research. *Journal of Nursing Administration, 37*(10), 432–435.

Newhouse, R. P., Dearholt, S. L., Poe, S. S., Pugh, L. C., & White, K. M. (2007). *Johns Hopkins Hospital Nursing Evidence-based Practice Model and Guidelines.* Retrieved from http://nursing. jhu.edu/news-events/news/archives/2009/evidence_based_model.html

Oermann, M. H., Turner, K., & Carman, M. (2014). Preparing quality improvement, research and evidenced-based manuscripts. *Nursing Economics, 32*(2), 57–69.

Perrin, K. M. (2015). *Principles of evaluation and research for health care programs.* Burlington, MA: Jones & Bartlett Learning.

Polit, D., & Beck, C. (2017). *Nursing research: Generating and assessing evidence for nursing practice* (10th ed.). Philadelphia, PA: Lippincott Williams & Wilkins.

Portela, M. C., Pronovost, P. J., Woodcock, T., Carter, P., & Dixon-Woods, M. (2015). How to study improvement interventions: A brief overview of possible study types. *BMJ Quality & Safety, 24,* 325–336.

Purvis, S., Kaun, A., McKenna, A., Viste, J. W., & Fedorov, E. (2018). Outcomes of clinical nurse practice in the implementation of video monitoring at an academic medical center. *Clinical Nurse Specialist, 32*(2), 90–96. doi: 10.1097/NUR000000000000356.

Rosswurm, M. A., & Larrabee, J. (1999). A model for change to evidence-based practice. *Journal of Nursing Scholarship, 31*(4), 317–322.

Rycroft-Malone, J. (2004). The PARIHS framework: A framework for guiding the implementation of evidence based practice. *Journal of Nursing Care Quality, 19*(4), 297–304.

Sackett, D. L., Rosenberg, W. M., Gray, J. A., Haynes, R. B., & Richardson, W. S. (2000). *Evidence-based medicine: How to practice and teach EBM* (2nd ed.). London, UK: Churchill Livingstone, p. 1.

Schaffer, M. A., Sandau, K. E., & Diedrick, L. (2012). Evidence-based practice model for organizational change: Overview and practical applications. *Journal of Advanced Nursing, 69*(5), 1197–1209. doi: 10.1111/j.1365-2648.2012.06122x

Shirey, M. R., Hauck, S. L., Embree, J. L., Kinner, T. J., Schaar, G. L., Phillips, L. A., . . . McCool, I. A. (2011). Showcasing differences between quality improvement, evidenced-based practice and research. *Journal of Continuing Education in Nursing, 42*(2), 57–68.

Spurrier, A. E., Suttle, C., Matheson, L., & Baker-Watson, A. (2018). The effects of a health promotion program on rural West Virginia adults. *Family and Community Health, 41*(2), 95–104. doi: 10.1097/FCH.0000000000000179

Stetler, C. B. (2001). Updating the Stetler model of research utilization to facilitate evidence-based practice. *Nursing Outlook, 49,* 272–278.

Stevens, K. R. (2004). *ACE Star model of EBP: Knowledge transformation. Academic Center for Evidence Based Practice.* The University of Texas Health Science Center at San Antonio. Retrieved from http://www.acestar.uthscsa.edu

Stufflebeam, D. L. (1983). The CIPP model for program evaluation. In G. F. Maddaus, M. Scriven, & D. L. Stufflebeam (Eds.). *Evaluation in Health and Human Services* (Vol. 6, pp. 117–141). Boston, MA: Kluwer-Nijhoff Publishing.

Sundberg, M. J., Parver, S., Morin, M., & Stack, A. M. (2017). An intervention to improve caregiver adherence to oral rehydration therapy. *Pediatric Quality & Safety, 2*(3), e020. doi:10.1097 /pq9.0000000000000020

Titler, M. G., Kleiber, C., Steelman, V., Goode, C., Rakel, B., Budreau, G., . . . Goode, C. J. (2001). The IOWA model of evidence based practice to promote quality care. *Critical Care Nursing Clinics of North America, 13*(4), 497–509.

Titler, M. (2011). Nursing science and evidenced based practice. *Western Journal of Nursing Research, 33*(3), 291–295.

Toles, M., & Barroso, J. (2018). Introduction to qualitative research. In G. Lobiondo-Wood & J. Haber, *Nursing research: Methods and critical appraisal for evidence-based practice* (9th ed., pp. 88–101). St Louis, MO: Elsevier.

United States Department of Health and Human Services. Office of Human Research Protection. (2009). *Protection of human subjects. Title 45 Code of Federal Regulations. Part 46.* Washington, DC: Department of Health and Human Services. Retrieved from http://www.hhs.gov/ohrp /humansubjects/regbook2013.pdf.pdf

United States Department of Health and Human Services. Health Resources and Services Administration. (2011). *Quality Improvement.* Retrieved from http://www.hrsa.gov/quality /toolbox/methodology/qualityimprovement/

Vejar, M. V., Makic, M. B., & Kotthoff-Burrell, E. (2015). Medication management for elderly patients in an academic primary care setting: A quality improvement project. *Journal of the American Association of Nurse Practitioners, 27,* 72–78. doi:10.1002/2327-6924.12121

Weimer, D. L., & Vining, A. R. (2017). *Policy analysis: Concepts and practice* (6th ed.). New York, NY: Routledge.

Helpful Resources

Evidence-based Practice Resources

Joanna Briggs Institute (JBI) Resources

Overview of JBI. http://joannabriggs.org/jbi-approach.html
Critical appraisal tools. http://joannabriggs.org/research/critical-appraisal-tools.html
Levels of evidence. http://joannabriggs.org/assets/docs/approach/JBI-Levels-of-evidence_2014.pdf
The JBI model. http://joannabriggs.org/assets/docs/approach/The_JBI_Model_of_Evidence_-_ Healthcare-A_Model_Reconsidered.pdf

Johns Hopkins Nursing Evidence-based Practice Tool Kit

Provides resources including guides for appraising research and non-research evidence for nursing practice. https://www.hopkinsmedicine.org/evidence-based-practice/ijhn_2017_ebp.html

Critical Appraisal Tools for Study Types

All guidelines are now housed on the EQUATOR network at www.equator-network .org

Study Type	Manuscript or Guideline Format
Randomized trials	CONSORT
Observational studies: cohort, case control, cross-sectional	STROBE
Systematic reviews & meta-analysis	PRISMA
Qualitative Research	COREQ, SRQR
Case Reports	CARE
Quality Improvement project	SQUIRE 2.0
Clinical Practice Guidelines	AGREE-II
Economic evaluations	CHEERS
Evidence-based practice project	EPQA*

*The EPQA guidelines are available in the following journal article:
Lee, M. C., Johnson, K., Newhouse, R. P., & Warren, J. I. (2013). Evidence-based practice process quality assessment: EPQA guidelines. *Worldviews on Evidence-Based Nursing, 10*(3), 140–149. doi: 10.1111/j.1741-6787.2012.00264.x

National Data Registries

Agency for Healthcare Research and Quality (AHRQ): Medical Expenditure Panel Survey. Online query system for the Medical Expenditure Panel Survey data maintained AHRQ. Available at http://www.meps.ahrq.gov/mepsweb/data_stats/meps_query.jsp

AHRQ: Healthcare Cost and Utilization Project data. Online query system for the Healthcare Cost and Utilization Project data. Available at http://hcupnet.ahrq.gov/

American Fact Finder—U.S. Census Bureau. A source for population, housing, economic, and geographic information. Available at http://factfinder2.census.gov/faces/nav/jsf/pages/index.xhtml

CDC Wonder. Online query system for data maintained by the Centers for Disease Control and Prevention. Available at http://wonder.cdc.gov/

National Center for Health Statistics. This site has links to survey instruments, methods, public use data sets, online data summaries, and reports. Available at http://www.cdc.gov/nchs/

United Kingdom (UK) Data Archive. Collection of digital research data in the social sciences and humanities. Available at http://www.data-archive.ac.uk/

Program Evaluation Resources

Centers for Disease Control. Several resources on models for program development and evaluation on a variety of health initiatives. Available at http://www.cdc.gov/eval/resources/

RAND Corporation. Provides exemplars of evaluation of health care programs Available at. http://www.rand.org/topics/health-care-program-evaluation.html

Quality Improvement Resources

Agency for Healthcare Research and Quality (AHRQ). (2017). *The CAHPS ambulatory care improvement guide: Practical strategies for improving patient experience.* Retrieved from https://www.ahrq.gov/cahps/quality-improvement/improvement-guide/improvement-guide.html

Institute for Healthcare Improvement. Available at http://www.ihi.org/

U.S. Department of Health and Human Services, Health Resources and Services Administration (HRSA). *Quality Improvement Tools and Resources.* https://bphc.hrsa.gov/qualityimprovement/index.html

Survey Resources

Agency for Healthcare Research and Quality (AHRQ) Surveys. Available at http://www.ahrq.gov/data/Centers for Disease Control Division of Adolescent and School Health. Available at http://www.cdc.gov/HealthyYouth/data/surveillance.htm

National Behavioral Risk Factor Study Survey. Available at http://www.cdc.gov/brfss/

National Center for Health Statistics, Surveys and Data Collection Systems. Available at http://www.cdc.gov/nchs/express.htm

RAND Corporation. Health surveys are available from RAND, a nonprofit institution that helps improve policy and decision making through research and analysis. Available at http://www.rand.org/health/surveys_tools.html

Survey Monkey. Free for 10 questions per survey with 100 responses per survey; $17/month for unlimited questions and unlimited responses. Available at http://www.surveymonkey.com

CHAPTER 8

Interprofessional and Intraprofessional Collaboration in the DNP Project

Dianne Conrad

CHAPTER OVERVIEW

As the doctor of nursing practice (DNP) student formulates the question for the scholarly project, additional resources will be needed to assist in assessment, planning, implementing, and evaluating the outcomes of the project. This process allows the student to practice the skills outlined in *The Essentials of Doctoral Education for Advanced Nursing Practice* (American Association of Colleges of Nursing [AACN], 2006) related to organizational and systems leadership, as well as forming and leading collaborative teams. This chapter will define collaboration with professionals within nursing and other professions. Nationally, nurses are called to actively collaborate within interprofessional teams to improve quality, provide cost-effective and efficient care, and improve outcomes (Institute of Medicine [IOM], 2003). The *Future of Nursing* report (IOM, 2010) stated that developing well-functioning teams with coordination of care among multiple providers is a crucial objective to address the complexities of care across a wide range of settings throughout the healthcare system. Specific to the nursing practice doctorate, the Implementation of the DNP Task Force (AACN, 2015) emphasized that organizational and systems leadership knowledge and skills are critical for the DNP-prepared nurse to develop and evaluate new models of care delivery. The DNP project provides students the opportunity for attaining and refining the competencies needed for collaborative team participation and leadership.

CHAPTER OBJECTIVES

After completing the chapter, the learner will be able to:

1. Discern the difference among the terms *interdisciplinary collaboration,* *interprofessional collaboration,* and *intraprofessional collaboration.*
2. Discuss the importance and value of interprofessional and intraprofessional collaboration in the DNP project and in clinical practice settings.
3. Identify the competencies needed for the DNP leader in an interprofessional team.

▶ Gathering Resources for the DNP Project

Developing the DNP project is a comprehensive and rigorous process. As the clinical question for inquiry develops, the DNP student may find gaps in knowledge and skill sets to carry out the project. The student will require assistance not only from DNP faculty, but also from key players in the college of nursing or university and the organizational setting in which the clinical question is studied. Other collaborative efforts may be needed to effectively implement the project and develop an appropriate evaluation strategy. Finally, the DNP student may require assistance from appropriately qualified personnel to disseminate the results. This process will involve gathering not just one, but perhaps several teams consisting of members from nursing and other disciplines.

Clearly, the DNP project is not accomplished by the DNP student without guidance, but it is an opportunity for the student to experience and, in particular, refine the skills required for DNP *Essential* II: Organizational and Systems Leadership for Quality Improvement and Systems Thinking and *Essential* VI: Interprofessional Collaboration for Improving Patient and Population Health Outcomes (AACN, 2006). DNP *Essential* II involves the ability of the DNP graduate to organize care to address emerging practice problems, as well as collaborate with others to manage risks ethically, based on professional standards. *Essential* VI delineates the components of interprofessional collaboration and states that the DNP graduate should be able to:

- Effectively communicate and collaborate with others to develop and implement practice models, peer review, practice guidelines, health policy, standards of care, and/or other scholarly products.
- Develop the ability to lead interprofessional teams in an organization to address complex practice issues.
- Demonstrate the skills required to lead and collaborate with intraprofessional and interprofessional teams to address the change needed in health care and complex healthcare delivery systems (AACN, 2006).

Since the inception of the DNP degree, a critical component of DNP education was that it should include opportunities for students to form interprofessional teams (Draye, Acker, & Zimmer, 2006). This experience allows students to refine skills in effective team leadership and communication, and in guiding team members to the highest level of function to effectively improve health outcomes for patients and populations. The profession of nursing also benefits by the DNP student modeling to other members of the team and organization the behaviors of doctoral-level nursing leadership and collaboration in scholarly practice inquiry. The DNP graduate is equipped to serve on leadership teams with other practice doctorates in healthcare systems to address the complexities of health care.

▶ Definitions

The origin of the word *collaborate* comes from the Latin word *collabratus*, meaning to labor together. *Collaborate* is defined as "to work jointly with others or together especially in an intellectual endeavor" ("Collaborate," 2018, para. 1). Ash, Miller, and Zaccagnini (2017) noted that the concept of collaboration in successful business and management fields that includes "strategic alliances" and "interpersonal networks" can be transferred to the health sector. Collaborative partnerships that allow interaction between health professionals to share ideas and knowledge, as well as shared decision making, can improve quality and cost-effective care. Processes of collaboration include communicating, cooperating, transferring knowledge, coordinating, problem solving, and negotiating. Collaboration can occur within the framework of formal and informal teams that the DNP student may encounter during the DNP project process. The DNP student may work with formally identified teams during the project, such as his or her project team or other teams of professionals within the clinical site. The student may also use the same skill set in communicating and working with informal team members such as statisticians or other experts needed for consultation on specific aspects of the project.

The concepts of *interdisciplinary* and *interprofessional, multiprofessional* and *multidisciplinary* have been used interchangeably in the literature and often refer to types or processes within teams (Nancarrow et al., 2013). Using the term *interdisciplinary* or *multidisciplinary* can limit the concept to knowledge ascribed to a particular discipline. The term *interprofessional* or *multiprofessional* offers a broader definition than *interdisciplinary*; interprofessional or multiprofessional collaboration refers to the interactions among individual professionals who may represent a particular discipline or branch of knowledge but who *additionally* bring their unique educational backgrounds, experiences, values, roles, and identities to the process. The collaboration with other professionals is enriched with shared or overlapping knowledge, skills, abilities, and roles (Ash, Miller, & Zaccagnini, 2017).

To enhance the understanding of the phenomenon of interprofessional collaboration, D'Amour and Oandasan (2005) proposed the concept of *interprofessionality*. They defined *interprofessionality* as:

> . . .the process by which professionals reflect on and develop ways of practicing that provides an integrated and cohesive answer to the needs of the client/family/population. . . . [I]t involves continuous interaction and knowledge sharing between professionals, organized to solve or explore a variety of education and care issues all while seeking to optimize the patient's participation. . . . Interprofessionality requires a paradigm shift, since interprofessional practice has unique characteristics in terms of values, codes of conduct, and ways of working. (p. 5)

Interprofessional collaboration will be the term used in this text to refer to interactions with nursing and other health team members who do not belong to the nursing profession. The concept of *intraprofessional collaboration* is defined as interactions among colleagues *within the nursing profession* who share nursing professional education, values, socialization, and experience. However, the term interdisciplinary may be used at times in the discussion to accurately cite work from other authors.

▶ Components of Collaboration in the DNP Project: Who, What, Where, When, and How

The process of developing the DNP project will require collaboration with members of the nursing profession as well as other health professionals. Members of the team a DNP student gathers to complete a DNP project can include, but are not limited to, nursing and other disciplinary faculty project team members, organizational leadership and healthcare workers, business and management personnel, experts in informatics, statisticians, and the patients who are part of the intervention. To explore the components of collaboration with different professionals and members of scholarly project teams, the framework of *Who, What, Where, When, and How* will be used.

Whom to Collaborate With?

When the DNP student gathers resources needed for the scholarly project, *who* will be needed to assist in assessment, planning, implementing, and evaluating the process may include members from the nursing profession as well as members from outside the profession, including patients and populations served.

Intraprofessional Collaboration

The DNP student will find resources within the profession from both faculty and other nursing professionals in the clinical setting. Nursing faculty are the primary role models and resources for collaboration for the DNP student. The Implementation of the DNP Task Force recommended a doctorally prepared faculty member to help guide the student (AACN, 2015). Cronenwett and colleagues (2011) described the optimal learning environment for DNP students as "one in which doctorally-prepared faculty members are actively engaged in teaching, clinical practice, translational science and systems improvement, preferably within an environment characterized by robust interprofessional learning opportunities" (p. 14). Identifying faculty as mentors as well as content and research consultants in identified areas of the project is important

> Who *will be needed for the scholarly project team can include members from the nursing profession as well as members from outside the profession.*

early in the DNP project work. These faculty members may also serve as part of the DNP project team to guide the work of the student during the project. Carlson, Staffileno, and Murphy (2017) have outlined the value of PhD- and DNP-prepared faculty member collaboration, along with the organizational representative in project teams, to provide an environment that:

1. Leverages the potential of both DNP- and PhD-prepared faculty members' knowledge and expertise.
2. Encourages mutual respect and a vibrant intellectual community.
3. Promotes the scholarly formation of students while exemplifying the value of collaboration. (p. 4)

For more on the project team and their functions, see Chapter 9, The DNP Project Team.

As practice doctorate programs in nursing continue to grow, the collaboration of PhD- and DNP-prepared nurses in contributing to evidence-based practice will be realized. Many universities already have both nursing research and nursing practice doctorate programs. This is an ideal setting for PhD and DNP students to collaborate in research and/or projects from their respective viewpoints of research and practice for nursing knowledge generation. DNP students collaborate with their PhD-prepared nursing faculty, but the potential for collaboration between nursing PhD students and DNP students provides a multifaceted approach to healthcare problems.

Clinton and Sperhac (2009) stated that the two doctoral degrees in nursing are complementary and overlap. The interaction between the research and practice degrees in nursing can be applied to projects in which research questions are generated by the practice doctorate from clinical questions and then tested in the practice environment for application and evaluation with the assistance of the research doctorate. The process can be reversed in that the nurse researcher coming from a particular field of interest can enlist the aid of the practice doctorate in the clinical environment to test theory. In all, the nursing profession benefits from the collaboration of the practice and research doctorates in the generation of knowledge applied to evidence-based practice.

The opportunities for collaboration also occur with other nurses in the clinical setting where the scholarly project takes place. DNP students can model doctoral nursing leadership skills with other nurses—such as nursing administration, nursing staff, and nursing informatics experts involved in their project—and include them in their project team when appropriate. DNP students in administrative advanced practice roles can influence institutional policy with projects, such as instituting a new program to benefit a specific population. For example, the administrative DNP student might gather a team of nursing administrators, clinicians, and other departments, such as pharmacy and information technology, to inform a project

The nursing profession benefits from the collaboration of the practice and research doctorates in the generation of knowledge applied to evidence-based practice.

aimed at serving the local uninsured population. The DNP student can model leadership behaviors in a project proposal for his or her university and also present the project to the board of the institution to implement the innovative change.

The opportunity for intraprofessional collaboration can also occur with DNP students working with each other to complete different aspects of a project topic, such as diabetes care. See Chapter 3, Scholarship in Practice, for a discussion of scholar teams of DNP students working together on a DNP project.

Interprofessional Collaboration

In the 2001 report *Crossing the Quality Chasm: A New Health System for the 21st Century*, the IOM outlined aims for healthcare improvement that included care that is safe, effective, patient centered, timely, efficient, and equitable. To provide that care, the IOM, in *Health Professions Education: A Bridge to Quality* (2003), called for a change in how healthcare providers are prepared to meet these challenges that includes working in teams. Many health professional programs are now collaborating to educate students to learn by, with, and from others from outside their own profession. Interprofessional education is the interactive learning and collaboration of students from different health and social professions "for the explicit purpose of improving interprofessional collaboration or the health/well-being of patients/clients (or both)" (Reeves, Perrier, Goldman, Freeth, & Zwarenstein, 2013, p. 4).

Educational preparation for multiple professions working in teams often begins with simulation exercises to develop interprofessional team communication skills (Wagner, Liston, & Miller, 2011) and interprofessional mentoring in the clinical setting (Lait, Suter, Arthur, & Deutschlander, 2011).

To fully operationalize the concept of interprofessional collaboration in practice, the Robert Wood Johnson Foundation (RWJF) (2015) states that:

> Effective interprofessional collaboration promotes the active participation of each discipline in patient care, where all disciplines are working together, fully engaging patients and those who support them, and leadership on the team adapts based on patient needs.
>
> Effective interprofessional collaboration enhances patient- and family-centered goals and values, provides mechanisms for continuous communication among caregivers, and optimizes participation in clinical decision-making within and across disciplines. It fosters respect for the disciplinary contributions of all professionals. (p. 1)

Dr. Abby Winterberg illustrates the value of DNP education in the areas of interprofessional collaboration and information technology in **EXEMPLAR 8-1**.

Interprofessional Clinical Models

Traditionally, healthcare professionals have practiced in the silos of their perceived professional boundaries. Lack of communication and coordination of care has led to fragmentation, excess cost, and a healthcare system that is disease oriented rather than health oriented. In 1983, Bonnie Wesorick began work to address these issues, developing the Clinical Practice Model (CPM) Framework™ to create the best places to give and receive care. One goal of the CPM Framework was to unravel the complexity of factors impacting healthcare culture in a holistic framework with an

EXEMPLAR 8-1 The Impact of Interprofessional Collaboration and Information Technology Innovation to Improve Healthcare Outcomes

Abby Winterberg, DNP, APRN, FNP-BC

As a nurse practitioner in a pediatric preanesthesia consult clinic, I am passionate about ensuring that each patient has the best perioperative experience and outcome. With my prior background as a research assistant in the basic sciences, I aspired to not only deliver exceptional care, but also to develop new solutions that would improve patient experiences, quality of care, and outcomes. The DNP program offered the perfect opportunity to develop skills for my ideal role through mastery of the DNP *Essentials*, particularly interprofessional collaboration and information technology. My DNP project focused on the development and implementation of an electronic tool for documenting pediatric behavioral responses to anesthesia inductions. This initially seemed like a simple challenge with a straightforward solution. In reality, effective execution of the project required in-depth knowledge of the scientific literature, collaboration with experts in the field of anesthesia, development of staff education, partnering with a PhD researcher to develop a staff survey/metrics, and collaboration with our electronic health records team. The interprofessional approach to development was successful, as the tool was recently validated and it continues to be a sustainable method for electronic documentation nearly 4 years after implementation.

I wanted to continue the type of work I was doing during the DNP program after graduation, but found there was no role in my department for an advanced practice registered nurse (APRN) doing this type of work. Towards the end of my doctoral program, I requested a one-on-one meeting with the anesthesia chief. I shared the in-depth project work that was completed during my DNP program and highlighted the skills that could benefit our department. I expressed my desire to continue working in our department, but that I aspired to have a combined role in clinical care and quality improvement/research. After a few additional discussions with the anesthesia chief and our director of research, we created an innovative role for an advanced practice DNP-prepared nurse.

Since graduating in 2015, I have been principal investigator on five grants that have spanned many clinical-practice focused projects. Projects have included conducting multiple studies, including validation of the tool developed during my DNP program and an observational study to generate practice guidelines for patients with developmental/behavioral diagnoses. Studies have been accomplished through partnerships with PhD-prepared scientists, statisticians, and anesthesiologists with expert practice knowledge. Currently I am leading a project that focuses on developing a new application (app)/device for patient use preoperatively. This project has required internal and external collaborations, including team members with expertise in anesthesia, design, videography, engineering, and computer programming.

While working with colleagues from many different professions, I have often had to adapt to using new technologies. I have also had to develop creative ways to share my ideas. My DNP program placed a strong emphasis on the use of technology in our coursework, making the process of learning new technologies second nature. The ability to quickly learn new technologies, particularly different apps, has been exceptionally useful. Apps have enabled me to create short movies, develop animations and storyboards, and even learn basic computer coding skills to create a prototype app. The technology and informatics skills acquired during my DNP program have undoubtedly enabled success in my current role.

(continues)

EXEMPLAR 8-1 The Impact of Interprofessional Collaboration and Information Technology Innovation to Improve Healthcare Outcomes   *(continued)*

The unique preparation acquired during the DNP program enables DNP-prepared nurses to be leaders and strong collaborators across many disciplines. As front-line clinicians, DNP-prepared nurses have an optimal vantage point to develop and implement innovative solutions to complex healthcare challenges. The competencies and skills learned during the DNP program are key components that allow clinicians to adapt and effectively lead in an ever-changing technological and healthcare environment.

integrated team approach rather than focusing only on individual issues in patient care (Elsevier Professional Practice Services, 2018).

Today, the Elsevier CPM Framework™ is implemented in hundreds of acute care settings in North America. Elsevier's CPM Framework is founded on core beliefs, healthcare-related theories, and principles that describe the nature of the work and the actions steps necessary to transform health care at points of care (Wesorick & Doebbeling, 2011). The patient, family, community, and caregiver are at the core of the model because they are impacted by transformational change and their stories live at the center of the healthcare experience (see **FIGURE 8-1**). This framework is designed to assist practitioners to focus on practice priorities, evidence-based clinical decision support, and practice expertise to ensure improved patient outcomes, compliance with national patient safety standards, and an overall improvement in interprofessional staff collaboration and satisfaction. The CPM Framework also contains a health informatics model and includes more than 400 evidence-based clinical practice guidelines, which are rigorously researched and leveled to support professional scopes of practice and care processes across health professions (Troseth, Mayo, Nieves, & Lambrecht, 2017). The CPM Framework provides a way to document professional processes of care and creates practice and content interoperability. Collaboration on driving big data analysis will become more valuable as the ability to perform data extraction from electronic health records evolves. The value of this framework is that it is scalable, data driven, and replicable, and supports sharable and comparable data (Christopherson, Troseth, & Clingerman, 2015).

Fundamental knowledge used in the CPM Framework that enhances interdisciplinary communication and influences cultural and practice transformation includes dialogue, partnership, and polarity management. Many problems plaguing health care today are considered persistent, reoccurring, dilemmas, paradoxes, dualities, tensions, or *wicked problems*, and contain more than one right answer. It is important to prioritize polarity management as a first step in managing healthcare issues that are not actually problems to solve (Johnson, 1992). Polarities involve interdependent pairs of values or points of view. Polarity thinking invites the various disciplines to look at a health dilemma from different, often opposing, points of view when there is tension between two "sides" and when the issue cannot be fixed by choosing one or the other. This way of thinking encourages professionals to consider a "both/and" perspective and enhances communication as team members appreciate and work through paradoxes or dilemmas (see **TABLE 8-1**).

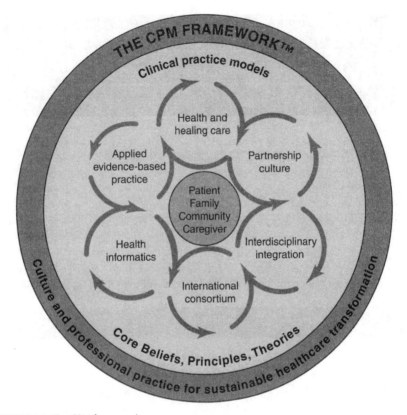

FIGURE 8-1 The CPM framework.

Reproduced from The CPM Framework™: (Professional Practices Services, 2018) Culture and professional practice for sustainable healthcare transformation [Brochure], Elsevier CPM Resource Center. Copyright Elsevier (2011).

Many of the cultural shadows that haunt us today and prevent us from reaching a higher ground of a healthy work culture and integrated care are the result of trying to fix problems that are really polarities (Wesorick, 2002). Wesorick also encourages the DNP-prepared nurse to be aware of the polarity of individual "task" AND "scope of practice," which can divide members from different health professions who are trying to work together. The team leader must be clear on each profession's scope of practice to effectively lead the team (Wesorick, 2014, 2016).

This is a challenge for the team leader but it is essential to break silos of professionals trying to protect their domains, yet attain an integrated competency of working together as a team. The ultimate goal is to bring each profession's expertise together to benefit the individual patient, society, and the healthcare delivery system (Wesorick, 2014).

Bonnie Wesorick is a pioneer in interprofessional nursing practice and embodies the leadership reflected in the DNP *Essentials* that enhances the nursing profession. Her work began and continues in the clinical setting and reflects the impact of scholarly practice.

The RWJF (2015) has identified exemplar healthcare organizations that have embraced interprofessional collaboration and published best practices in their report *Lessons from the Field: Promising Interprofessional Collaboration Practices*. Key

TABLE 8-1 Polarity Thinking™	
Polarity Thinking	
"LIFE" Polarities	
Home life	Work life
Activity	Rest
Self	Others
Candor	Diplomacy
Gentle love	Tough love
Yin	Yang
"Healthcare" Polarities	
Framework-driven change	Project/Initiative-driven change
Autonomous care	Standardized care
Integrated competency	Individual competency
Mission	Margin
Hospital interest	Physician interest
Staff satisfaction	Patient satisfaction
Patient safety	Staff freedom

Reprinted with permission from Elsevier CPM Resource Center and Polarity Management Associates. All rights reserved.

findings from the report show that successful interprofessional collaboration models include:

- Putting patients first
- Demonstrating leadership commitment to interprofessional collaboration as an organizational priority through words and actions
- Creating a level playing field that enables team members to work at the top of their license, know their roles, and understand the value they contribute
- Cultivating effective team communication
- Exploring the use of organizational structure to hardwire interprofessional practice

DNP students can use these principles of integrated clinical models and interprofessional collaborative best practices during their immersion experiences and in implementing their DNP projects.

What Type of Information is Needed?

The gathering of resources includes identifying the gaps in knowledge that the student may need to inform the DNP project. The DNP student may need to look outside the nursing profession to other disciplinary fields to inform the development of the DNP project question. For example, in preparing for this author's DNP project regarding the use of standardized nursing language in the electronic health record (EHR), independent study was needed in the area of nursing standardized language, healthcare informatics, and the development and function of the EHR. This preparation involved collaborating with nursing informatics experts in an independent study class, as well as working with information technology experts at a national conference of EHR vendors. Nursing informatics is a rapidly developing field, and the independent study allowed an in-depth exploration of the current status of the visibility of nursing practice reflected in electronic documentation. Learning the new technical language of information technology allowed dialogue with EHR vendors to understand how advanced practice nurses can be involved in asking for the tools, such as reference terminologies available in EHRs, to reflect nursing language and nursing care. This DNP project was published in the *Journal of the American Academy of Nurse Practitioners* (Conrad, Hanson, Hasenau, & Stocker-Schneider, 2012).

Other types of information needed by the DNP student can be provided by business, management, and statistical professionals, as well as professionals in other healthcare disciplines. For example, to explore the feasibility of purchasing new equipment to relieve pressure ulcers in the hospitalized patient used in a safety study, the DNP student may need to gather information from equipment vendors, budget office personnel (for funding), and clinicians who may use the equipment on the clinical units. The DNP student will need a broad lens to explore his or her chosen field of study to narrow down the clinical question to be studied. Gathering the resources and interacting with other members of the identified team provide an opportunity for the DNP student to practice interprofessional competencies, including leadership and communication skills. Faculty mentors and the DNP student's project team can assist in identifying and linking the student with the appropriate resources needed to inform the project. The DNP student will continue to perfect these skills as the project matures in the context of his or her clinical immersion experiences.

> *What type of information is needed to complete the DNP project? Answering this question may involve investigation and study in other disciplinary fields.*

Where and When Does Collaboration Take Place?

Gathering the team together, particularly in the planning and implementation phases of the project, will likely take place during the immersion experience in the facility chosen to implement the DNP project. During this time, the DNP student will use the organizational evaluation techniques learned in DNP core courses, as well as implement change theory techniques if the project involves a practice intervention.

Evaluation of the culture of the organization is critical to not only identifying clinical problems, but also to designing and implementing a successful clinical intervention. Several tools are available for assessing organizational culture (see Chapter 13, The DNP Project Toolbox, for organizational assessment tools). These types of tools assign a score to organizations for current and future assessments in areas such as organizational

> *When and where to implement an intervention in a DNP project may be guided by the collaborating team.*

leadership, management of employees, and strategic emphases. Organizational assessments are essential for the student to evaluate the phenomenon of interest or problem in the context of the organizational need. The organizational assessment also includes determining organizational potential for change with a DNP project intervention. The DNP student will need to approach the organizational assessment with a broad lens by first identifying the key stakeholders in the organization. Engaging key members of an organization such as administrators, financial personnel, providers, and staff is important to the success of a project. For example, a DNP student who is working with a home healthcare organization for implementation of a nurse practitioner on staff will need to not only evaluate the existing organizational structure for support for the new position, but also assess financial viability, the collaborative resources available to the advanced practice nurse, and needs of the population to be served (See Chapter 6, Developing the DNP Project, for more information on performing an organizational assessment).

The team that the DNP student gathers can have a formal or informal structure. An example of a formal team is the DNP project team (see Chapter 9, The DNP Project Team). Informal members of the team can be people whom the DNP student consults to plan and implement a project within an organization. This could be the nursing manager of a unit or a nurse informatics specialist whom the student will consult to inform various aspects of project implementation.

After identifying the organizational structure and the individuals who will be part of the collaborating team for the DNP project, the student then embarks on implementing the project. Change theory can guide the DNP student in planning

> *The DNP project allows the DNP student to practice and refine skills on how to lead a collaborative team.*

TABLE 8-2 Examples of Change Theory	
Model	**Components of the Change Theory**
Lewin/Schein's Change Theory (Wirth, 2004)	Stage 1: Become motivated to change (unfreezing). Stage 2: Change what needs to be changed (unfrozen and moving to a new state). Stage 3: Make the change permanent (refreezing).
Kotter's 8-Step Change Model (Kotter, 1996)	Step 1: Create urgency. Step 2: Form a powerful coalition. Step 3: Create a vision for change. Step 4: Communicate the vision. Step 5: Remove obstacles. Step 6: Create short-term "wins." Step 7: Build on the change. Step 8: Anchor the change in corporate culture.

and implementing the intervention. **TABLE 8-2** features just two examples of many change theories that can be used in understanding the process of change.

When and where to implement the change may be influenced by the DNP student's collaborating team based on the assessment of the organization. Ash, Miller, and Zaccagnini (2017) cautioned that even a desirable change can meet resistance by the team members and other members of the organization. DNP-prepared nurses must be change agents for successful collaboration and understand and apply various change theories to accomplish collaborative team goals.

How to Accomplish a Successful DNP Project Using Collaboration

The skill set of leading successful interprofessional teams is multifaceted and involves specific competencies to be attained by the DNP student.

In response to the IOM's (2001) call for improvement by the healthcare professions in addressing the American healthcare delivery system, the National Center for Healthcare Leadership (2017) defined leadership competencies for medicine, nursing, and administration. The model consists of three domains—*transformation, execution,* and *people*—that "capture the complexity and dynamic quality of the health leader's role and reflect the dynamic realities in health leadership today" (p. 3). Each domain has specific competencies related to that domain to further outline the specific skill set needed by the healthcare leader (see **FIGURE 8-2**).

In 2011, the Interprofessional Education Collaborative (IPEC) first released *Core Competencies for Interprofessional Collaborative Practice,* a report that outlined action strategies to support implementation of the interprofessional education competencies. In 2016, the report was updated to organize the competencies within a singular domain of Interprofessional Collaboration, encompassing the topics of

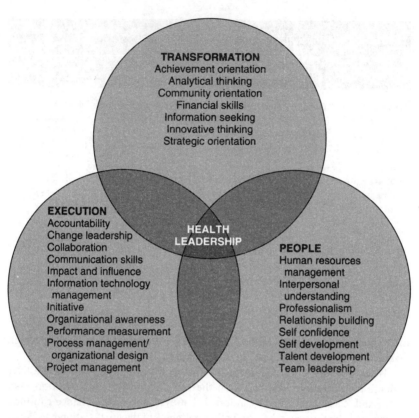

FIGURE 8-2 NCHL Health Leadership Competency Model™.
Reproduced with permission from the National Center for Healthcare Leadership.

values and ethics, roles and responsibilities, interprofessional communication, and teams and teamwork. The IPEC competencies also reflect the IOM's goals for interprofessional care delivery and include:

Competency 1: Work with individuals of other professions to maintain a climate of mutual respect and shared values. (Values/Ethics for Interprofessional Practice)

Competency 2: Use the knowledge of one's own role and those of other professions to appropriately assess and address the healthcare needs of patients and to promote and advance the health of populations. (Roles/Responsibilities)

Competency 3: Communicate with patients, families, communities, and professionals in health and other fields in a responsive and responsible manner that supports a team approach to the promotion and maintenance of health and the prevention and treatment of disease. (Interprofessional Communication)

Competency 4: Apply relationship-building values and the principles of team dynamics to perform effectively in different team roles to plan, deliver, and evaluate patient/population-centered care and population health programs and policies that are safe, timely, efficient, effective, and equitable (Teams and Teamwork). (IPEC, 2016, p. 10)

The opportunity to develop and practice these competencies arises within the process of the DNP project. Developing a successful collaborative team requires progress through various stages of team development, according to Tuckman and Jensen (1977). The stages include teams progressing through phases of *forming, storming, norming, performing,* and *adjourning.* See Chapter 10, Creating and Developing the Project Plan, for a detailed discussion of each phase.

The DNP student can address the following factors to assist the team to achieve the DNP project goals:

- *Shared purpose, goal, and buy-in of members:* The DNP student must be clear on articulating the purpose of his or her project in relation to the benefits to the patients, members of the team, and organization.
- *Reciprocal trust in team members:* The DNP student will utilize the immersion experience in the organization to foster a culture of trust and transparency.
- *Recognition and value of the unique role or skills each team member brings:* Respect for team members and modeling this behavior by the DNP student allows for successful interaction with and among team members.
- *Functioning at the highest level of skill, ability, or practice:* The DNP student has the opportunity to utilize clinical expertise in formulating and implementing a scholarly practice innovation and can model the aim of the *Future of Nursing's* (IOM, 2010) call for nurses to practice to the full extent of their education and training.
- *Clear understanding of roles and the responsibilities of team members to meet goals:* The DNP student must use high-level communication skills throughout the project to ensure that each team member understands his or her role in completing the project. This can decrease conflict and uncertainty among team members and enhance timely completion of the project.
- *Work culture and environment that embrace the collaborative process:* The DNP student's evaluation of organizational culture and environment is necessary to identify barriers to implementing and completing the project and enlist the help of the team to overcome the barriers.
- *Collective cognitive responsibility and shared decision making:* The DNP student is the leader of his or her project team but must enlist the aid of team members for timely and appropriate decision making during all aspects of the project process.

The DNP core courses provide the opportunity to explore leadership competencies. The DNP student will refine leadership skills in clinical practice as well as in the completion of the scholarly project. Dr. Stephanie Brady outlines many of these competencies in the following description of her DNP project (see **EXEMPLAR 8-2**).

EXEMPLAR 8-2 The Impact of Mindfulness Meditation on a Culture of Safety on an Inpatient Psychiatric Unit

Stephanie Brady, DNP, APRN-BC

My project, "The Impact of Mindfulness Meditation on a Culture of Safety on an Inpatient Psychiatric Unit," involved the implementation of a 6-week program on mindfulness meditation for a multidisciplinary team that worked on an inpatient adult psychiatric unit. The premise was that if we could teach the multidisciplinary teams how to be present for patients, we would see a decrease in the number of falls, a reduction in the number of patient incidents of aggression, and an increase in patient satisfaction. The mindfulness meditation class was conducted weekly for an hour along with daily homework assignments. The class size was limited to a maximum of 15 participants. Staff were required to attend every session for the 6-week time frame. The multidisciplinary team included physicians, nurses, social workers, mental health technicians, and recreational therapists. The outcome metrics were gathered for the period 6 months before the class and the 6 months post-class. I was able to demonstrate a clinically significant reduction in patient falls, a decrease in the number of patient aggressive incidents, and a significant increase in patient satisfaction.

This project required me to work closely with the nurse manager of the inpatient unit to facilitate the scheduling of the interested staff, the psychologist who was teaching the class, the nurse who is the risk manager for the facility, the recreational therapist for the room space, and the psychiatrists for their buy-in to the project. Although advice was provided by my DNP committee, the operational perspective of the project really fell to me for implementation. In my role in behavioral health within our health system, I interact on a daily basis with the interdisciplinary team.

This study was published in the *Perspectives of Psychiatric Care* in 2012 (Brady, O'Connor, Burgermeister, & Hanson, 2012). As a result, there has been continued interest in this topic from other health professionals. A replication study was completed on a child and adolescent inpatient unit and was published in 2014 in the *Journal of Child and Adolescent Psychiatric Nursing* (Hallman, O'Connor, Hasenau, & Brady, 2014). While my work in the organization is now in other areas, clinicians have embraced the topic of mindfulness and the culture of safety and expanded the focus to many other areas of health care.

▶ Summary

The complexity of health care requires innovative approaches to solve the multifaceted health issues of individuals and populations. Healthcare professionals must work together to change the current linear disease-oriented care system to new models in which all disciplines are contributing specialized skills and abilities that allow them to practice to the full scope of their education and training. However, high-level communication and leadership skills are needed to form and guide the team to function at each individual professional's highest level to accomplish a goal. See **TABLE 8-3** for interprofessional and leadership resources. In this way, the collaborative team can contribute to high-quality, cost-effective, and safe patient-centered care (Ash, Miller, & Zaccagnini, 2017). The DNP-prepared nurse begins to actualize this skill set in carrying out the DNP project in the context of interprofessional and intraprofessional collaboration.

Resource	**Purpose**	**For More Information**
Robert Wood Johnson Project on Interprofessional Collaboration: Promising Interprofessional Collaboration Practices (2015)	Identifying and spreading practices to enable effective interprofessional collaboration	www.rwjf.org/en/library /research/2015/03/ lessons-from-the-field .html
Clinical Practice Model (CPM)	A clinical framework to integrate evidence-based practice with multiple disciplines to improve patient care	www.elsevier.com /solutions/care-planning
NCHL Health Leadership Competency Model	Defined health leadership competencies for multiple health disciplines	http://nchl.org/static .asp?path=2852,3238
Texas A&M Health Science Center Interprofessional Education & Research: Core Competencies for Interprofessional Collaborative Practice	Defined interprofessional education competencies	www.tamhsc.edu/ipe /research/ipec-2016 -core-competencies.pdf

TABLE 8-3 Interprofessional and Leadership Resources

Impact

- Successful interprofessional, collaborative teams are transforming healthcare delivery. Dissemination of DNP projects incorporating evidence-based interventions can lead to replication in other organizations and populations, generating evidence-based knowledge.
- Read more about mindfulness-based stress reduction (MBSR) classes for interprofessional staff to decrease stress levels and improve their self-care, resulting in improved patient care, in:
  - Brady, S., O'Connor, N., Burgermeister, D, & Hanson, P. (2012). The impact of mindfulness meditation in promoting a culture of safety on an acute psychiatric unit. *Perspectives of Psychiatric Care, 48*(3), 129–137. doi: 10.1111/j.1744-6163.2011.00315.x
  - Hallman, I. S., O'Connor, N., Hasenau, S., & Brady, S. (2014). Improving the culture of safety on a high-acuity inpatient child/adolescent psychiatric unit by mindfulness-based stress reduction training of staff. *Journal of Child and Adolescent Psychiatric Nursing, 27*(4), 183–189. doi: 10.1111 /jcap.12091

- Read more about Dr. Winterberg's development and implementation of an electronic tool for documenting pediatric behavioral responses to anesthesia inductions in:
  - Winterberg, A. V., Colella, C. L, Weber, K. A., & Varughese, A. M. (2018). The child induction behavioral assessment tool: A tool to facilitate the electronic documentation of behavioral responses to anesthesia inductions. *Journal of Perianesthesia Nursing, 33*(3), 296–303.e1. doi: 10.1016/j.jopan.2016.10.004

Key Messages

- The DNP student is expected to model doctoral-level leadership skills in forming and leading interprofessional and intraprofessional teams to accomplish the DNP project.
- *Who* will be needed for the DNP project team can include members from the nursing profession and members from outside the profession.
- *What* types of information are needed to complete the DNP project may involve investigation and study in other disciplinary fields.
- *When and where* to implement an intervention in a DNP project may be guided by the collaborating team.
- The DNP project allows the DNP student to practice and refine skills and competencies on *how* to lead a collaborative team.

Action Plan—Next Steps

1. In selecting the phenomenon of interest or the DNP project, identify gaps in the knowledge and skills needed to formulate the question and design, implement, and evaluate the scholarly practice inquiry.
2. Gather resources and faculty members who can assist in filling the knowledge and skill gaps, keeping in mind that consultation with other disciplines and organizational members will be needed.
3. Consider professional development in other areas of study to broaden the knowledge base needed to complete the project.
4. Study and practice the leadership skill competencies needed to participate and lead interprofessional teams.
5. Formalize the relationship of faculty mentors and other team members with the formation of the DNP project team or other advising structure recommended by the university or college of nursing.
6. Begin relationship building with potential team members within the immersion experience organization.

References

American Association of Colleges of Nursing (AACN). (2006). *The essentials of doctoral education for advanced nursing practice.* Retrieved from http://www.aacnnursing.org/Portals/42/Publications /DNPEssentials.pdf

American Association of Colleges of Nursing (AACN). (2015). *The doctor of nursing practice: Current issues and clarifying recommendations.* Retrieved from https://www.pncb.org/sites/default /files/2017-02/AACN_DNP_Recommendations.pdf

Ash, L., Miller, C., & Zaccagnini, M. E. (2017). Interprofessional collaboration for improving patient and population health. In S. M. DeNisco & A. M. Barker (Eds.), *Advanced practice nursing* (3rd ed., pp. 123–152). Burlington, MA: Jones & Bartlett Learning.

Brady, S., O'Connor, N., Burgermeister, D., & Hanson, P. (2012). The impact of mindfulness meditation in promoting a culture of safety on an acute psychiatric unit. *Perspectives of Psychiatric Care, 48*(3), 129–137. doi: 10.1111/j.1744-6163.2011.00315.x

Carlson, E. A., Staffileno, B. A., & Murphy, M. P. (2017). Promoting DNP-PhD collaboration in doctoral education: Forming a DNP project team. *Journal of Professional Nursing.* Retrieved from https://doi.org/10.1016/j.profnurs.2017.12.011

Christopherson, T., Troseth, M., & Clingerman, E. (2015). Informatics-enabled interprofessional education and collaborative practice: a framework-driven approach. *Journal of Interprofessional Education in Practice,* 1(*1*),10–15. doi.org/10.1016/j.xjep.2015.03.002

Clinton, P., & Sperhac, A. M. (2009). The DNP and unintended consequences: An opportunity for dialogue. *Journal of Pediatric Health, 23*(5), 348–351. doi:10.1016/ j.pedhc.2009.06.004

Collaborate. (2018). *Merriam-Webster's Online Dictionary.* Retrieved from http://www.merriam -webster.com/dictionary/collaborate

Conrad, D., Hanson, P. A., Hasenau, S. M., & Stocker-Schneider, J. (2012). Identifying the barriers to use of standardized nursing language in the electronic health record by the ambulatory care nurse practitioner. *Journal of the American Academy of Nurse Practitioners, 24*(7), 443–451. doi:10.1111/j.1745-7599.2012.00705x

Cronenwett, L., Dracup, K., Grey, M., McCauley, L., Melies, A., & Salmon, M. (2011). The doctor of nursing practice: A national workforce perspective. *Nursing Outlook, 59,* 9–17. doi:10.1016/j .outlook.2010.11.003

D'Amour, D., & Oandasan, I. (2005). Interprofessionality as the field of interprofessional practice and interprofessional education: An emerging concept. *Journal of Interprofessional Care, 19*(Suppl 1), 8–20.

Draye, M. A., Acker, M., & Zimmer, P. A. (2006). The practice doctorate in nursing: Approaches to transform nurse practitioner education and practice. *Nursing Outlook, 54*(3), 123–129.

Elsevier Professional Practice Services (2018). *The Elsevier clinical practice model framework.* Retrieved from https://www.elsevier.com/solutions/care-planning/professional-practice-services

Hallman, I. S., O'Connor, N., Hasenau, S., & Brady, S. (2014). Improving the culture of safety on a high-acuity inpatient child/adolescent psychiatric unit by mindfulness-based stress reduction training of staff. *Journal of Child and Adolescent Psychiatric Nursing, 27*(4), 183–189. doi: 10.1111/jcap.12091

Institute of Medicine (IOM). (2001). *Crossing the quality chasm: A new health system for the 21st century.* Washington, DC: National Academies Press. Retrieved from http://www.nationalacademies.org /hmd/~/media/Files/Report%20Files/2001/Crossing-the-Quality-Chasm/Quality%20Chasm%20 2001%20%20report%20brief.pdf

Institute of Medicine (IOM). (2003). *Health professions education: A bridge to quality.* Washington, DC: National Academies Press. Retrieved from http://www.nap.edu/openbook.php?record_id =10681&page=45

Institute of Medicine (IOM). (2010). *The future of nursing: Leading change, advancing health.* Washington, DC: National Academies Press.

Interprofessional Education Collaborative (IPEC) (2016). *Core competencies for interprofessional collaborative practice: 2016 update.* Retrieved from https://www.tamhsc.edu/ipe/research/ipec -2016-core-competencies.pdf

Johnson, B. (1992). *Polarity management, identifying and managing unsolvable problems.* Amherst, MA: HRD Press.

Kotter, J. P. (1996). *Leading change.* Boston, MA: Harvard Business School Press.

Lait, J., Suter, E., Arthur, N., & Deutschlander, S. (2011). Interprofessional mentoring: Enhancing students' clinical learning. *Nurse Education in Practice, 11,* 211–215. doi:10.1016/j.nepr.2010 .10.005

Nancarrow, S., Booth, A., Ariss, S., Smith, T., Enderby, P., & Roots, A. (2013), Ten principles of good interdisciplinary work. *Human Resources for Health, 11*(19). doi: 10.1186/1478-4491-11-19

National Center for Healthcare Leadership (NCHL). (2017). *National Center for Healthcare Leadership competency model summary.* Retrieved from http://www.nchl.org/static.asp?path =2852,3238

Reeves, S., Perrier, L., Goldman, J., Freeth, D., & Zwarenstein, M. (2013). Interprofessional education: Effects on professional practice and healthcare outcomes (update). *Cochrane Database of Systematic Reviews,* CD002213. doi: 10.1002/14651858.CD002213.pub3

Robert Wood Johnson Foundation (RWJF). (2015). *Lessons from the field: Promising interprofessional collaboration practices.* Princeton, NJ: Author. Retrieved from https://www.michigan.gov /documents/mdch/Lessons_from_the_Field-Promising_Interprofessional_Collaboration _Practices_486256_7.pdf

Troseth, M., Mayo, D., Nieves, R., & Lambrecht, S. (2017). Case Study 12.1: Clinical practice model (CPM) framework approach to achieve clinical practice interoperability and big data comparative analysis. In C. W. Delaney, C. A. Weaver, J. J. Warren, T. R. Clancy, and R. L. Simpson (Eds.). *Big data enabled nursing: Education, research and practice* (pp. 244–251). Cham, Switzerland: Springer International Publishing. doi: 10.1007/978-3-319-53300-1

Tuckman, B. W., & Jensen, M. A. C. (1977). Stages of small-group development revisited. *Group & Organizational Management, 2*(4), 410–427. doi:10.1177/105960117700200404

Wagner, J., Liston, B., & Miller, J. (2011). Developing interprofessional communication skills. *Teaching and Learning in Nursing, 6,* 97–101. doi:10.1016/j.teln.2010.12.003

Wesorick, B. (2002). 21st century leadership challenge: Creating and sustaining healthy healing work cultures and integrated service at the point of care. *Nursing Administration Quarterly, 26*(5), 18–32.

Wesorick, B. (2014). Polarity thinking: An essential skill for those leading interprofessional integration. *Journal of Interprofessional Healthcare, 1*(1), 1–17. Retrieved from http://www.jihonline.org/jih /vol1/iss1/12.

Wesorick, B. (2016). *Polarity thinking in healthcare: The missing logic to achieve transformation.* Amherst, MA: HRD Press.

Wesorick, B., & Doebbeling, B. (2011). Lessons from the field: The essential elements for point-of-care transformation. *Medical Care, 49*(12, Suppl 1), S49–S58.

Winterberg, A. V., Colella, C. L, Weber, K. A., & Varughese, A.M. (2018). The child induction behavioral assessment tool: A tool to facilitate the electronic documentation of behavioral responses to anesthesia inductions. *Journal of Perianesthesia Nursing, 33*(3), 296–303.e1. doi: 10.1016/j.jopan.2016.10.004

Wirth, R. A. (2004). *Lewin/Schein's change theory.* Retrieved from http://www.entarga.com /orgchange/lewinschein.pdf

CHAPTER 9

The DNP Project Team

Marisa L. Wilson, Shannon Idzik, and Dianne Conrad

CHAPTER OVERVIEW

According to the American Association of Colleges of Nursing (AACN), as of 2017, 344 programs were enrolling students into doctor of nursing practice (DNP) programs with 124 programs in the planning stages (AACN, 2018). In 2017, approximately 29,000 students were enrolled in DNP programs nationwide (AACN, 2018). Some of these students are progressing from baccalaureate preparation, earning an advanced specialty as they move through their course work (see Chapter 2, Defining the Doctor of Nursing Practice: Current Trends); others are entering DNP programs after having earned a master's degree. All of these programs produce nurse leaders who are uniquely prepared to bridge the gap between the discovery of new knowledge and the scholarship of translation, application, implementation, evaluation, and dissemination of impact (AACN, 2006). The DNP project is a demonstration of what the DNP student has achieved with his or her newly acquired skills and knowledge. The breadth of the project must be distinguishable from projects conducted by baccalaureate and master's students. Guiding and assisting these students to achieve this goal is a responsibility of faculty members.

Many DNP programs require faculty members and other disciplinary experts to serve on a project team to guide the student through the DNP project process. According to the AACN (2015), the project team should consist of a DNP student or group of DNP students with a minimum of a doctorally prepared faculty member (project faculty mentor) and a practice mentor. The project faculty mentor, along with the project team, will oversee the project, ensuring that the topic, processes, and timelines stay within school policy and procedure and that the final product is at an acceptable level of rigor for the degree and the program. This chapter outlines the purpose, roles, and function of the DNP project team. The DNP student's role in refining the leadership competencies and collaborating with members within and outside the nursing profession, beginning with the DNP project team members, is discussed. Finally, alternatives to the traditional academic committee structure are presented, as outlined in the DNP Task Force recommendations, (AACN, 2015) to provide efficient use of resources and support student learning.

CHAPTER OBJECTIVES

After completing the chapter, the learner will be able to:

1. Discern the differences between a DNP project and a dissertation or thesis.
2. Explore the role of the DNP project team and project faculty mentor in the project completion process.
3. Formulate plans for project team and project faculty mentor interactions and management.

▶ Thesis, Dissertation, and the DNP Project

A graduate student demonstrates mastery of the core essentials of a program of study in a variety of ways. Presentation, scholarly writing, and article development are just a few. The thesis, dissertation, and DNP project are usually culminating demonstrations of knowledge, competencies, and skills attained through a program of study. Some DNP students may be familiar with a master's thesis, having completed one during a previous program of study. DNP students are also usually familiar with doctoral dissertations because they probably see the rigorous process their PhD peers undergo as they pursue completion of this work. In addition, DNP students must demonstrate proficiency and integration of required competencies in the completion of a rigorous DNP project. Both the student and the faculty guiding these graduate students can find themselves having difficulty with differentiation between these products. What are the purposes of and differences among the thesis, dissertation, and DNP project? The detailed answers lie in the individual university or college student handbook. Students are encouraged to review and discuss that information with their project faculty mentor or advisor; however, there are some basic purposes and differences.

In the context of academic studies, the definition of *thesis* and *dissertation* is a written, formal document that supports the student's candidacy for a degree. The *thesis* may be the term used for this product at the master's level in some universities, whereas the term *dissertation* often refers to a written document produced in the framework of doctoral studies, advancing a new point of view resulting from research (DifferenceBetween.net, 2018). The DNP project is the deliverable that demonstrates the student's achievement of the eight DNP *Essentials of Doctoral Education for Advanced Nursing Practice*, as outlined by the American Association of Colleges of Nursing. The final DNP project should demonstrate "synthesis of the student's work" and lay the groundwork for future scholarship (AACN, 2006, p. 20). The common theme is that the main purpose of the thesis, dissertation, and DNP project is to serve as a tangible demonstration of skills and competencies that integrates each through a culminating experience.

The products of a program of study move the frontiers of knowledge and answer a contestable question.

The competencies to be demonstrated in the final work are different among the nursing practice, doctorate, and the research doctorate. Gardenier and Stanik-Hutt (2010) explain that DNP students are prepared to transform health through leadership and evidence-based practice within a transdisciplinary environment. Therefore, in order to make an impact in health care delivery and health outcomes, DNP students need to be able to analyze and use evidence, use clinical information systems, influence health policy, and lead teams. Since nurse researchers are educated as scientists, they need preparation in theory construction, research methodology, and must have a comprehensive understanding of statistics.

Therefore, the purpose and content of a product to demonstrate the competencies of a research versus a practice doctorate can be different, but equally rigorous. The thesis, dissertation, and DNP project are also used as a means for faculty to judge whether a student has mastered a body of knowledge. Each is meant to provide novel intellectual contributions to a field. Each of these products of a program of study moves the frontiers of knowledge further and answers a contestable question.

A major difference among a thesis, a dissertation, and a DNP project in some cases lies in the method of inquiry. In a thesis or dissertation, graduate students propose a research study in which data are collected, analyzed, and reported in the final product. With a dissertation, one is engaged in original research work, whereas a thesis can require an analysis of secondary information (perhaps faculty provided). The dissertation is based on the student's own background research about a topic, whereas a thesis provides arguments to defend a standpoint or hypothesis. The thesis or dissertation will often have a broader scope than a DNP project. The DNP project may have a more narrow area or topic because of its practice and translation nature. The thesis and dissertation are also solo activities, whereas the DNP project may be accomplished in a group. See Chapter 3, Scholarship in Practice, for an in-depth discussion of what qualifies as a DNP project.

The DNP project also must address a complex practice, process, or system problem in a real-world practice setting that is having a deleterious effect on patients or populations (AACN, 2006). The DNP student must evaluate the impact of the intervention on the target group. Waldrop, Caruso, Fuchs, and Hypes (2014) offer that this project must do the following:

1. Enhance health outcomes, practice outcomes, or health policy.
2. Reflect a culmination of practice inquiry with the student becoming an expert on the problem.
3. Require engagement of partnerships.
4. Implement and translate evidence into practice.
5. Evaluate health care, practice, or policy outcomes.

This will require that the project team consist of those faculty who are, first and foremost, secure in the parameters of the DNP project, but who also understand the problem being addressed. In addition, the faculty team mentor must be able to advise the student in the evidence-based practice process, through organizational change and leadership of interprofessional teams, and on evaluation processes. The complexity and scale of these projects will vary, but the faculty lead has a responsibility to ensure that every graduate will have the skills and experience needed to bridge the research practice gap.

The DNP project starts with a thorough literature review that addresses a problem or issue. This literature synthesis is followed by a discussion describing the unique contribution that the student intends to make in addressing the problem or issue in his or her professional endeavors. The student then describes a translational process meant to address the problem or issue (the project plan), implements the plan, and follows this with an evaluation of the implementation and a plan for disseminating the findings. (See Chapter 10, Creating and Developing the Project Plan.) Often the DNP project includes specific recommendations or offers materials that can be used in implementing the proposed method of addressing the problem or issue. The average length of time required to complete the DNP project will vary, but it may take a year or longer to complete. However, the DNP student must note that some colleges and universities require the project to be completed in a prescribed number of semesters. The DNP student should carefully ascertain his or her university's requirements for project completion.

▶ Choosing the DNP Project Faculty Mentor and Project Team Members

Composition of the team of individuals responsible for mentoring the doctoral student through their final scholarly academic work varies depending on degree and college/university policy. The challenges associated with mentoring DNP students and PhD students differ. The number of students seeking the DNP degree has grown exponentially over the past 10 years, with over four times as many students enrolled in DNP programs (29,093) as are enrolled in PhD programs (6090) (AACN, 2018). Simply identifying an adequate number of qualified faculty to mentor DNP student projects has become a challenge for many DNP programs. In many schools, the admission criteria are less likely to require that the student be matched exactly with a faculty member's area of scholarship. This is an advantage for the admission process but has led to DNP cohorts with diverse practice interests that are more difficult to match to the skills of the current faculty.

Membership also varies between DNP project teams and PhD committees. Research can often be done without significant community partnerships. For example, PhD students have opportunities to do bench research or secondary data analyses within the confines of the school. Nearly all DNP projects require community partners. Finding and forging these relationships can be a challenge for some practice doctoral students, although many DNP students may have practice connections that will overcome these difficulties. PhD committees almost always require the expertise of a statistician. Although some DNP projects require statisticians, it is less likely that they will be formal members of the DNP project team. If needed, a statistician may be an ad hoc member, a consultant, or a staff resource at the school. However, it is important to have current practice experts on DNP project teams, which may not be necessary on PhD committees. Because many DNP projects involve community partners, it is almost always necessary to have organizational members outside the school of nursing on DNP project teams.

It is important that all doctoral students be mentored through this rigorous process by experienced faculty mentors, both from the academic and practice sites.

The development of the project team (student and mentors) is a crucial part of the student's success. For some students, this mentoring will be formalized through a committee structure and process that may be regulated by the school of nursing or the graduate school, depending on which school awards the degree. Not all schools use a committee structure, and the student will be guided by the individual policies of the institution. However, for those that do, the size, requirements, and composition of this committee or project team are outlined in the doctoral student handbook and will vary from one school or university to another. According to AACN (2015), "the DNP Project team should consist of a student or a group of students with a minimum of a doctoral prepared faculty member and a practice mentor who may be from outside the university" (p. 5). The practice mentor is from the organization where the project will be implemented. The practice mentor provides organizational context to the project and guides the student through potential organizational hurdles. The practice mentor should have knowledge of the problem being addressed, but more importantly, should be someone with influence in the practice site.

▶ Forming the Project Team

Of utmost importance, the project team needs to be able to function as a whole, with each member bringing a skill set that will support the student to achieve the goal. Forming a cohesive and collegial team whose members will work together is vital to the success of the student. The first step is selecting the appropriate DNP project faculty mentor, who, as mentioned, should be a doctorally prepared member of the graduate faculty of the school of nursing. The student should consult the DNP project guidelines in their respective school for all requirements related to timing and selection criteria for the project faculty mentor and project team members. However, one of the first considerations, aside from the expertise of the faculty mentor, is that the student and the faculty mentor should have mutual respect for one another and should have positive regard toward each other (Magnan, 2019). Magnan (2019) indicated that the faculty member fulfilling this role must possess an interest in the topic; theoretical, methodological, or content expertise; and the wherewithal to get the student through the final project on time (p. 132).

The next step is for the student and the project faculty mentor to determine the skills and expertise needed within the project team to complete the DNP project and ensure success. The specific talents that will be needed are directly determined by the nature of the student's proposed work. Some questions to consider are:

1. Will this work be done in a specific organization?
2. Will a specific population be affected by the project?
3. Will the student need to implement certain tools, technologies, or guidelines?
4. Will there be a methodological or analytical process that requires certain expertise?
5. Will there be a need for statistical consultation?

The student will want a well-rounded team whose members have complementary areas of expertise. Choosing team members carefully will ensure that the student has the depth of knowledge available for a successful completion. The project faculty mentor and the student should also be familiar with the school policies regarding faculty affiliation when choosing members. Often schools will impose a maximum number of team members whose primary affiliation is outside the school or university.

"How does one find project team members?" is a question that a doctoral student may ask. Many schools have a list of faculty and their stated areas of expertise available

Forming a cohesive and collegial project team whose members will work together is vital to the success of the student.

for students to review. The doctoral student should review this list and then do some further investigation by looking at publications, presentations, and the teaching expertise of the potential team members. Often schools will offer opportunities for students to meet faculty and hear about their areas of expertise. When inviting new team members, it is important for students to take a professional approach. The invitation should be a formal email or letter introducing themselves, describing their proposed project, and identifying other members serving on the project team. The request should include how the potential project team member's expertise would benefit the team.

Schools typically require a member of the organization where the project will be implemented to be part of the project team to assist the student in navigating the facilitators and/or barriers of project implementation. Getting buy-in and interest from nonfaculty can often be challenging for students. It is critical for students to identify individuals in the organization to be part of the project team who are truly interested in the project. Much of this work starts long before the team is selected and should be considered early on when the project itself is being identified. Students should consider:

1. Is there overall organizational support for this project?
2. Is there someone in this organization who can help navigate organizational challenges?
3. Is there someone interested in and willing to be part of this project team?
4. Is there someone willing to sustain this work after the project is complete?

In some programs, the director may team a student with a faculty mentor based on expertise of that faculty and the interests of the student early in their academic career. However, as the student progresses, it is not uncommon for goals to change, and this may call for a change in the faculty mentor. As a potential student in a DNP program, it would serve the interested student well to inquire about the process used in their DNP program.

▶ Roles and Expectations of Project Team Members

The role of the project faculty mentor is to act primarily as the scholarly advisor to the student. The project faculty mentor must be prepared to evaluate the process and progress of the project. In addition, the project faculty mentor is usually responsible for evaluation of all written work, ensuring that the project and process come to completion in a timely manner. The project faculty mentor is usually a member of the graduate faculty. The specific school expectations of the project team are often described in the doctoral student handbook.

> *The specific school expectations of the project team are often described in the doctoral student handbook.*

The project team members, on the other hand, have the primary roles of lending their expertise to help develop the ideas, to direct specific aspects of the work, to serve as mentors through the DNP project process, and to evaluate the project as a whole. The DNP project team members will be responsible for helping to craft and approve the project, for participating in the completion of a defense or comprehensive examination testing overall student knowledge of the domain, and for approving the final product. Because the DNP student is pursuing a practice doctorate, one member of the team should serve as an organizational practice mentor who will guide and advise the student through the DNP project process at a particular site. As mentioned, the practice mentor should be from within the organization where the project will be implemented, giving the student access to organizational leaders with whom he or she might not otherwise engage in the translation process.

In addition, when putting together the project team, it is important that the student and the project faculty mentor consider looking outside the discipline of nursing. Creating an interprofessional committee with representation from medicine, business, public health, law, the allied health sciences, and research can help to shape a very rich DNP project. This interprofessional team has the potential to influence other members of the healthcare team and can assist the DNP student in developing leadership skills and competencies as outlined in *Essential* VI. Chapter 8, Interprofessional and Intraprofessional Collaboration in the DNP Project, provides additional information and guidance in forming quality interprofessional and intraprofessional collaborations that can be manifested through the DNP project.

An important role in the project team is that of the student. This is not a passive role. In many schools, it is expected that the student will take an active role in selecting a project faculty mentor (i.e., based on expertise, in vetting team members, and in managing the team activities). However, in some schools, the project faculty mentor is assigned by the college of nursing. Therefore, it is important for the DNP student to check with the DNP handbook or advisor before seeking a DNP project faculty mentor. The DNP student must use communication and leadership skills to keep all activities moving toward completion of the final DNP project. Moreover, it is the responsibility of the student to stay in close contact with the project faculty mentor to apprise him or her of progress.

▶ Defining the Timeline for the DNP Project

A very important role of the project faculty mentor and the project team is to assist the DNP student in developing a project that can be completed within the time frames outlined by the school or university. It is not uncommon for doctoral students to propose a grandiose project that would take much longer than time permits. Team members and the project faculty mentor often must help the student to narrow the focus to meet a reasonable time frame while maintaining a high level of rigor and scholarly outcome.

The student and the project faculty mentor must be aware of any constraints placed on the timeline by the plan of study, and together they must formulate a schedule to meet those targets. See Chapter 13, The DNP Project Toolbox, for scheduling tools such as the project timeline. Meetings should be set up in advance between the student and the project faculty mentor, and subsequently between the project faculty mentor and other team members, at regular intervals so that adequate control and appraisal of progress may be maintained. Doctoral students must be aware that most project faculty mentors and team members will require several weeks or longer to review work and provide feedback, so the student must build this time into the plan.

> *The project team members and the project faculty mentor must help the student to narrow the focus of the project to meet a reasonable time frame while maintaining a high level of rigor and scholarly outcome.*

▶ Enhancing Team Productivity

Leadership skills, including the ability to facilitate effective and productive meetings, are an essential attribute of DNP graduates. Learning meeting productivity and facilitation skills starts during the educational process. Doctoral students should prepare for and lead their own project team meetings as a demonstration of this competency. In many ways, doctoral project team meetings are no different from most other meetings. Sometimes early in this process, doctoral students feel that they are being shuttled back and forth by the opinions and experiences of the project faculty mentor and the project team members. As doctoral students become confident in their skills and knowledge, it is incumbent on them to step up and lead their project with the project faculty mentor and project team members providing guidance.

Preparation is essential. Key components in preparing for a project team meeting are meeting necessity, purpose, and outcomes; inviting the right people; agenda; logistics, including room and equipment; and proper lead time (**BOX 9-1**).

The first step in preparation is determining whether a meeting is actually necessary. Meetings should not just be automatic events. What are the purpose and outcome of the project team meeting? If the meeting is only scheduled to share information, could an email suffice? Meetings may need to be held at various times throughout the DNP project. Meetings held during the formative

> *Leadership skills, including the ability to facilitate effective and productive meetings, are an essential attribute of DNP graduates.*

BOX 9-1 Key Components of a Project Team Meeting

- Meeting necessity, purpose, and outcomes
- Inviting the right people
- Agenda
- Logistics
- Proper lead time

---

stages of the project and those held during summative stages may have very different purposes and outcomes. For example, a formative meeting may be necessary to discuss a major change in the student's implementation plan, while a summative meeting may be held for the student to present the final proposal of his or her implementation plan for approval. As the number of doctoral students increases, the toll on faculty workload will become evident. Not all meetings require all members to be present, and it is important to invite only relevant members. Initial meetings may include only the student and the project faculty mentor, whereas meetings in which project approval is needed may require all members. Keep in mind that there are alternative technologies available that allow for team members to attend by conference call or virtual meeting computer applications, when necessary. There may also be times when ad hoc members are needed for problem solving, or the student may be working directly with one team member who possesses expertise that is needed for a certain section.

Once it has been determined that a meeting is needed, a purpose and outcome have been identified, and participants have been selected, an agenda should be created. The agenda should be detailed and include the outcome expected for each topic, the person responsible for each topic, and the amount of time allotted to each. See Chapter 13 for tools such as a meeting agenda template. The agenda should be distributed in advance of the meeting to allow the participants to prepare. The project faculty mentor and the student should be familiar with the school policies on reserving rooms and equipment. Although this is a seemingly simple step, being caught without a room or proper equipment can be disastrous for a meeting.

Facilitating a meeting is a learned skill and can be difficult even for expert leaders. Early in the project, the project faculty mentor may need to assist the DNP student. Janice Francisco (2007), a change facilitator, suggested four steps to facilitating a meeting:

1. Get everyone on the same page.
2. Strike a balance between creative and critical thinking to productively support discussion and decisions.
3. Document the meeting and its accomplishments by capturing meeting minutes and actions.
4. Evaluate the effectiveness of the meeting.

A formal approach to meetings sets the stage for an effective meeting. All meetings should start with ground rules for how the meeting will be conducted. A brief introduction of new members and the role of each and a review of the agenda should follow.

Project team members are often chosen because of their diversity and variety of expertise. Although this leads to an improved product, conflict can result from differences. The best way to resolve conflict within the committee is to prevent it

(Mind Tools Limited, 2015), and the best way to prevent conflict is to be prepared for the meeting and reduce the opportunity for conflict. Spotting potential conflicts early and managing them can prevent them from becoming problematic. If a conflict does arise, conflict management skills are essential. Depersonalizing, questioning, removing/reducing the perceived threat, and taking issues offline are all conflict management skills to use. Depersonalizing involves making the conflict about the issue rather than about the person raising the issue. Questioning involves asking the members with the conflict for specific details about the concern and suggestions for resolution. Conflict in meetings can arise when a member perceives a threat to his or her reputation or success. For example, if a team member disagrees with the path that the project faculty mentor has recommended for the student, the project faculty mentor may feel that his or her reputation is being threatened. Removing or reducing the perceived threat by supplying the correct information or clearing up unknowns may help to resolve the conflict. The DNP student must realize that it is the duty of the project faculty mentor to manage these high-level conflicts with team members, and the project faculty mentor may need to have a one-on-one discussion with the team member or replace a team member who is blocking progress. This can be a difficult discussion, particularly for a doctoral student. It is very important for the student to have a mentor as a member of the project team who can guide him or her through this process. It may be difficult for the doctoral student to take an active role in negotiating disagreements to consensus, but it is necessary. This process prepares students for their eventual responsibilities as a DNP-prepared nurse, which will require them to be tactful but direct with those they may view as having more experience or authority. However, most team interactions are productive in moving the student toward the goal of completing the project. See Chapter 11, Driving the Practicum to Impact the DNP Project, for a discussion of the importance of developing the emotional competence that enables a leader to manage the relationships between individuals and groups.

Once the meeting is over, the real work often begins. The most important component of a meeting is the follow-up and follow-through. All members who attended the meeting should understand the action plan at the end of the meeting. Additionally, meeting minutes and action items should be sent out right away to the appropriate people. See Chapter 13 for tools to help in managing and communicating your project, as well as Chapter 10, Creating and Developing the Project Plan. If possible, the action plan items should be addressed before the next meeting to ensure timely progression of the DNP project.

▶ Alternative Approaches to a Traditional Committee for Project Supervision

Many schools began DNP programs as post-master's programs and implemented committee structures similar to the traditional PhD programs. Although that structure is the standard for traditional PhD programs, the structure for DNP programs is evolving. For example, some schools have implemented alternatives to the committee structure. As the number of students in DNP programs grows exponentially and faculty resources to supervise projects become stretched, it will become necessary for schools to investigate and implement alternative structures. Recognizing this mounting concern, the Implementation of the DNP Task Force (AACN, 2015) has recommended that the traditional committee designations and structures be replaced with the concept of the DNP project team to minimize confusion between the PhD dissertation committee and the faculty and mentors who oversee the final DNP project.

Alternative approaches to the traditional committee structure are becoming more prevalent and new models are being tested. One variation from the traditional approach is to assign each student (or a team of students) to a single project mentor. In place of multiple faculty on a team, some schools are developing a project oversight team to review all proposed and completed projects. This DNP project process is being used particularly in schools where students progress from a bachelor of science in nursing (BSN) to DNP. It is not uncommon to see students working on projects in teams or on group projects in these programs.

Kirkpatrick and Weaver (2013) discuss the option of the small group approach to the DNP project. This could be accomplished with several students exploring different aspects of a complex project, with independent clinical questions explored. Another option presented by the authors was one project addressing a single clinical problem that could be implemented at different sites. However, in group projects, the faculty must assure individual student accountablility for attaining the DNP competencies as outlined in the *Essentials* (AACN, 2006).

Another alternative approach in well-established programs is using a faculty member as the primary advisor and DNP alumni as project team members and community partners.

Brown and Crabtree (2011) have proposed a seminar course series approach for group mentoring of DNP projects. This approach has eased faculty workload connected to the increasing numbers of DNP students and project team responsibilities. Core DNP courses are the prerequisites to the seminar course series. One faculty member is responsible for the same cohort of DNP students for an academic year. The faculty member establishes an ongoing relationship with the students working in groups on projects on a similar topic. It is important that the cohort be a manageable size, usually fewer than 10 students. The goals of the seminar course series are to develop, implement, and evaluate the DNP project in a group format in a quality, cost-effective way. This is an innovative approach to addressing the concern expressed regarding faculty workload and the length of time required to complete the DNP project.

> *Alternative approaches to traditional committee structure are evolving.*

The various approaches to creating project teams to guide the student through the DNP project have pros and cons. The traditional approach of assembling a project mentor and several members provides a team with a strong understanding of the student's project, but the faculty workload for this type of structure is significant. Because of the amount of interaction with team members and the significance of their input, students can sometimes be pulled in many directions. Having a sole advisor and then having the project go out to a project review team decreases the faculty workload, but also decreases the amount of input from experts in the student's project. Having only one faculty member responsible up to the point of proposal could result in wide variability in projects, as well as the student needing to make significant revisions once the project is reviewed by the project team. Using DNP alumni as part of the project team structure is a promising avenue, because DNP alumni are often excited to share their knowledge and practice expertise. This method again reduces the number of faculty on project teams but may increase the amount of work for the project faculty mentor because the alumni may need to be coached regarding the DNP project process.

Innovative models of team structure and support continue to evolve, especially with larger cohorts of students in DNP programs. The benefits of DNP–PhD collaboration in doctoral education as applied to DNP project teams was addressed by Carlson, Staffileno, and Murphy (2017). Purposefully pairing the expertise of PhD- and DNP-prepared faculty team members assists the student with differing approaches to project work and establishes future collaboration expectations based on faculty-modeled behaviors. The structure of the DNP project team to include the expertise of DNP- and PhD-prepared faculty, along with intentional development of an academic-practice partnership with a major health system, was studied by Vanderkooi, Spoelstra, and Conrad (2018). They found that this structure improved time-to-complete assignments, defense, and graduation, along with student, mentor, and faculty satisfaction. It also strengthened academic-practice partnerships, leading to additional student placements. See Chapter 16, The Rest of the Story—Evaluating the Doctor of Nursing Practice, for more information on this exemplar from the authors.

As mentioned in Chapter 2, the Implementation of the DNP Task Force recommendations related to designing DNP programs with attention to program efficiency include the following (AACN, 2015):

- Consider new models and processes for implementing DNP project teams that provide efficient use of resources and support student learning.
- Adopt a process that allows for oversight and evaluation of DNP projects that ensures quality and equity of resources.
- Provide faculty development to ensure quality student learning outcomes to include:
  - Curricular design of DNP programs.
  - Development of new, innovative teaching strategies.
  - Development of innovative, new practice opportunities to support achievement of the DNP *Essentials* learning outcomes.
  - Strategies to support and evaluate the DNP project.
  - Implementation of quality improvement processes.
  - Interprofessional education and practice experiences.

▶ Crediting the Project Team

After completion of the project, the deliverables for communicating the results may include DNP project submissions to the college or university, a manuscript submitted for publication, public presentations of the result of projects, or practice portfolios. (See Chapter 15, Disseminating the Results.) Because the project team has provided substantial guidance regarding process and content for the DNP project, crediting the project faculty mentor and/or project team members in the publications and presentations is a way to recognize their contributions.

The DNP student should seek guidance from his or her doctoral student handbook and/or the project faculty mentor for the school's policy or usual procedure on crediting the project team and other acknowledgments of significant contributors to the DNP project when communicating results.

▶ Summary

Schools and universities operationalize their DNP project oversight teams in various ways. Many schools began by modeling the traditional PhD dissertation committee structure of one chair and committee for each doctoral student, but are finding that they must develop new ways to manage clinically based projects because of different complex clinical issues, student demand, and faculty workload. The prudent DNP student should investigate the practice doctorate requirements at the beginning of the program of study or while making decisions about programs.

The DNP student must also be aware of and familiar with policies, directions, and procedures that guide and impact the doctoral student in his or her school or university. The DNP student handbook for each school must be reviewed frequently and followed to ensure successful completion of the DNP project. All DNP students (or teams of students) should understand that they will be guided in their project work by more experienced faculty and clinical mentors. Their purpose is not to do the work for the student or to impede progress, but to ensure that the product and demonstrations of work of the DNP student truly represent the synthesis of all required competencies and that the student is prepared to confidently and capably move forward to doctoral-level scholarly practice after completion.

The following excerpt by Dr. Katie Alfredson highlights the value of the DNP project team and the impact on the overall project quality (see **EXEMPLAR 9-1**).

EXEMPLAR 9-1 My Experience with the DNP Project Team

Katie Alfredson, DNP, RN, AGNP-C

Throughout my DNP project, the support and contributions of my committee members were vital to its success. My project examined the structures and processes used at a private, primary care practice identified as a Patient-Centered Medical Home (PCMH) that enabled successful outcomes, particularly the success realized in the Meaningful Use Incentive Program. This practice had successfully attested for Meaningful Use Stage 2 during the first quarter of 2014 while the rest of the nation continued to struggle to meet Stage 2 requirements. I wanted to know what enabled this practice to be so successful in this program so I could recommend a framework for others to replicate and potentially experience similar benefits.

As my project developed, it was clear the nursing staff, as members of the interdisciplinary team, played a pertinent role in conducting the processes that were required to meet the Meaningful Use objectives. I struggled, however, in determining how their essential roles could be quantified. This is where my committee proved to be invaluable.

I originally thought I could quantify the value of nurses in the primary care setting by literally timing their productivity as they completed tasks requiring the nursing skill

(continues)

EXEMPLAR 9-1   My Experience with the DNP Project Team   *(continued)*

set, versus the skill set of a medical assistant or other unlicensed personnel. I thought I would then quantify the reimbursement realized as a result of these tasks and determine the return on investment for incorporating nurses in the primary care setting. This turned out to be a laborious and impossible feat.

Upon this realization, I consulted with my committee, which was composed of a DNP-prepared nurse practitioner, a physician, a business doctorate, and a PhD-prepared nurse. It was because of breakthrough conversations with these committee members that I realized one component of the interdisciplinary team could not be separated from the rest. Each team member was needed for the others to be successful. Placing a price-tag value on an individual team member was not possible or desirable, as it breaks down the system to a nonbeneficial level.

As a result of the crucial conversations with committee members, project development and evolution occurred, which led to the eventual success of the final project. Once I realized that the project could not be broken down to the individual team member level, I changed the project methodology and began tracing processes that were vital to Meaningful Use Stage 2 attainment. Contributions from various members of the interdisciplinary team were identified as they were required for each process. In doing so, processes enabling the success of the practice in the Meaningful Use program were described and a case was made for the inclusion of key team members used for the completion of these processes.

Collaborating with committee members not only helped guide the direction of my project, but also provided me with a broader understanding of what is needed to conduct a successful project. It was through this collaboration that I developed an understanding regarding the fluidity of a project. A project cannot be approached with a concrete plan. There must be flexibility to adapt and alter original plans and perspectives.

I also came to the first-hand realization that so much more can be accomplished through the use of an interdisciplinary project team. Each committee member brought their unique experience and background to the table. This created an environment rich in creativity for project development. My project ended up being so much more than it ever could have been if I had completed it independently or from the perspective of a single discipline. Collaboration with committee members enriched the entire experience.

Impact

- Support for the student in completing the DNP project is provided by the project team mentor and team members, contributing diverse expertise and creating an environment for the development of clinical scholars.
- Development of practice-academic partnerships is occurring as healthcare systems realize the value-added impact of DNP student projects.
- Terhaar and Sylvia (2016) state: "The DNP has the potential to improve clinical, operational and financial outcomes. Population demographics require it, complexity of health care demands it, success of healthcare reform depends on it and pressure to realize meaningful quality improvement will fail without it" (p. 173).

Key Messages

- The DNP project differs from a master's thesis and PhD dissertation in scope as well as method of inquiry and has a practice focus. The final product should reflect the mastery of the practice doctorate competencies within a rigorous and scholarly process.
- Forming a cohesive and collegial team whose members will work together is vital to the success of the student.
- The project faculty mentor and project team members guide the DNP student during the DNP project and provide expertise needed to help develop the ideas, direct specific aspects of the work, serve as mentors through the DNP project process, and evaluate the project as a whole.
- Leadership skills, including the ability to facilitate effective and productive meetings, are an essential attribute of DNP graduates.
- As DNP programs mature, alternative approaches to the traditional committee structure for project supervision are evolving.
- DNP students must familiarize themselves with their institution's DNP student handbook to ensure that they understand the particulars about the project team structure, function, and timing; this will greatly impact successful completion.

Action Plan—Next Steps

1. Review your university's requirements for the DNP project team, if any, including composition requirements (i.e., for the project faculty mentor and other team members).
2. Check the timeline for completion of the DNP project according to university policies.
3. Choose the project faculty mentor and other team members who will provide the expertise, guidance, and mentoring needed to complete the project (if part of the process in your program).
4. Practice the leadership skills required of doctoral students in working with the project team members and other collaborators during the DNP project.
5. Make sure all interactions between you and the oversight committee are executed in an efficient and effective way; be prepared.

References

American Association of Colleges of Nursing (AACN). (2006). *The essentials of doctoral education for advanced nursing practice.* Retrieved from http://www.aacnnursing.org/Portals/42/Publications/DNPEssentials.pdf

American Association of Colleges of Nursing (AACN). (2015). *The doctor of nursing practice: Current issues and clarifying recommendations.* Retrieved from https://www.pncb.org/sites/default/files/2017-02/AACN_DNP_Recommendations.pdf

American Association of Colleges of Nursing (AACN). (2017). *DNP fact sheet.* Retrieved from http://www.aacnnursing.org/News-Information/Fact-Sheets/DNP-Fact-Sheet

American Association of Colleges of Nursing (AACN). (2018). *2017–2018 enrollment and graduations in baccalaureate and graduate programs in nursing.* Washington, DC: Author.

Brown, M. A., & Crabtree, K. (2011, November 15). *Maturational issues in DNP practice inquiry/improvement projects* [Webinar]. National Organization of Nurse Practitioner Faculties. Retrieved from http://www.nonpf.org/displaycommon .cfm?an=1&subarticlenbr=64

Carlson, E. A., Staffileno, B. A., & Murphy, M. P. (2017). Promoting DNP-PhD collaboration in doctoral education: Forming a DNP project team. *Journal of Professional Nursing*. Retrieved from https://doi.org/10.1016/j.profnurs.2017.12.011.

DifferenceBetween.net. (2018). *Difference between thesis and dissertation*. Retrieved from http://www.differencebetween.net/language/difference-between-thesis-and-dissertation/

Francisco, J. (2007). How to create and facilitate meetings that matter: Learn how to plan and run a successful meeting using crucial checklists. *Information Management Journal*, 54–58.

Gardenier, D., & Stanik-Hutt, J. (2010). Should DNP students conduct original research as their capstone projects? *The Journal for Nurse Practitioners*, 6(5), 364–365.

Kirkpatrick, J. M., & Weaver, T. (2013). The doctor of nursing practice capstone project: Consensus or confusion? *Journal of Nursing Education*, 52(8), 435–441. doi:10.3928/01484834-20130722-01

Magnan, M. A. (2019). The DNP: Expectations for theory, research, and scholarship. In L. A. Chism (Ed.), *The doctor of nursing practice: A guidebook for role development and professional issues* (pp. 117–148). Burlington, MA: Jones & Bartlett Learning.

Mind Tools Limited. (2015). *Mind tools: Essential skills for an excellent career* (6th ed.). Retrieved from http://www.mindtools.com

Terhaar, M. F., & Sylvia, M. (2016). Scholarly work products of the doctor of nursing practice: One approach to evaluating scholarship, rigour, impact and quality. *Journal of Clinical Nursing*, 25(1–2), 163–174. doi: 10.1111/jocn.13113.

Vanderkooi, M., Spoelstra, S., & Conrad, D. (2018). An enhanced actualized DNP model to improve DNP projects. *Nursing Education Perspectives*, 39(5), 299–301.

Waldrup J., Caruso, D., Fuchs, M. A., & Hypes, K. (2014). EC as PIE: Five criteria for executing a successful DNP project. *Journal of Professional Nursing*, (30)4, 300–306.

CHAPTER 10

Creating and Developing the Project Plan

Rosanne Burson and Katherine Moran

CHAPTER OVERVIEW

It is important for the doctor of nursing practice (DNP) student to have an appreciation of doctoral work, which is not linear, but rather more circular or spiral in nature. Much of the cognitive work that occurs as the student explores an area of interest will be reworked through the process of developing the DNP project. The phenomenon will continue to be contemplated, the proposal will develop, literature will continue to be reviewed, and the methodology for the design will evolve.

If one considers the DNP project development process holistically, it is very similar to the nursing process—assess, diagnose/determine the problem, plan how to manage the problem and measure the outcomes, implement the plan, then evaluate (see **Figure 10-1**). All DNP projects should have a planning, implementation, and evaluation phase (American Association of Colleges of Nursing [AACN], 2015). The DNP student will select a phenomenon of interest, identify a problem or opportunity for improvement, develop a clinical question, develop a project plan, implement the plan, monitor the implementation to ensure that the process is working as intended, and then evaluate the outcome to determine if the goal has been met. Indeed, the DNP project is the ultimate nursing *practice* activity because it utilizes the nursing process at the doctoral level.

The DNP project plan is a formal document used to plan and design the scholarly project in preparation for implementation. Successful project

> *The DNP project is the ultimate nursing practice activity because it utilizes the nursing process at the doctoral level.*

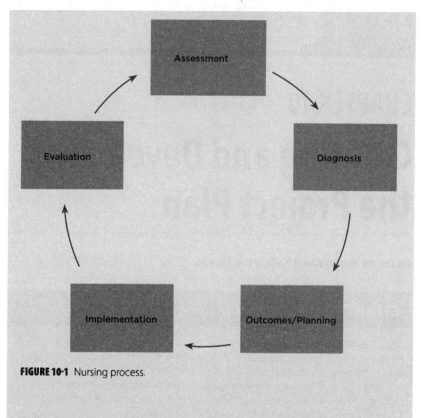

FIGURE 10-1 Nursing process.

implementation depends on a carefully considered plan, with attention to detail. This process is just as important as planning the initial proposal, because if significant problems occur during implementation, it can lead to unsuccessful outcomes. The intent of this chapter is to present a broad overview of points to consider in creating an innovative project and developing a plan to successfully prepare for project implementation.

CHAPTER OBJECTIVES

After completing the chapter, the learner will be able to:

1. Create alternate strategies for potential innovation implementation.
2. Choose a best solution based on a cost–benefit analysis.
3. Develop an understanding of the various components of a project plan, for use in planning project implementation.
4. Analyze which components may be helpful for the individual project.
5. Consider aspects of the institutional review board (IRB) approval process that will impact the timeline of the project.

▶ Creation of Innovation

Once the phenomenon of interest has developed, the student will have a deep understanding of the topic of interest. The literature review will build on the understanding of the phenomenon, which leads to new ideas and innovations that could improve care or make a contribution to nursing. As mentioned in Chapter 6, Developing the DNP Project, it will be important to commit to a general concept that will continue to evolve and mature as the student encounters additional coursework and applies new knowledge to the understanding of the phenomenon. Through this process, the student will also acquire new skills that can be applied to the development of a project.

Within each phase of the project development process, the DNP student is able to use more concepts to expand the process to incorporate health systems and populations of patients. For instance, in the *assessment* phase, the DNP student explored the information at hand. Factors included in this phase are the necessity that goals and outcomes of the project are aligned with the organization's strategic plan, development of project specifications, financial analysis, and the identification of the team that will be able to move the project forward (Waxman, 2018). An assessment was critical and helped define the issues that will now guide decisions in the project planning phase (see Chapter 6). Tools to help the student with the assessment phase can be found in Chapter 13, The DNP Project Toolbox. It is in this phase that the commitment of the organization to the project should be clarified. The student should work within their school guidelines to formalize the implementation site for the project.

The *diagnosis* phase of the nursing process translates to the development of a problem statement based on all the information that was pulled together when the student identified the issues surrounding the problem. Here is where framing the problem occurs. In Chapter 6, the DNP student chose the appropriate data that highlighted the specific issues surrounding the problem and presented this information in a problem statement.

The *planning* phase includes the determination of potential alternative solutions with pros and cons. The student must describe how each solution will address the identified need and consider the feasibility and impact potential of each solution. Creative thinking and innovative ideas are a part of this phase.

A cost–benefit analysis can be an effective tool to present the financial aspects of the project. In this analysis, the project team (1) identifies the costs of the project, (2) identifies the benefits, and (3) compares costs and benefits. All potential costs of the project should be brainstormed, which include one-time costs such as equipment and training, as well as recurring costs such as payroll. Nonmonetary costs should also be considered and given a monetary value. This may include issues related to productivity, as well as risks to the project outcomes. Including the costs of not doing the project may be effective as well.

In determining the benefits, accurate projection of revenue can be challenging. It is best to forecast using conservative figures. Dollar amounts on the intangible benefits need to be incorporated as well. Examples of benefits include direct profits, increased production, and increased employee/patient satisfaction.

Identify the optimal solutions based on analysis of the costs and benefits. There are many sample tools available to develop the cost–benefit analysis (Smartsheet, n.d.). As the team compares the costs and benefits, consider the time it will take for the benefits to repay the costs. The project plan is developed based on the identified optimal solution. If the project involves large sums of money, the team will want to consider net present value (NPV) and/or internal rate of return (IRR) to more accurately examine the financial decision (Mind Tools Limited, n.d.). The DNP student working with financial experts within the organization collaboratively prepares the assessment. In this way, the DNP student brings the understanding of the clinical environment and consideration of aspects that will influence costs, while the financial experts can work with appropriate tools to determine calculations to support the project.

Part of the planning phase will also include planning for *implementation*—developing the project plan and determining outcome measures and metrics for the project. Well-defined outcomes and metrics are developed prior to implementation. When outcomes are specific, meaningful, and measurable, expectations of the project are described.

Evaluation incorporates the measurement of all metrics/identified outcomes. Successful outcomes deliver a recognized and successful project.

TABLE 10-1 identifies the various components in each phase. See Chapter 13, The DNP Project Toolbox, for a closer look at items that can assist in each phase.

TABLE 10-1 Developing Project Innovations

Phase	Tools
Assessment	SWOT analysis Force field analysis Community analysis Needs assessment Organizational data
Diagnosis	Framing the problem Problem statement
Planning	Potential alternative solutions Cost–benefit comparisons Optimal solution identified Plan for implementation (project plan) Metric/outcome development
Implementation	Project plan in process
Evaluation	Metrics Satisfaction (patient/staff/provider) Clinical outcomes Cost outcomes Other measures

▶ The DNP Project Plan

Once a basic project concept has developed, the focus moves to preparing for the specifics of the project. There is extensive environmental planning required that includes identifying the setting, collaborating with a content expert, and interfacing with the DNP project team and/or faculty mentor. In addition, written work is required for developing the proposal, obtaining institutional review board (IRB) approval (if needed), submitting a grant proposal to support the project (if applicable), and, finally, developing the project plan. The DNP student will need to select the most appropriate items to use for his or her project planning—*not every item is needed for every project.*

The DNP student will need to select the most appropriate items to use for his or her project planning—not every item is needed for every project.

Identifying the Setting

As the project plan takes shape, identifying the setting is an important aspect that must be considered early in the plan development. Will this project be applied in the acute care, primary care, community, or another environment? The student will need to investigate options and secure a location to move forward in the project plan development process. For students who are interested in implementing their project in a setting outside their work environment, it is important to schedule extra time for the approval process. This is especially true in the corporate setting, where multiple levels of approval may be required. As academic practice partnerships are developing, there may be additional avenues for the student to systematically pursue project opportunities.

Once the setting is secured, it is time to begin the development of the project plan. To help the student through this process, the following information is presented using an example of an actual project plan template in an annotated format. The student should keep in mind that this is just one of many project plan formats available. It is best to check with the DNP project team or project faculty mentor to determine the format used by the university or college prior to beginning the planning process. Although a multitude of topics are presented here, the DNP student will want to *choose* the aspects *specific* to his or her project.

When reading this section, note that each part of the plan includes section descriptions, and some sections point out additional documents that may be needed to complete the plan. See Chapter 13, The DNP Project Toolbox, for a project plan template. This plan is designed to address most project sizes; however, smaller projects may not require completion of the entire plan. What follows is the plan example.

(Project Name)

Project Plan

(Student Name)

(University)

(Date)

Table of Contents

1. Introduction

1.1 Purpose of the Project Plan

In this section, describe the purpose of the project. When a project charter is used to gain organizational approval for the project, the description of the purpose from the project charter can be used in this section. See Chapter 13, The DNP Project Toolbox, for a description of the project charter. It is helpful to identify the intended audience of the project in this section as well.

2. Executive Summary

This section is used to give a quick preview of the project plan. It is a high-level overview of the project that should include a brief description of the project scope, deliverables, required resources, scheduling requirements, budget, and any reference material necessary to fully understand the project. The goal is to grab the attention of readers by providing them with enough information to gain a reasonable understanding of the project, but not bore them with the specific details. It is best to limit the summary to one page. Again, if the student already developed a project charter, include a reference to the approved project charter.

3. Project Goals and Objectives

In this section, describe the overall project goals, and then describe in detail the objectives that will be used to reach the goals. See Chapter 6, Developing the DNP Project, for more information regarding the development of goals and objectives.

4. Scope

The project scope describes the breadth of the project—that is, what is relevant and what is not relevant to the project. As indicated in Chapter 6, it should include all the work that needs to be accomplished to successfully complete the project. Budgetary requirements and the time required to complete the work should be considered in the scope.

5. Project Administration

The project administration section is used to describe the overall project structure, how the project is organized in relation to team member responsibilities, and how the project interfaces with the organization and potentially other organizations—especially related to organizational boundaries.

5.1 Structure

An organizational chart can be used to describe the management structure of the project, including lines of authority (where applicable) and responsibility. See Appendix A.

5.2 Boundaries

When the project includes more than one organization or team, the boundaries of each are identified in this section. This helps everyone understand the organizational and/or team expectations right from the beginning.

5.3 Roles and Responsibilities

The roles and responsibilities of each team member are briefly described in this section.

6. Project Management

The management process section includes the project assumptions, risks/constraints, risk management plan, monitoring plan, staffing plan, and communication management plan.

6.1 Assumptions and Risks/Constraints

Assumptions

Project assumptions include those items that are assumed to be provided so that the project will move forward—for example, access to the setting, access to participants where applicable, use of equipment, etc.

Risks/Constraints

Project constraints include any event that could potentially have a negative impact on the project objectives—for example, lack of staff, subjects, or material resources.

6.2 Risk Management Plan

To successfully manage any potential project risks/constraints, a risk management plan should be developed. This section should describe the identification and potential impact of the risks and how they will be mitigated. The improvements made can be documented as lessons learned. If a project charter was developed, a reference to the project charter is appropriate. See Chapter 13 for an example of a risk assessment tool.

6.3 Monitoring Plan

The monitoring plan should include those tools that will be used for monitoring or tracking adherence to the project plan. This section should also include a description of how information will flow, how change will be approved and implemented *(if warranted), and how progress is reported. See Chapter 13 for examples of project management tools.*

6.4 Staffing Plan

In this section, indicate the total number of people who will be required to complete the project objectives.

6.5 Communication Management Plan

The purpose of the communication plan is to describe how communication will occur during the project. This plan includes how and when information will be communicated (i.e., meetings, email, memorandums, etc.), who communicates the message (based on roles), and what is communicated. See examples of a communication plan, project agenda/minutes, status report, and issues log template in Chapter 13.

7. Software and Hardware Requirements

Describe any software and hardware requirements for the project. For example, describe the computer software system that will be used (if applicable), what it will be used for (e.g., documentation), and who will have access to the software. Any policy or procedure required to implement or utilize this software should be described in this section as well.

7.1 Security

Specify security requirements that will be needed to both support the project and access the specific software (where applicable), for example, such as if any special login and password are required. For example, perhaps only a few key team members will have access to all the software features, whereas others may have only limited access based on what is needed for their role.

8. Work Breakdown Structure

This section of the project plan will specify the work structure, identify the relationships among them, state the project resource requirements, provide a cost management plan, and establish a project schedule.

8.1 Work Structure

A description of the work breakdown structure (WBS) for all activities is required to complete this section. An example of a WBS is provided in Chapter 13.

8.2 Relationships

This section should describe the relationships between various aspects of the work needed to complete the project. It should include any dependencies or interdependencies among the various tasks, as well as any external dependencies or interdependencies.

8.3 Resources

A list of all the resources required to complete the project is included in this section. Included are all material resources, such as computers and computer software and hardware, training time, travel, and maintenance requirements.

8.4 Cost Management

In this section, clearly describe the project budget and how the project costs will be managed. The project budget should include specific information on the financing required to complete the project from start to finish. This section identifies the person responsible for the budget plan, discloses how changes are made to the budget and who has responsibility for those changes, describes how cost variances will be managed and who has responsibility for those variances, and discusses how and when costs will be reported. An example of a project budget is provided in Chapter 13.

8.5 Schedule/Time Management

This section describes the project schedule, including all activities, milestones, and team member roles and responsibilities in relation to time to complete. An example of a project schedule is provided in Chapter 13.

9. Quality Management

The quality management section describes the project milestones/key deliverables and quality indicators.

9.1 Milestones

Milestones are important events or key deliverables that are completed during the life cycle of the project. A table can easily be utilized to describe and track the estimated time of completion for each milestone (see **TABLE 10-2***).*

TABLE 10-2 Project Milestones

Milestones	Description	Estimated Completion Date

9.2 Quality Indicators

Quality indicators are those items that are considered desirable and promote project success. Examples include staying within the projected budget and meeting project milestones. It is helpful to indicate the desired quality baseline in this section to use as a point of reference throughout the project and to describe measures that will be taken to ensure that the desired quality is met and maintained (e.g., audits, inspections) (see Chapter 6 for more information on quality indicators).

10. Project Initiation Plan

In this section, describe how the project will be rolled out. Provide a detailed description of each step in the process, from securing the setting to delivering the end project.

11. Training Plan

Most projects will require some type of training. When considering the training plan, it is important to describe the training process in as much detail as possible. Include information on who will provide the training, who will be trained, when the training will occur, the tools that will be used in the training process, the time required to provide the training, and where the training will be held.

12. Procurement Plan

This section describes how the resources for the project will be acquired—that is, hardware, software, licenses, and any other resources needed to successfully complete the project.

13. Appendices

Include any appendices to the project in this section. Items to consider for this section include those that add meaning or that may help one understand the project plan.

13.1 Appendix A—Organizational Structure

13.2 Appendix B—Definition of Key Terms

Any terms or acronyms used in the plan or by the organization are listed in this appendix.

13.3 Appendix C—References

List any documents referenced in the plan and where they are located.

Appendix A

Organizational Structure

Appendix B

Definition of Key Terms

The following table provides definitions for terms and acronyms that may be used throughout the project plan.

Term/Acronym	Definition
Budget	An itemized summary of planned income and expenditures over time
Customer	The individual or group for which a project is designed
WHO	World Health Organization

Appendix C

References

The following table includes all the documents referenced within the project plan.

Name	Description	Location

This plan (pp. 194–208) was adapted from the Centers for Disease Control (n.d.), North Carolina Enterprise (2004), and Project Management Docs (n.d.).

▶ Collaborating with Content Experts

As the project plan becomes clearer, it will be important to collaborate with content experts and begin interfacing with the identified DNP project faculty mentor (see Chapter 9, The DNP Project Team). The DNP student should assess the areas in which he or she has expertise and the areas in which a content expert may be required. It may be helpful to consider the multiple aspects of the general plan in the assessment. For example, in a health policy project, the DNP student may be a content expert on the impact of the advanced practice nurse (APN) in reducing costs in transitional care. In addition, the DNP student may have considerable expertise interacting with legislators on this same topic. However, the DNP student may need assistance in the area of policy development. If this is the case, the DNP student could seek out a policy expert to further explore the content required for the project and its success. An important part of doctoral work is *collaboration*, which assists the student in growth and adds to the richness of the project (see Chapter 8, Interprofessional and Intraprofessional Collaboration in the DNP Project).

> *An important part of doctoral work is collaboration, which assists the student in growth and adds to the richness of the project.*

▶ Institutional Review Board Approval

As part of the project development, consideration should be given to human subject approval. The student should note that acceptance of the proposal by the DNP project team may occur prior to institutional review board (IRB) application submission. Therefore, thinking about the IRB process in the project development stage is important. It is imperative that the student ascertains the policy of the college or university regarding DNP projects and the IRB.

However, when the IRB application is required, the process can be daunting for doctoral students. Incomplete or flawed submissions have the potential to slow down the progress of the project. This can be a problem because of the short time frame the DNP student may have to complete the program. Understanding the IRB process and addressing potential areas of concern will help ensure a smooth, efficient, and more predictable outcome.

All projects may need to be reviewed by the IRB. Typically, the proposal will initially be reviewed by the IRB chair to determine the type of review required. There are three categories of review: (1) exempt, (2) expedited, and (3) full review. If an IRB application is exempt, no formal IRB review is required because there is no risk for human subjects. Typically, this is reserved for projects that use surveys, noninvasive procedures, secondary documents, or methods in which the data are deidentified (Houser, 2018). Expedited review occurs when there is minimal risk to human subjects, described as discomfort or risk that is not greater than that encountered in daily life. The expedited review is usually completed by one or two members of the committee. A full review is completed by the entire committee and is done for projects that do not qualify for exempt or expedited review (Houser, 2018). The type of review that is determined by the IRB will affect the timeline. Often, committees meet at predetermined monthly times, so if a full review is required, the time from application to approval could be lengthy.

In previous years, quality improvement (QI) projects did not require IRB review. However, today, QI projects may be included in an IRB review. Currently, there have been discussions regarding when to consider a project a research study, as opposed to a QI project. QI did not use research methods and always aimed to directly benefit participants, and the work was not published. Today, the distinction between research and QI has become more blurred, with many projects being published. In addition, QI projects now may use research methods (Weiserbs, Lyutic, & Weinberg, 2009). As a result, some IRBs have instituted IRB-QI subgroups to fast-track QI projects. Defining QI projects and policies regarding protection of human subjects can be reviewed at the U.S. Department of Health and Human Services Office for Human Research Protection website (www.hhs.gov/ohrp/).

Understanding IRB-related requirements ahead of time will help prepare the DNP student for the process. For instance, in addition to IRB approval at the site of the project, approval through the university IRB may be required. Also, in preparation for IRB application, accrediting processes ensure the understanding of human subject protection. The student can complete these certifications ahead of time. Typically, a module review, test, and printed certifications are included in the IRB application packet.

Identifying which IRBs will be needed and the requirements of each can smooth the process. "One of the most important steps that a new investigator can take regarding the IRB process is to schedule a meeting with an IRB representative to learn about the institution's IRB processes" (Weber & Cobaugh, 2008, p. 2062).

Some of the questions to consider include:

1. Is there a contact person who may be helpful for answering questions?
2. What is the process of application?
3. Is there a template to be used for the application?
4. What are the educational/certification requirements? Can these be completed ahead of time?
5. How will the completed application be forwarded to the committee?
6. Will the university IRB work with the format of any other IRB committees (especially those in the organizations where projects occur), or is a separate application process required?
7. What is the usual time frame for IRB approval in each institution?

Remember that the IRB is not there to block research or QI, but to "help researchers by looking for risks in a research proposal that the investigator may have overlooked or underemphasized, thereby protecting the researcher, the institution, and all potential research subjects" (Colt & Mulnard, 2006, p. 1607). Federal regulations require that any research on human subjects be approved by an IRB. The IRB committee must complete a very detailed review to accept the proposal. Understanding the components of the review will assist the DNP student in preparing for the application.

Pech, Cob, and Cejka (2007) outlined the areas that the IRB committee must review. A project needs to ensure that:

1. Risks to the subjects are minimized.
2. Risks are reasonable in relation to anticipated benefits.
3. There is equitable selection of subjects.

4. There is informed consent.
5. There is monitoring of data to ensure safety of subjects.
6. Protection of subject privacy and data confidentiality is safeguarded.

The role of the investigator is to "explain in simple terms the reason for the research and its risk to human subjects, and to clearly demonstrate how those subjects will be protected" (Colt & Mulnard, 2006, p. 1605). There are many types of people on IRB committees, so simplicity and clarity are of particular importance. The student will need to describe each of the preceding areas of concern in the IRB application.

Typically, the format of the application process will include an institution-specific application and a narrative proposal that incorporates the purpose, clinical question, and procedures that will be utilized for the project. All forms are submitted, such as consent, surveys, tools, and questionnaires. Because many IRB applications are now web based, they can be accessed and developed over time. The goal for the student when preparing the IRB submission is to submit a thorough application to reduce approval delay and to maintain subject protection.

Here are some tips to prepare well for IRB submission:

1. Avoid an incomplete or flawed submission. This includes:
   - Proofread for content and grammatical errors.
   - Be sure that all elements of the form are completed.
   - Ensure that all signatures are completed.
   - Provide complete information in all required documents.
2. Be consistent in all documents: Ensure that the information provided is the same across all documents.
3. Provide all survey tools that will be used.
4. Be in contact with your assigned IRB member: Identify potential areas of concern and usual questions prior to the submission.
5. Consider the audience: Use simplified, easy-to-understand language.
6. Prepare a thorough application to reduce time to approval.
7. Keep requirements in mind to justify the project.
   - Provide rationale for the study and the design.
   - Describe the risk to subjects.
   - Describe how subjects are protected throughout the research.
8. Allow for a realistic time frame (Colt & Mulnard, 2006; Greaney et al., 2012).

The IRB committee will review the application and make a decision. There may be full or conditional approval. In the case of conditional approval, revisions may need to be made prior to initiating the project. There is also the possibility of the committee denying approval, in which case, the student should work carefully with the IRB representative to identify the changes that need to be made prior to resubmission. Of course, the project cannot be implemented prior to approval (see the Helpful Resource section at the end of this chapter for IRB resources).

▶ Submitting for Grant Support

An additional area of consideration is submitting a grant proposal. Small grants can provide financial assistance for the project. The process of applying for a grant can encourage the writer to work on clarity of the project problem statement, goals, and objectives. Look for available small grants in areas of one's specialty, such as perianesthesia nursing, or within nursing organizations, such as local chapters of Sigma Theta Tau. Also, consider grants available for novice researchers or students, such as the Blue Cross Blue Shield of Michigan Foundation Student Award. Walsh and Bowen (2012) have provided the following suggestions for writing a grant:

1. Tailor the grant to the funding agency's mission.
2. Showcase your expertise and the environment.
3. Minimize the reviewer's work by having a clear, concise, and well-organized application.
4. Follow instructions exactly.
5. Take advantages of any resources for preparing and submitting the grant.
6. Contact the funding agency's program officer with any questions.
7. Be sure the application tells an interesting story (p. 22).

Obtaining a grant can lend credibility to the project, assist with the budget, and build experience for future grant opportunities.

▶ Preparing for Implementation of the DNP Project

Once the project plan has been finalized with your project team, the proposal has been defended and approved, and IRB status has been approved (if needed), the implementation process will commence. The following items should be considered prior to the initiation of the project.

Earlier in this chapter, the student learned about key points to consider when developing a project plan. Although the project plan provides the framework for success, what constitutes a successful project is dependent on several variables: (1) completing the project on time, (2) completing the project within budget, (3) achieving the intended goals, and (4) achieving stakeholder satisfaction (Pinto & Slevin, 1987). Therefore, careful attention will be needed when implementing the plan.

Clearly, project implementation will involve more than simply dropping the project in place. The implementation phase of the project is complex and may require "simultaneous attention to a wide variety of human, budgetary, and technical variables" (Pinto & Slevin, 1987, p. 167). The student will need to consider the environment where the project will be implemented, as well as the processes involved for training. "If you think through implementation from a holistic approach and communicate well, there is a much greater likelihood that your project will end as a win" (Mochal, 2003, para. 5). It is clear that the implementation of the project will require not only project

The implementation phase of the project is complex and may require "simultaneous attention to a wide variety of human, budgetary, and technical variables" (Pinto & Slevin, 1987, p. 167).

management, but also change management. These are two distinct disciplines that are integrated for the purposes of achieving a project goal.

Project management involves planning, organizing, acquiring, managing, leading, and controlling resources to achieve the overall project goal(s) ("Project management," 2018). Project management begins long before the implementation of the project; it begins with the planning and designing of the project. As discussed earlier in the chapter, first the project goals are determined, objectives are outlined, specific activities to achieve the objectives are developed, and so forth.

Change management, on the other hand, focuses on helping the people involved in the process make the changes required effectively and efficiently. For example, change management begins with gaining buy-in from stakeholders, but also includes training of individuals involved in the project implementation phase. As one can imagine, much of the work involved in change management includes effective communication. See Chapter 8 for information regarding how change theory can be used to guide the DNP student in planning and implementing the project.

> *Change management focuses on helping the people involved in the process make the changes required effectively and efficiently.*

Both project management and change management techniques and processes are useful and help the student implement the project successfully. Another important point to consider when implementing a project is that it is often a circular process. For example, as is the case with most projects, the process will involve continued monitoring that may result in further project refinement and/or adjustments to the plan. **FIGURE 10-2** illustrates the project implementation process.

Project Structure

Now that the process is understood and the tools are in place to help ensure a positive outcome, it is time to look at the project structure. This includes finalizing project implementation details with the project setting, which encompasses coordinating

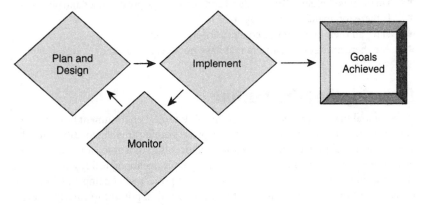

FIGURE 10-2 Project implementation flowchart.

with the organizations that are involved in the project, preparing the infrastructure for implementation, identifying the participants and covariables, and, finally, implementing the training (if applicable).

Coordinating with Organizations

Regardless of the type of project being implemented, successful implementation will require activities such as coordinating schedules and resources with organizations involved in implementation. This may require simple one-time communication efforts to confirm that the affiliation agreement is in place, or it may involve several meetings to ensure that everyone involved is on the same page. The goal is to coordinate efforts with everyone or every group with a role in the project. For example, for information technology solutions, there may be an operations group and several infrastructure groups that will need to be communicated with prior to implementing the project (Mochal, 2003). The student should recognize that failure to plan ahead and coordinate efforts with those involved leads to increasing levels of frustration and roadblocks and may lead to a lack of commitment to completing the project.

. . . Failure to plan ahead and coordinate efforts with those involved leads to increasing levels of frustration and roadblocks and may lead to a lack of commitment to completing the project.

The following focus questions will help the student coordinate and communicate project plans.

Focus Questions

- Who are the people or groups that touch the project in some way or form?
- Have all the required relationships been established?
- Has the project implementation plan been communicated effectively?
- Do the stakeholders all understand and agree on the project goals and objectives?
- Is there top management support?
- Have all their questions or concerns been addressed?
- Are there any hidden barriers that have not been uncovered?

Preparing the Infrastructure

It is essential that the characteristics of the DNP project environment be considered and that the project infrastructure be in place prior to implementation. In other words, successful project implementation requires the student to gather the support he or she will need, including resources (i.e., people, technological resources, materials, and supplies). Although in many cases, the project will be implemented in an organization that is familiar to the student, it is still important to carefully review the resources that are available to support the project. For example, the student may need to conduct a review of computer hardware or software, or review the documentation and communication tools to confirm that the information technology infrastructure (databases) will support the project as intended. In doing so, the student is able to identify potential issues and problem solve before they become a barrier to implementation. Chapter 11, Driving the Practicum to Impact the DNP Project, discusses how to evaluate and prepare the environment for the DNP project.

A few questions to consider follow.

Focus Questions

- Are the needed documentation tools in place?
- Does the documentation system capture the data needed for the project?
- Are there any security or access issues that have not been addressed?
- Are the data secured?

Forming the Team

Building a successful organizational project team is critical to a successful project outcome. All of those within the organization that will impact the implementation of the DNP project should be considered as project team members. The DNP student should identify all stakeholders as potential team members dependent on the specific project. Examples of team members may include providers, clinical and administrative staff, management, and patients. To ensure that all members of the team are appropriately invested, and to improve the likelihood of the project's success, the DNP student project manager should be cognizant of the team's development stages. This information will help the DNP student project manager resolve problems early and keep the project moving forward. Typical group development stages include *forming, storming, norming,* and, finally, *performing* (Tuckman & Jensen, 1977).

The *forming* stage occurs when the team comes together before project implementation. There may be several opportunities for forming to occur: during the initial meeting when the project is introduced, during project implementation planning meetings, during project training meetings, and during other meetings designed to help ensure the project's success. Throughout this stage, some team members meet other team members for the first time; people start to understand the project's objectives, become engaged in the process, and come to understand their role in the process; team member relationships are developed; and members' strengths, weaknesses, and authority are recognized. The DNP student project manager will direct the team at this stage of team orientation.

The next group development stage is *storming*. During this stage, team members may compete for specific roles or responsibilities, there may be disagreements over how to get things done, and individual hidden agendas may become more evident. The DNP student project manager will need to lead the group by example, keep on top of issues between members, and implement problem-solving strategies and conflict management techniques to keep the project moving forward.

The *norming* stage of team development is characterized by congruent team behavior. During this stage, specific rules are developed (either formally or informally), and each team member's role and responsibility are established. The team becomes more efficient and productive. There is a sense of comradery. The DNP student project manager should focus on facilitating group meetings and including everyone's perspective when possible.

The *performing* stage occurs when the team is working well together and objectives are being met. Team members rely on each other to perform their roles and responsibilities to the standard established by the group and help each other where possible. At this stage of team development, the team is cohesive, and there is a sense of unity. The DNP student project manager focuses on meeting the project objectives.

Training the Team

Most projects will require some form of team member training or coaching prior to implementation. This training should occur close to the time the project is ready to start. If a significant amount of time passes between the initial training and the project implementation, there is a risk that the critical elements required for implementation may be forgotten.

The focus of the training is on key functions of each team member. During training, team members should be provided with a document that summarizes the project training key elements and identifies a contact person for questions or problem-solving during implementation. By the end of the training, members should understand what will be required to implement the project and be comfortable performing their roles. Pre- and post-tests of knowledge gained in training sessions can be part of project deliverables.

In some cases, a dress rehearsal may be feasible. This can be a very valuable exercise because modifications to the plan can be incorporated that address problems identified in this process. Rehearsing the project prior to implementation also serves to decrease team member performance anxiety and builds confidence.

Once the training is complete, the student should ask the following questions.

Focus Questions

- Are the members of the team clear on the purpose of the project?
- Are they clear on the project goals and initiatives?
- Do the team members understand the objectives and how they will be measured?
- Were team members' questions answered sufficiently?

▶ Summary

In summary, as the DNP student progresses through coursework, the project plan and proposal will continue to develop. Expect to continue to work through more details of the project plan as time progresses. The practicum is an opportunity to work some elements of the DNP project into place and will be discussed in Chapter 11.

The following excerpt from Dr. Michele Corker highlights the planning experience for the DNP Project (see **EXEMPLAR 10-1**).

EXEMPLAR 10-1 Evaluation of an Army Regulation Electronic Contingency Notebook as a Process Improvement Tool During the Soldier Readiness Process

Michele Corker, DNP, FNP-BC, AN/Maj

My DNP QI project was to evaluate and analyze the effectiveness and ease of use of a technological electronic database repository. The database repository would be used as a tool to improve the Soldier Readiness Process (SRP) at a large military multiforce installation. Planning the evaluation included identification of all stakeholders, review of deployment medicine and military fit for duty standards, and an evaluation of consistency in practice and provider accountability. Development of an interview tool, which involved collaboration between military and civilian providers, was included in the plan.

The student must have an awareness of all required processes for approval in the environment where the project will be implemented. In this case, applications and approvals from multiple sources such as the Soldier Readiness Center (SRC) Medical Officer in Charge (OIC), Deployment of Medicine Chief Officer, university IRB, and the Army Medical Center IRB were obtained.

Following the Institute for Health Improvement (IHI) model, planning the "how" of the evaluation was initiated by using process mapping and the logic model as a planning tool framework to show clarity of purpose, organization of actions, and outcomes of the project, and to obtain the support of leadership. Process mapping provided a visual display or outline of the project focus, helped keep the ultimate mission in mind, and was used to track progress. The logic model is a visual outline to display inputs (what is needed to perform the project), outputs (activities to perform QI, participation of stakeholders), and outcomes (short, medium, and long: goal of QI). An interview tool for evaluation of the project was authored to determine if the outcomes were met.

Finally, planning also included the Plan-Do-Study-Act (PDSA) model to test effectiveness of the electronic database (notebook) through comparison of the expected and actual outcomes and continuous evaluation of rapid cycle change. Modifications were made through observation and experiences from the team as they used the notebook. The PDSA model allowed for continuous flexibility, improvements, and reevaluations during the evaluation process. The notebook continues to be revised, which contributes to the relevance and sustainability of the project.

Now, 3 years later, the *Army Regulation Electronic Contingency Notebook* is the *Soldier Readiness Process Standard Operating Procedure (SOP) Electronic Notebook*. This database of all updated deployment and Army information continues as a validated repository of information. The original purpose was to develop and field a sustainable, specific, and comprehensive resource as a training tool for current and future incoming military and civilian providers, and to support the execution of complex deployment and redeployment SRP policies.

Some of the original stakeholders identified during the qualitative improvement project process are still employed at Fort Hood Soldier Readiness Center. There have been three U.S. Reserve Units who have since passed through, along with many new government and contracted employees. At least 90% of current providers utilize and assess the notebook for information and communication.

The consensus from current providers is that the notebook continues as a valuable, irreplaceable, easily accessible tool. It is easily placed into department specific computer hard drive for ready access when updated. Currently, it has been requested, forwarded,

(continues)

EXEMPLAR 10-1 Evaluation of an Army Regulation Electronic Contingency Notebook as a Process Improvement Tool During the Soldier Readiness Process   *(continued)*

and received by other Army deployment platforms (Fort Bliss, Fort Drum) and reserve component commanders across the U.S. by a unique, military Safe Access File Exchange, not previously available. It has been, and will continue, to require constant updates as the Army, Fort Hood, and OCONUS (outside the continental United States) Areas of Responsibility (AOR) update regulations and policies. In conclusion, this DNP project, at the time an innovative technological project, continues with revisions that contribute to the relevance and sustainability of the project.

Impact

- The impact of a well-planned project cannot be overemphasized.
- The attention to detail allows for implementation to proceed in an organized fashion.
- Plans that are well designed and communicated maintain transparency and the integrity of the team.
- Competencies of the doctoral nursing practice student are utilized to bring together teams, innovate, and evaluate results in sustainable projects that contribute to organizations.

Key Messages

- Use the nursing process at a doctoral level to refine your innovation and project plan based on assessment data.
- Successful project implementation depends on a carefully thought-out plan, with attention to detail.
- Multiple tools are available to assist in the development of the innovation idea and the project plan.
- Collaborate with content experts to build a team for the project.
- Understand all the specific requirements of the college or university and the organization where the project will be implemented.

Action Plan—Next Steps

1. Create alternative solutions to the identified problem.
2. Choose the best solution as the innovation.
3. Prepare for implementation using appropriate components of the project plan document.
4. Be aware of all requirements within the university and the organization.
5. Consider using the practicum as a stepping stone for project implementation.

References

American Association of Colleges of Nursing (AACN). (2015). *The doctor of nursing practice: Current issues and clarifying recommendations.* Retrieved from https://www.pncb.org/sites/default/files/2017-02/AACN_DNP_Recommendations.pdf

Colt, H. G., & Mulnard, R. A. (2006). Writing an application for a human subjects institutional review board. *Chest, 130*, 1605–1607.

Greaney, A. M., Sheehy, A., Heffernan, C., Murphy, J., Mhaolrunaigh, S. N., Heffernan, E., & Brown, G. (2012). Research ethics application: A guide for the novice researcher. *British Journal of Nursing, 21*(1), 38–43.

Houser, J. (2018). *Nursing research: Reading, using and creating evidence.* Burlington, MA: Jones & Bartlett Learning.

Mind Tools Limited. (n.d.) *Cost benefit analysis.* Retrieved from https://www.mindtools.com/pages /article/newTED_08.htm

Mochal, K. (2003). *Project implementation: Eight steps to success.* Retrieved from https://www .techrepublic.com/article/project-implementation-eight-steps-to-success/

Pech, C., Cob, N., & Cejka, J. T. (2007). Understanding institutional review boards: Practical guidance to the IRB review process. *Nutrition in Clinical Practice, 22*, 618. doi:10.1177 /0115426507022006618

Pinto, J. K., & Slevin, D. P. (1987). *Critical success factors in effective project implementation.* Retrieved from https://www.researchgate.net/publication/260621619_Critical_Factors_in_Successful _Project_Implementation

Project management. (2018). *Wikipedia.* Retrieved from http://en.wikipedia.org/wiki/Project _management

Smartsheet. (n.d.). *Cost benefit analysis template.* Retrieved from https://www.smartsheet.com /free-cost-benefit-analysis-templates

Tuckman, B. W., & Jensen, M. A. C. (1977). Stages of small-group development revisited. *Group & Organizational Management, 2*(4), 410–427. doi:10.1177/ 105960117700200404

Walsh, M. M., & Bowen, D. M. (2012). An introduction to grant writing: De-mystifying the process. *Canadian Journal of Dental Hygiene, 461*(1), 17–48.

Waxman, K. T. (2018). *Financial and business management for the doctor of nursing practice* (2nd ed.). New York, NY: Springer Publishing Company.

Weber, R. J., & Cobaugh, D. J. (2008). Developing and executing an effective research plan. *American Journal of Health-Systems Pharmacy, 65*, 2058–2065.

Weiserbs, K. F., Lyutic, L., & Weinberg, J. (2009). Should QI projects require IRB approval? *Academic Medicine, 84*(2), 153. doi:10.1097/ACM.0b013e3181939881

Helpful Resources

Grant Resources

Blue Cross Blue Shield of Michigan Student Award. Available at https://www.bcbsm.com/content /dam/microsites/foundation/student-award-program.pdf

Fastweb. *Scholarships.* Available at http://www.fastweb.com/content/featured_scholarships

Institutional Review Board Resources

CITI Program (Collaborative Institutional Training Initiative). *Research ethics and compliance training.* Available at https://www.citiprogram.org/Default.asp

U.S. Department of Energy. *Human subjects protection resource book.* Available at https://science. energy.gov/~/media/ber/human-subjects/pdf/education-and-resources/doe-resources/DOE _HSR_Resource_Book_2012_Update.pdf

U.S. Department of Health and Human Services, Health Resources and Services Administration (HRSA). *Protecting human subjects training.* Available at https://www.hrsa.gov/public-health /clinical/human-subjects/index.html

CHAPTER 11

Driving the Practicum to Impact the DNP Project

Rosanne Burson

CHAPTER OVERVIEW

The practicum is a unique opportunity to plan field experiences that support the development of doctor of nursing practice (DNP) competencies and professional scholarly growth. Immersion experiences provide an opportunity to apply, integrate, and synthesize the DNP *Essentials* necessary to demonstrate achievement of desired outcomes in an area of advanced nursing practice (American Association of Colleges of Nursing [AACN], 2015). There is also the potential to use the practicum in preparation for implementation of the DNP project. This chapter presents a process to focus and organize plans for an effective practicum with the designed outcomes. The practicum plan is driven by the DNP student's identified needs in collaboration with faculty and mentors.

CHAPTER OBJECTIVES

After completing the chapter, the learner will be able to:

1. Assess professional growth needs in relation to the DNP *Essentials* and the project needs.
2. Develop objectives for the practicum to successfully attain goals for professional development.
3. Identify an appropriate site and effective mentor for the practicum in collaboration with the faculty.
4. Use the opportunities within the practicum for professional growth and to prepare for DNP project implementation.

▶ Practicum Purpose

As the time for the practicum course approaches, DNP students may be at very different points in their preparation for the DNP project. The DNP student may have developed a keen view of the phenomenon and reviewed many aspects of the literature surrounding the phenomenon. There may be an understanding of the clinical question and the process that will be used for outcome improvement. Some of the integral structural parts of the plan may be in place, such as potential nursing theories that will support the project, or there may be some early thoughts on the methodology that will be utilized in the DNP project.

At this point in the curriculum, the student may have completed the DNP program coursework, which undoubtedly strengthened the student's skill set related to the DNP *Essentials*. The student should also be deciding on a project type and should begin thinking about all the components that will be required to complete the project successfully. It is important that the student understand that the DNP project team members and faculty support is available for assistance. (See Chapter 9, The DNP Project Team, for specific information related to relationships with the project team members.)

The practicum is another opportunity for the student to hone skills within the DNP *Essentials*. However, this course can also be used to further networking relationships and assess the organizational climate as a precursor to the implementation of the DNP project. The practicum is an ideal location to build the required skill set of the student and develop the setting for the project. This field time is also an opportunity to showcase the abilities of the DNP student and market the potential of DNP education to assist organizations in transition driven by data.

> *The practicum is an ideal location to build the required skill set of the student and develop the setting for the project.*

▶ Identifying the Setting

The DNP student should consider the potential setting of the DNP project as he or she plans for the practicum. For instance, a project that will improve the quality of care delivered to ventilated patients in the intensive care unit will require an acute care setting. Does the student have access to an acute care organization? The student may be working within an acute care organization, or he or she may have a professional contact within another organization.

Some universities have been strengthening their practice partnerships to enhance learning for DNP students and commit to strategic organizational goals related to health care. This approach provides an environment and key stakeholders who are committed to the project. Academic practice partnerships (APP) are intentional relationships based on shared vision, goals, knowledge, and respect (AACN/ American Organization of Nurse Executives [AONE], 2012). Chapter 3, Scholarship in Practice, discusses academic practice partnerships in more detail. The APP creates a system for doctoral nurses to achieve their goals for project development, implementation, and evaluation within the practicum and during project completion.

It is important for the DNP student to have a full understanding of the college or university requirements of the practicum. Some universities do not allow practicum hours within the organization of their place of work; others require that the student not work within the confines of his or her current role in the organization.

It is important for the student to have a full understanding of the college or university requirements of the practicum.

Each practicum setting choice has distinct positives and negatives. A practicum in an organization of which the student is not a member or employee offers a new lens that can broaden understanding of the project topic. The DNP student may identify issues within the practicum organization that align with the student's experience, or issues may be considerably different. The organization may benefit from a fresh pair of eyes viewing areas in which the organization has an interest, as well as expert hours offered to work on these specific aspects of the organization.

If the student is completing a practicum within his or her organization, one can assume that a relationship and a level of trust has developed. A good reputation can take one far. The student may have knowledge of different departments with which he or she will need to work to complete practicum and project objectives. The student may be knowledgeable about the organization and the current environment. Although this knowledge is helpful, it is important for students to separate themselves from their usual workday competencies. The student should keep in mind that it may be difficult for others with whom the student works on a daily basis to relate to him or her in another capacity.

Regardless of employment status, the bulk of the practicum can be positioned in the organization where the DNP project will be implemented. In this way, understanding the organization and developing relationships and trust, which are critical features that have already been established, will help the student successfully implement the project. Caution should be exercised, however, because the organization and the student may have competing goals. Further, the practicum design should incorporate specific experiences and deliverables that will give the student the opportunity to demonstrate the development of relationships and networks to facilitate the DNP project. For instance, as discussed in Chapter 10, Creating and Developing the Project Plan, identifying the institutional review board (IRB) representative and spending time asking specific questions related to the organization's IRB application process will develop a collaborative relationship and smooth the way for this part of the process. Practice experiences may include direct patient care but should also include indirect care practices in healthcare environments (AACN, 2015) to attain DNP competencies.

The student is demonstrating the DNP Essentials to the organization and so may be "sowing seeds" for potential roles suitable for the DNP-prepared nurses.

Finally, the student must remember several items. The student is demonstrating the DNP *Essentials* to the organization, and so may be "sowing seeds" for potential suitable roles for the DNP-prepared nurses. The student is marketing not only himself or herself but also the value-added benefits of the DNP-prepared nurse. Expect many opportunities within the practicum to discuss what the DNP-prepared nurse is all about and why the student has chosen this path. Preparing an "elevator speech" ahead of time can assist the student to respond in a logical, consistent, and concise manner. It is necessary to be able to respond in various time frames—a very short 1-minute response, as well as responses that are afforded more time.

Sometimes a student will identify the need for an independent study to become further immersed in a specific topic. An example is the DNP student who completed an informatics independent study to become more fully informed regarding available software and information technology (IT) issues to implement a project. As the DNP student considered the project scope, his or her realization of the need for additional understanding of informatics evolved. Many DNP programs have elective courses built into the curriculum and encourage independent studies that will strengthen the project.

▶ Matching Student Competency with Project Needs

An assessment of the student's current skill set prior to the onset of the practicum is essential in developing a practicum plan that will address strengthening core competencies. A recommended approach is to review each of the DNP *Essentials* competencies (AACN, 2006). The DNP student will identify specific areas for one's professional growth. For example, consider *Essential IV: Information Systems/Technology and Patient Care Technology for the Improvement and Transformation of Health Care.* One of the identified competencies is to demonstrate the conceptual ability and technical skills to develop and execute an evaluation plan involving data extraction from practice information systems and databases. The student may choose to design a plan for the practicum hours that will incorporate experiences to strengthen this core competency by spending time within the IT department or with the informatics nurse.

> *An assessment of the student's current skill set prior to the onset of the practicum is essential in developing a practicum plan that will address strengthening core skills.*

In addition to identifying learning needs for the student, an assessment of the competencies that will be needed specifically for the DNP project is in order. For example, the student may determine that outcome data for a population will need to be extracted as a step in the project. So, within the practicum, the student will want to identify a specific outcome or deliverable that will assist him or her in the project. Examples of deliverables may include defining data sets that are applicable for the DNP project, or it may be identifying and working with the data or IT department within the organization. Both of these outcomes will assist in moving the project forward through the practicum.

The student should move through each of the DNP *Essentials* competencies and determine what additional experiences will be needed for the project, differentiating current student strengths from competency areas that will be attained in the practicum (see **TABLE 11-1**).

Move through each of the DNP Essentials competencies and determine what additional experiences will be needed for the project— differentiating areas of student strength with what will need to be pursued in the practicum.

In this table, column 1 describes the specific competencies for this *Essential*. Column 2 is a self-rating by the student of his or her current competency on a scale based on Benner's (1984) novice to expert 1–5 competency levels. An asterisk (*) in column 3 indicates that this particular skill set is needed for the project. All competencies needed for the project, regardless of level of student competency, should be included in the practicum plan and identified by an *. If the student identified a professional growth need that is also needed for the project, column 4 will identify the need for practicum time in this area, identified by an additional *.

The practicum can also be used to strengthen a student's skill set that may not be required for the DNP project. The ^ sign will map this out as well.

In the preceding competency assessment example, the DNP student is reviewing competencies within *Essential* II. The student has identified that he or she has advanced communication skills, as evidenced by the rating of high competency. This is a skill set needed for the project (as indicated in column 3*). Even though the student has a high competency in this area, practicum time will need to be incorporated to move the project forward. The networking and collaboration accomplished during the practicum will assist the student in completing the project within that specific organizational environment. For this reason, column 4 identifies an *, indicating that it is needed for the practicum.

In the second competency, the student identifies a growth need in the area of business and finance to implement a practice initiative (self-rating 3). This is also identified as a component needed for the project. For this reason, column 4 posts **. In this case, practicum time is needed for both professional development and the project. The student will need to incorporate the cost initiatives as part of the project, so he or she will need to understand specific costs. In addition, the practicum time can be used to develop networks within the financial teams of the organization. For example, time spent with the chief financial officer (CFO), the business manager, or the finance team will build relationships for use during the project, as well as an understanding of the cost factors that drive the organization.

In the final competency, the student again identifies a growth need in the area of budget monitoring. However, it is determined that this specific skill is not needed for the project. Here, the DNP student uses the opportunity within the practicum to improve on the budget monitoring skill set even though it is not specifically needed as a skill in the project. This time is identified with the ^ sign. The *competency assessment for practicum design* tool template is available in Chapter 13,

TABLE 11-1 Competency Assessment for Practicum Design

Essential II: Organizational and Systems Leadership for Quality Improvement and Systems Thinking	DNP Student Competency Rating (1–5: See key)	Needed for Project	Needed for Practicum
Competencies			
Use advanced communication skills/ processes to lead quality improvement and patient safety initiatives in healthcare systems.	5	*	*
Employ principles of business, finance, economics, and health policy to develop and implement effective plans for practice-level and/or systemwide practice initiatives that will improve the quality of care delivery.	3	*	**
Develop and/or monitor budgets for practice initiatives.	1		^

Key:
Assessment 1–5

Explanation (based on Benner's *Novice to Expert*)
Student self-rated competency

- 5 = **Expert**: Highly competent or expert demonstration of competency.
- 4 = **Proficient**: Understands a situation as a whole, but not yet an expert with the competency.
- 3 = **Competent**: Does not yet have enough experience to recognize a situation in terms of an overall picture, but has an understanding of the competency.
- 2 = **Advanced Beginner**: Able to demonstrate marginally acceptable performance of the competency.
- 1 = **Novice**: No experience of the competency in which they are expected to perform.

*   Competencies needed for the scholarly project

**   Identified professional growth need for the project

^   Additional identified professional growth need

Reprinted with permission from the American Association of Colleges of Nursing (AACN). (2006). *The essentials of doctoral education for advanced nursing practice*. Retrieved from http://www.aacnnursing.org/Portals/42/Publications/DNPEssentials.pdf

The DNP Project Toolbox, Appendix A. It includes all the DNP *Essentials* and related competencies.

Once the student has worked through all the DNP *Essentials* and competencies in relation to the self-identified learning needs and project needs, he or she will be able to design an individualized plan for experiences within the practicum. The student will also be required to develop objectives and measurable outcomes for the practicum that address the self-identified assessment plan. The student collaborates with faculty in the assessment of learning needs and designing practice experiences to assure attention to all of the DNP *Essentials* (AACN, 2015). Also see Chapter 13 for use of the tool to identify competencies.

> *Once the student has worked through all the DNP Essentials and competencies in relation to the self-identified learning needs and project needs, he or she will be able to design an individualized plan for experiences within the practicum.*

▶ Site Agreements

It is important for the DNP student to understand that a site agreement may need to be in place prior to beginning the practicum. More information regarding the college- or university-specific process may be available in the DNP program policies. This is important to note because it can take time for the university to negotiate a new site agreement. Work closely with faculty and the DNP program director to be sure that the site agreements are in place prior to initiating field time within the institution. In addition, organizations may have varied requirements that must be met prior to the practicum. The college or university will most likely have requirements as well. These may include basic life support certification; tuberculosis test results, as well as proof of immunization or titers for varicella, MMR (measles, mumps, rubella), and hepatitis B; malpractice insurance; and others. These items may take time to procure, so be sure to allow for this time when planning your practicum.

> *Work closely with faculty and the DNP program coordinator to be sure that site agreements are in place prior to initiating field time within the institution.*

Practicum site decisions are a very important part of completing the *Essentials* competencies for the DNP student and for prepping for the scholarly project. Students should consider their personal needs assessment, their professional contacts, and the objectives for their practicum in making this decision. For some students, there may be multiple practicum sites to accomplish the determined objectives. Therefore, it is wise to check with an advisor early in the process to determine if the college or university will be making the contacts or if the student is expected to initiate contact with potential sites.

▶ Practicum Hours

DNP programs are accredited through a certification process administered by the Commission on Collegiate Nursing Education. The practicum requirement is based on AACN DNP *Essentials*, which require 1,000 hours of post-baccalaureate clinical hours in a practice setting. For post-master's DNP programs, each institution determines the number of relevant graduate hours required to have been attained per enrollee and how many additional hours are needed. A typical scenario is 500 hours post-master's of science in nursing (MSN) to be completed within the doctoral program. Advanced nursing practice hours are assessed individually by the program to determine the amount of required additional hours to develop DNP competencies (AACN, 2015). The DNP student should be well acquainted with all written descriptions and policies related to the practicum within one's university as well as documentation of practicum hours. A sample log for practicum hours (**TABLE 11-2**) is provided. Planning for these hours in one's life is very important. Therefore, the student should consider his or her fixed responsibilities (work, other courses, family, etc.) and the potential for reorganizing his or her life to commit to and complete the practicum and the DNP project. As rigorous as the process is, the student will want to be prepared to become immersed in the experience, grow as much as possible, and even enjoy it!

> *Consider reorganizing your life to commit to and complete the practicum and the DNP project.*

▶ Choosing a Mentor

Choosing a mentor is a critical feature of preparing for a successful practicum. "Mentoring is a developmental partnership through which one person shares knowledge, skills, information and perspective to foster the personal and professional growth of

TABLE 11-2 Practicum Tracking				
Date/Topic	**Description**	**Course Objective**	**DNP Essential**	**Hours**

Modified from Madonna University, Livonia, MI.

someone else. The power of mentoring is that it creates a one-of-a-kind opportunity for collaboration, goal achievement and problem-solving" (Stone, n.d., para. 1).

In a qualitative analysis of the characteristics of outstanding mentors, Cho, Ramanan, and Feldman (2011) identified the following attributes:

- Exhibits enthusiasm, compassion, and selflessness.
- Acts as a career guide, tailored to the mentee.
- Is able to make a time commitment.
- Supports personal/professional balance.
- Has effective communication skills.
- Is respected in the workplace by peers and senior administrators.
- Is politically astute.
- Is highly knowledgeable in the field.

When considering a mentor, the student should be sure to understand the requirements of the mentor in the specific DNP program. Many programs identify formal and professional experience as a requirement for the professional role, preferring a graduate degree in a specialty area of practice. For example, if the DNP student is working with the chief financial officer, it is expected that the CFO has a graduate degree in finance.

Often, the written descriptions of the practicum and the mentor–mentee relationship will set the stage for a successful practicum. This may include clearly defined roles and expectations of the mentor. Mentor–mentee expectations are particularly important because the DNP student may be rather new to the healthcare scene and unlikely to have an in-depth understanding of the DNP degree and the potential associated roles. Taking the time to review the expectations of both the mentor and mentee will lay the groundwork for a mutually respectful relationship.

> *Taking the time to review the expectations of both the mentor and the mentee will lay the groundwork for a mutually respectful relationship.*

As the student considers potential mentors, he or she should think about the expertise the mentor possesses as well as the opportunity to think differently and achieve the next stage of growth. The following characteristics of the mentor should be considered in relation to the specific needs of the student. The mentor should:

- Understand the nuances of the organization.
- Hold a position in the organization that matches the student need.
- Be able to network with multiple departments and high-level executives.
- Have expertise in an area that the DNP student requires.
- Be willing to share time and knowledge with the student.

In considering mentors, review the primary areas that have been identified for professional growth and project requirements. For instance, a DNP student who is studying to become a primary care nurse practitioner may be expert in the management and care of patients with asthma. The identified goals of professional growth may include informatics, the use of technology to reach patients, data mining, and the budgetary process for office management. The DNP student may consider a mentor who is in the finance or informatics area to develop a deeper understanding of these areas. The DNP student will also use the skills learned to apply to the project. In addition, when the project is completed within this organization, the DNP student will have developed relationships in these areas to assist with data or finance issues specific to the project.

Sometimes it may be difficult for the DNP student to identify an appropriate mentor. Discussing one's specific goals and objectives for the practicum with faculty, student peers, and work colleagues may elicit a potential list of mentor candidates for consideration.

While working with the mentor, the DNP student may require additional contacts to fulfill all the defined objectives. A mentor who is respected within the organization, networks well, and has a good understanding of the corporate dynamics will be able to advise the student on additional experiences and follow-up contacts. The DNP student in this example may wish to spend time with the director of the primary care practices or the IT department that works directly with the primary care office. Because the practicum plan is driven by the objectives, the additional contacts and experiences are unique and individualized to each student's identified needs.

Grossman (2007) described a *multiple mentoring model* whereby "the mentee can seek out advice from more than one mentor as well as use the most qualified mentor for each need" (p. 9). The DNP student may very well seek out multiple mentors to achieve the identified goals of the practicum. Various mentors will offer very different perspectives and be able to coach with different skill sets. In addition, at this time, many DNP students are being mentored by people who are not DNP-prepared nurses. Because of the lack of DNP mentors, the student may choose to seek out multiple mentors with various specific characteristics and skill sets. This is evolving as more DNP-prepared nurses become a part of organizations and offer the specific skill sets that the student is seeking. Even as the DNP mentor becomes a reality, the student will selectively choose additional mentors to focus on areas they wish to develop.

> *The DNP student may very well seek out multiple mentors to achieve the identified goals of the practicum.*

Reverse mentoring is defined as the mentee mentoring the mentor (Grossman, 2007). Sometimes the student will be able to offer expertise and mentoring in an area the mentee would appreciate. Of course, this varies based on the expertise of both mentor and mentee. For instance, the DNP student may bring a wealth of clinical background that can be used by the mentor. Mentoring is often thought of as a synergistic relationship in which all concerned learn, develop, and share.

As the DNP student considers the practicum experience in the mentee role, it is advantageous to reflect on the *Essentials* competencies of the mentee:

- Internal locus of control
- Interest in learning
- Emotional competence
- Achievement focused

For the practicum to yield maximum results, the DNP student needs to drive the experience, seeking out people and situations that will serve to meet the identified objectives. These characteristics exemplify internal locus of control and achievement focus. Further, an attitude that exemplifies an interest in learning will encourage the mentor and others that one meets to develop new relationships and share pearls from their experience. In essence, the DNP student must showcase emotional competence.

Emotional competence is defined as a "collection of perceptions, behaviors, knowledge, and values that . . . enable a leader to manage meaning between individuals and groups within an organization" (Porter-O'Grady & Malloch, 2015, p. 396). Emotional competence is critical in a new environment, where having a sense of appropriate behavior within the setting can make or break the experience. Some of the attributes of emotional competence include self-awareness, mindfulness, openness, appreciation of ambiguity and paradox, appreciation of knowledge, compassion, passionate optimism, and resilience (Porter-O'Grady & Malloch, 2015).

The following excerpt by Dr. Lisa Zajac demonstrates all these attributes as she describes her practicum experience (see **EXEMPLAR 11-1**).

> *For the practicum to yield maximum results, the DNP student needs to drive the experience, seeking out people and situations that will serve to meet the identified objectives.*

> *Emotional competence is critical in a new environment, where having a sense of appropriate behavior within the setting can make or break the experience.*

EXEMPLAR 11-1 DNP Practicum Reflection

Lisa M. Zajac, DNP, RN, ANP-BC, OCN

In my DNP program, our first practicum experience was in the policy course. Looking back, I remember how uninterested I was with policy in general. I always associated policy with lobbying and knew that I was not the type to march on Capitol Hill or influence legislators; I was fully content letting others speak on my behalf. However, after being immersed in the course content, spending 2 days at our state capitol meeting legislators, and meeting with my city councilwoman at a local town hall meeting, I learned that I did have a voice. I shared my concerns regarding community health issues and made suggestions for improvements, and they wanted to hear it. I realized that I could positively impact the health of my community, and that motivated me to do more.

(continues)

EXEMPLAR 11-1 DNP Practicum Reflection *(continued)*

The momentum continued in my epidemiology and population health course. My practicum experience in this course included conducting a windshield survey, which I chose to conduct in several zip codes in Detroit. Through this first-hand experience I was able to see the great aspects of the community, but also the incivilities and lack of healthcare resources in some of the neighborhoods. After researching the literacy, employment, crime, and healthcare statistics for the city, I realized that the residents could benefit from healthcare education as well as other resources. I took advantage of an opportunity that presented itself to talk to the residents in the community about their health concerns. They were open and honest and willing to share, and at the top of their list was the need to improve the safety of their neighborhoods.

This led me to attend a public "Conversations with the Councilwoman" forum focusing on public lighting. Approximately 150 residents attended the session. Representatives from the regional electric company were asked to attend the meeting to inform the residents of their plan to update all of the residential street lighting. While the residents were pleased to hear that residential street lights would be replaced, they were concerned because alley lighting was not included in the plan, which would be needed to deter crime. After hearing their concerns, the representatives from the electric company agreed to replace the alley lights for free; however, the cost of maintaining the alley lights would fall on the resident where the light was located. The representatives estimated that the cost would be about $15 a month to maintain one alley light. The residents were visibly disturbed by this. In a district where approximately one-third of the residents are living in poverty, it was clear that this would be difficult for residents to sustain.

After the meeting, I introduced myself to the councilwoman, told her I was a DNP student, and asked if she would be willing to meet with me to discuss the data I had collected that related to the health and welfare of the district that she represented. She agreed. While I was pleased to gain the interest of the councilwoman, I knew that I needed to come up with a feasible alternative that would address the residents' concerns about safety. This was the beginning of my community healthcare recommendation focusing on safety and security: the most basic healthcare need. A couple of weeks later, I walked into the city council office and presented my "Adopt an Alley" lighting initiative. She was impressed with my plan and offered her full support. The councilwoman quickly arranged a meeting with the executives from the electric company and asked me to present the "Adopt an Alley" lighting initiative. While they were initially resistant to the plan, after I addressed their concerns and presented a proposed operationalized plan, they agreed to support the initiative.

My final practicum course began the following term, which allowed me the opportunity to continue to work on my policy initiative. I was able to secure my practicum placement with the director of the Office of Nursing Policy for the state of Michigan. When I met with my mentor the first time, I shared my "Adopt an Alley" initiative and briefed her on what had transpired to date. She quickly connected me with key stakeholders in Michigan who she thought would have interest in my work, and the potential for dissemination began.

While the initiative began as a recommendation in my population health course, it was during my final practicum experience that I was able to see how all of the DNP *Essentials* (AACN, 2006) were incorporated and how all of my previous practicum experiences had laid the foundation to move this initiative forward. For example, early in the process my advanced nursing skills were used to assess the needs of the community, develop a plan to address the identified needs, and guide individuals and groups through the transition (*Essential* VIII). To accomplish this, I first analyzed both nursing and public health research to determine the nature and significance of the health problem. Since nearly all policy directly or indirectly impacts health, it was clear that a policy change was needed that would address the community's concern about safety and their overall well-being. As a result, an innovation was designed to meet the community's needs that was mindful of the ethical principles of justice and fidelity (*Essentials* I, III, and V). Throughout my doctoral coursework, I took advantage of opportunities to enhance my skill sets in leadership, advocacy, and principles of negotiation. As a result of these advanced skills, I was able to capitalize on my capacity to facilitate interprofessional collaboration in order to address the needs of the community. Even though I was initially met with resistance, I was eventually able to convince the executives from the electric company of the merit of my recommendation (*Essentials* II, VI, and VII). While I already possessed advanced informatics skills, it was because of my ability to translate the potential use of technology from a conceptual to an operationalized plan that the executives from the electric company were even willing to listen (*Essential* IV).

To close, as future DNP students look toward planning their practicum, I urge them to fully embrace each hour, for had I not, I would not have had the experience I did in Detroit. For my final practicum, I looked for opportunities where I could strengthen my skill set as a DNP student; I did not seek experiences where I felt most comfortable. Because of this, I am fully confident as a nursing leader who can truly make a difference in both policy and population health.

Prior to meeting with the identified mentor, the DNP student must have a complete understanding of the practicum requirements, mentor–mentee expectations, and objectives for the practicum, from both a program perspective and a professional development perspective. This will serve to increase the DNP student's confidence and will start the experience off in the right direction, with all participants on the same page. Dye and Garman (2006) have suggested a few expert tips in relation to approaching a mentor:

- Convey that one is grateful for the help.
- Be well prepared.
- Honor the meeting arrangements.
- Use time efficiently.
- Make it a two-way relationship.

In that first meeting with the mentor, using the preceding tips will help the DNP student get off to a great start. For example, a "thank you for the opportunity" can be a good introduction and lead-in for the meeting. When the student is well prepared, is on time, and uses the meeting time efficiently, a message of respect, professionalism, and time well spent is conveyed. Finally, by asking questions, listening attentively, and being engaged in the conversation, the student demonstrates true interest in the mentor's perspective, which will help develop the relationship. All these behaviors demonstrate emotional competence, an important characteristic of a successful mentee in laying the groundwork for the practicum.

▶ Developing Objectives for the Practicum

After identifying the specific professional growth and project needs, the DNP student is responsible for developing objectives that will drive the experiences within the practicum. By way of review, the final outcome of the practicum experiences is the achievement of a goal (Bastable, 2014). Goals are typically broad and difficult to directly measure. To begin, the student should consider the overall goal that he or she would like to reach. For example, perhaps the student's goal is to develop an innovation that will improve asthma care in the primary care setting. In this case, the DNP student will require a working knowledge of the asthma database within the health system to obtain preliminary data. After the overall goal is identified, the student needs to determine related objectives that are more specific to help him or her reach the overall goal. In other words, the objectives will describe the steps needed to reach the goal. In this example, a few of the objectives might be to (1) meet with the informatics specialists to review the data system and to identify key aspects of asthma reports and (2) identify potential clinical areas that receive asthma reports and would be amenable to working on their current processes related to asthma care.

Mager (1997) identified three parts to the objective:

1. A measurable verb (what the learner should be able to do)
2. A condition that the performance will occur within (under what conditions the learner should be able to do it)
3. Criteria for acceptable performance (how well the learner should be able to do it)

Writing objectives provides the learner with a way to organize activities in order to reach a goal, communicates to the mentor and/or faculty the activities for the design of the practicum, and provides deliverables that indicate when the objectives have been accomplished. The process of developing and communicating objectives will ensure that the practicum time is well designed and goals are met.

For the DNP student, writing of objectives allows one to focus on self-assessment and to design activities that will allow attainment of objectives. Reviewing the DNP program objectives, the DNP *Essentials*, and the practicum course objectives will assist the student in maintaining congruence in expectations of doctoral study. Objectives are the measurable actions that result in goal achievement. They are the first step in designing an organized plan to ensure that the student will use time effectively in the field. For the faculty and the mentor, objectives describe the steps that the student will take to reach professional growth needs and to lay the groundwork for the practicum evaluation.

> *The process of developing and communicating objectives will ensure that the practicum time is well designed and goals are met.*

Higher-level objectives typical of doctoral study focus on application, analysis, evaluation, and creation. **TABLE 11-3** identifies verbs for each level objective based on the Iowa State University's model of learning objectives. The model was defined by Heer (updated in 2012) using Anderson and Krathwohl's 2001

TABLE 11-3	Level Objective Verbs				
Level Objective	**Verb**				
I. Remember	Recall	Retrieve	Recognize	Identify	
II. Understand	Illustrate	Categorize	Summarize	Explain	Describe
III. Apply*	Execute	Implement	Demonstrate	Employ	
IV. Analyze*	Distinguish Organize Compare	Discriminate Differentiate Appraise	Calculate Relate Contrast		
V. Evaluate*	Judge Appraise	Monitor	Critique	Detect	Test
VI. Create*	Hypothesize	Design	Construct		

* DNP level.
Data from Heer, R. (2012). *A model of learning objectives*. Ames, IA: Iowa State University, Center for Excellence in Learning and Teaching. Retrieved from www.celt.iastate.edu/wp-content/uploads/2015/09/RevisedBloomsHandout-1.pdf

revision of the original Bloom taxonomy. Compare the table's objective levels with the program objectives of one's DNP program. As one develops objectives, use verbs that are consistent with an appropriate level, such as analysis, evaluation, and creation.

The acronym SMART is a common format used to guide the development of objectives; SMART specifies that objectives should be:

- Specific—Be as concrete as possible, use action verbs to communicate effectively.
- Measurable—How will one know that the objective has been attained?
- Achievable—Within the allowed time frame.
- Realistic—The resources and the time allowed set one up for success.
- Timely—When will the objective be achieved?

Here is a sample for review:

1. Identify the overall goal related to the *Essentials*, professional growth, and the project:
    a. *Advance the use of information, IT, communication networks, or patient care technology in a particular patient practice setting.*
2. Identify specific objectives (steps) that will move toward goal achievement:
    a. *Analyze (verb—analysis level) current IT used in this practice setting (the setting in which this will occur) by field time with IT and the practice manager to observe practice specifics and compare with current literature (how this will occur).*

b. In SMART format, the objective would read as: *Analyze current technology utilized in this practice* (specific) *by field time with IT and the practice manager to observe practice specifics in comparison with current literature* (measurable *and* achievable *based on time frame, with appropriate* resources) *by the fifth week of the practicum* (timely).

3. The student may determine that a practicum deliverable will assist in meeting the identified goal.

▶ Practicum Deliverables

In determining the practicum deliverables, one must identify which of the developed objectives will have a concrete item to be delivered to the faculty/mentor or organization. The student will need to determine which items will be helpful in connecting the objectives and outcomes to the *Essentials* and the project. Here are some examples of practicum deliverables related to the objectives discussed in the previous paragraph:

> Analyze the current state of this practice's use of the electronic health record, database, and patient portal in comparison with the current IT availability and report to the practice, mentor, and faculty in a one-page summary by week 6 of the practicum.

Sometimes a practicum deliverable will expand beyond the immediate site to incorporate next steps that will develop the DNP student in preparation for the DNP project. Here are a few examples:

> Organize and complete a poster presentation on the Blue Cross quality incentive program for providers, including electronic reporting of quality measures. Present the poster at the local chapter of Sigma Theta Tau research conference on September 23, XXXX.
>
> Design an independent study proposal that will contribute to an understanding of the full scope of the DNP project, which is an exploration, analysis, and synthesis of the current state of standardized language of advanced nursing practice in electronic health records. The independent study elective application will be developed with faculty in nursing informatics by fall XXXX.

The next example relates to implementing a change process within a clinical area. In this case, an organizational assessment may be a concrete deliverable. By performing the assessment, the DNP student demonstrates the ability to operationalize this skill in order to determine feasibility for the project success. In addition, strengths and weaknesses can be determined prior to project implementation to develop plans based on the results. The process of being involved with the staff will also begin to solidify relationships prior to implementation. Following is an example of an objective related to these skills:

> Explore the status of the organizational culture with key stakeholders within the system in relation to transforming primary care offices,

specifically two employed physician practices. The results will be submitted in the form of SWOT (strengths/weaknesses/opportunities/threats) analyses specific to the overall system and to each of the two practices to faculty by 7/1/XX.

Note that in the next examples, the objective is also tied to course practicum objectives, DNP *Essentials*, and competencies:

Meet with key stakeholders within the organization to discuss the organizational structure and culture within the primary care setting. Effective communication skills will be utilized in these meetings, articulating the purpose of the project and collaborating where appropriate to meet the needs of the specific care settings where the pilot will take place. A summary paper will be submitted to faculty by June 28, XXXX, as evidence of meeting practicum objective numbers 4 and 8 and DNP *Essentials* II-2a and e; VI-1; VII-2, 3; and VIII-1, 3, and 7.

In exploring business and finance aspects of the environment, the following objectives have been defined:

Examine budgets utilized within the organization specific to two identified offices. The purpose of the examination is to identify line items to consider in implementing new programs within primary care offices. The knowledge will be used to develop a budget proposal to sustain the nurse certified diabetes educator (CDE) within the patient-centered medical home (PCMH). The budget will be submitted for review to faculty and the business mentor by 7/23/XX (*Essential* II-1, 2a, b, c).

Examine the cost effectiveness and financial sustainability of integrating the registered nurse (RN) CDE in the primary care setting by evaluating current reimbursement for education and specific care management within a sample of primary care practices. This will be accomplished by evaluating the patient education reimbursement, evaluation and management codes used, billing charges submitted, and reimbursement received within a sample of these practices. A budget that summarizes the costs for integrating a CDE in this setting and the potential reimbursement will be submitted to faculty by July 24, XXXX, as evidence of meeting practicum objective numbers 2 and 3 and DNP *Essentials* II-2b, c, and d; IV-3; and VIII-7.

The key aspects of the practicum objectives are that they are driven by the needs of the DNP student, are designed to incorporate growth in doctoral essential competencies, and prepare the student for implementation of the DNP project.

▶ Presenting the Practicum Plan

The DNP student will present the objectives and deliverable plan to faculty and mentor(s) prior to initiation of the practicum. Input from faculty and/or mentor(s) may identify additional networking opportunities with departments or key players within the organization. Concurrently, the student will plan with the faculty/mentor regarding how, when, and where time will be spent to achieve the objectives within the practicum time frame. Practicum experiences should be tied back to student-developed professional objectives, practicum course objectives, and DNP *Essentials*. Practice experiences should prepare the student with outcomes delineated in all of the DNP *Essentials* and should be integrated into the student's practice (AACN, 2015). Table 11-2 suggests a format for tracking the practicum hours.

> *Input from faculty and/or mentor(s) may identify additional networking opportunities with departments or key players within the organization.*

▶ Implementing the Practicum

As the practicum is implemented, evaluate the progress toward goals and be ready to adjust the plan as needed. Take advantage of opportunities that develop that were not originally discussed. The richer the practicum experience, the more informed the student will be regarding the phenomenon of interest and the organization as a potential project site.

Multiple areas within the practicum can make for a smoother transition to the DNP project. Exploring specifics to the environment, such as the organizational structure, can prepare the DNP student for the scholarly project. Conducting a SWOT analysis of the environment in preparation for the project and developing relationships with the key stakeholders in order to understand the structure is time well spent (see Chapter 6, Developing the DNP Project).

Potential barriers to the DNP project may be identified during the practicum experience as well. Recognizing real or potential barriers early on will give the student the opportunity to develop action plans to either remove the barriers or to alter the plan. This again can smooth the project implementation experience and save valuable time.

Learning the IRB process within the organization during the practicum can also help move the project forward. Understanding the process and making contacts with the key players in the process will smooth the transition for the project and save time. Review Chapter 10 for more detailed information on the IRB process.

▶ Practicum Evaluation— Were the Objectives Met?

At the completion of the practicum, an evaluation of the objectives should be undertaken. The evaluation is completed by both mentor and student. Completion is validated by the deliverables that were identified in the planning phase of the practicum. If an objective was not met, barriers to achieving the outcome should be identified.

▶ Setting the Stage for the DNP Project

With a well-planned practicum, the student will be able to (a) identify a project site that aligns the organizational need with the goals of the project, b) develop key relationships that will assist him or her in working within the system, (c) assess the organizational culture to determine probability of successful implementation, (d) consider potential barriers so that a plan to move forward can be realized prior to the implementation of the project, and (e) learn aspects of the organizational system, such as formal and informal reporting and the IRB process, for use during the project implementation.

The site of the practicum may continue as the site for implementation of the DNP project depending on university requirements for the project. As always, the student should be familiar with the approach and recommendations of the university. Utilizing one's mentor for a smooth transition to the project is essential for credibility and consistent messaging. The mentor may also continue to be a valuable resource during the project implementation.

▶ Closing Out the Practicum

As the practicum comes to a close, the DNP student will want to tie up loose ends by communicating with all key stakeholders. The method of communication should mirror the organization's preferred methods—verbal, email, or formal report.

Showing appreciation to the mentor for time spent and knowledge shared is part of the closure of the practicum. The DNP student will want to choose a way to thank the mentor and may also want to keep the lines of communication open for future networking opportunities.

Impact

- A successful practicum will impact the student, organization, and the project in many ways.
- For the student, networking within the institution can expand connections that may later affect opportunities and further growth.
- The chance to exemplify the DNP competencies in the field serves to strengthen the student skills as well as confidence in newly developed competencies.
- The use of educated clinicians with a focus on an organizational need can assist the organization by moving strategic priorities forward.
- In addition, by working with the student, administrative leaders may develop new ways to support graduates through the creation of new roles, to accommodate their skill set to the advantage of the organization.
- Finally, a well-planned practicum will move the project forward from proposal to implementation and evaluation.

Key Messages

- The practicum is an ideal location to build the student's required skill set and develop the setting for the project.
- It is important for the student to have a full understanding of the college or university requirements of the practicum.

- The student is demonstrating the DNP *Essentials* to the organization and so may be "sowing seeds" for potential suitable DNP roles.
- An assessment of the student's current skill set prior to the onset of the practicum is essential in developing a practicum plan that will address strengthening core skills.
- Taking the time to review the expectations of both the mentor and mentee will lay the groundwork for a mutually respectful relationship.
- For the practicum to yield maximum results, the DNP student needs to drive the experience, seeking out people and situations that will serve to meet the identified objectives.
- The process of developing and communicating objectives will ensure that the practicum time is well designed and goals are met.

Action Plan—Next Steps

1. Assess professional growth needs based on the DNP *Essentials* and practicum course objectives.
2. Assess specific skill set needs for the DNP project.
3. Develop overall goals for the practicum.
4. Identify SMART objectives to reach the goals.
5. Plan practicum experiences and deliverables around the objectives.
6. Choose the site and mentor for the practicum.
7. Present practicum plan to faculty and mentor, integrating additional suggestions and refining based on input.

References

American Association of Colleges of Nursing (AACN). (2006). *The essentials of doctoral education for advanced nursing practice.* Retrieved from http://www.aacnnursing.org/Portals/42/Publications/DNPEssentials.pdf

American Association of Colleges of Nursing (AACN). (2015). *The doctor of nursing practice: Current issues and clarifying recommendations.* Retrieved from https://www.pncb.org/sites/default/files/2017-02/AACN_DNP_Recommendations.pdf

American Association of Colleges of Nursing/American Organization of Nurse Executives (AACN/AONE) (2012). *AACN/AONE task force on academic practice partnerships: Guiding principles.* Retrieved from http://www.aacnnursing.org/Academic-Practice-Partnerships/The-Guiding-Principles.

Anderson, L. W., & Krathwohl, D. R. (Eds.). (2001). *A taxonomy for learning, teaching and assessing: A revision of Bloom's taxonomy of educational objectives.* New York, NY: Addison Wesley Longman.

Bastable, S. B. (2014). *Nurse as educator: Principles of teaching and learning for nursing practice.* Burlington, MA: Jones & Bartlett Learning.

Benner, P. (1984). *From novice to expert: Excellence and power in clinical nursing practice.* Menlo Park, CA: Addison-Wesley, pp. 13–34.

Cho, C. S., Ramanan, R. A., & Feldman, M. D. (2011). Defining the ideal qualities of mentorship: A qualitative analysis of the characteristics of outstanding mentors. *American Journal of Medicine, 124*(5), 453–458.

Dye, C. F., & Garman, A. N. (2006). Mentors: How to identify, approach and use them for maximal impact. In C. F. Dye & A. N. Garman (Eds.), *Exceptional leadership: 16 critical competencies for healthcare executives* (pp. 207–212). Chicago, IL: Health Administration Press.

Grossman, S. C. (2007). *Mentoring in nursing: A collaborative and dynamic process.* New York, NY: Springer Publishing Company.

Heer, R. (2012). *A model of learning objectives.* Ames, IA: Iowa State University, Center for Excellence in Learning and Teaching. Retrieved from www.celt.iastate.edu/wp-content/uploads/2015/09/RevisedBloomsHandout-1.pdf

Mager, R. F. (1997). *Preparing instructional objectives* (3rd ed.). Atlanta, GA: Center for Effective Performance.

Porter-O'Grady, T., & Malloch, K. (2015). *Quantum leadership: Building better partnerships for sustainable health* (4th ed.). Burlington, MA: Jones & Bartlett Learning.

Stone, A. (n.d.). *University of South Carolina College of Mass Communication and Information Studies, USC CMIS Alumni Society Mentoring Program handbook.* Retrieved from http://cmcismentorprogram.wordpress.com/mentoring-program- manual/definition-of-mentoring/

CHAPTER 12

The Proposal

Katherine Moran

CHAPTER OVERVIEW

Students enter the doctor of nursing practice (DNP) program with different levels of exposure to academic writing. As a result, writing proficiency can vary from student to student. For those students with limited writing experience, just the thought of writing a formal project proposal can be intimidating. To support the student in the project proposal writing process, this chapter (1) helps the student recognize early in the process when he or she may need some additional writing support, (2) introduces the student to the components included in a project proposal, and (3) provides a template for the student to refer to when beginning the process of writing the DNP project proposal.

CHAPTER OBJECTIVES

After completing the chapter, the learner will be able to:

1. Evaluate his or her writing skills.
2. Develop a proposal outline.
3. Recognize the potential components of a proposal.
4. Write a project proposal according to institutional guidelines.

▶ Professional Writing

Whether it is writing a proposal for doctorate work or writing for the purpose of publication, professional writing is part of the dissemination-of-knowledge process. In the case of the doctoral proposal, it represents the student's intellectual ability, knowledge in the subject area, and contributions to nursing. As a doctorally prepared nurse, there is an expectation from the profession that nursing knowledge will be distributed either in written form or through oral presentation; it is considered part of one's professional responsibility. In some ways, it can be equated to being accountable to nursing research, theory, and practice.

The doctoral proposal represents the student's intellectual ability, knowledge in the subject area, and contributions to nursing.

Evaluating Your Writing Skill Set

Writing is a foundational skill that involves application, analysis, synthesis, and practice, which follows skill acquisition, discipline, and coaching (Giddens & Lobo, 2008; Shirey, 2013). The capacity to engage in scholarly writing is no longer a skill set that should exist exclusively within the professoriate; it is a competency required of all nurses to move the profession forward (Shirey, 2013). However, students enrolled in doctoral programs today come with varying skill sets and writing experiences. Moreover, graduate students may lack the knowledge, experience, and/or confidence to engage in scholarly writing (Fauchald & Bastian, 2015). A study by Dols, Hernandez, and Miles (2017) revealed poor writing skills in doctor of nursing practice (DNP) students were compounded by the inability of the students to meet the level of scholarship expected throughout the development, implementation, and evaluation of the DNP project; writing difficulties occurred in anywhere from less than 5% of students to the majority of students (p. 90). If the student is not experienced in the writing process, basic writing skills should be evaluated. For example, novice writers may inadvertently use improper sentence structure or grammar, cite secondary versus primary sources, neglect foundational literature, or simply have difficulty writing succinctly. As a result of these insufficiencies, some advanced writing skills, such as organization, synthesizing research, and writing evidence-based literature, may also be lacking (Moos & Hawkins, 2009). A study by Morse (2009) of academic chairs and deans ($n = 704$) that examined academic writing (undergraduate and graduate level) revealed that formatting issues (punctuation, spelling, capitalization, and paragraph formatting) were of *moderate* concern; formatting of citations and references received a ranking of *very concerned*; and writing style (presentation of ideas, precision, and clarity) received a ranking of *moderately* to *very concerned*, indicating a need for improvement in these areas.

These concerns, however, can be overcome with faculty and institutional support. For example, most universities have a writing center to help the student with basic writing skills, grammar, formatting, and use of Microsoft Office Word software. Using simple writing strategies can make the process less arduous and help the student write more effectively. For instance, expert writers have long preferred strong use of nouns and verbs when composing a meaningful manuscript; nouns let the reader see whom the student is writing about, and the verbs show the reader the action taken (Leddy, 2011). Adverbs should be used only to add significant meaning.

The student should also seek guidance from his or her advisor and DNP project team members and feedback on his or her work from colleagues early in the process. Gaining this insight from the collegial perspective is invaluable. Even though it may be difficult for the student to receive constructive criticism, he or she should take it willingly because the intent is to help improve the final product. For example, some students become frustrated when revisions are made based on the feedback, only to be reversed at a later date. The student should

> *The student should seek feedback from colleagues early in the writing process.*

keep in mind that this is *a process* for everyone involved—the student and the reviewers alike. Remember, as the proposal develops, it changes and evolves; as this occurs, the true meaning of the proposal becomes more evident. An added bonus is that through this process, the student's writing skills become more refined. Generally, the more one writes, especially when completing doctoral work, the easier the process becomes. Although it may be a labor-intensive process, it will be worth it in the end.

Another writing strategy that may be helpful is to look at the situation from different perspectives. Roy Peter Clark, a renowned master writer, refers to this as writing *cinematically* (Leddy, 2011). The concept of writing cinematically is vital when describing the totality of the phenomenon of interest. Stop to think about what the main message is and how to say it effectively without using clichés or jargon. Resist the temptation to replace conversational language with complex, long-winded dialogue because of the perception that it sounds more academic (Lee, 2010). Even complex material should be presented in a straightforward and simple manner. Using appropriately labeled headings and bulleted points (where appropriate) will help with clarity and make the proposal easier to read and understand.

A key factor to successful writing is allowing sufficient time for the writing process. Insufficient time for creative thinking, analysis and synthesis of the literature, or even careful consideration of the main message can lead to fragmented thoughts that are difficult to follow at best. Starting the proposal early is advantageous because it leaves time for revisions and final polishing (Leddy, 2011). The student should factor in enough time to deal with unexpected changes recommended by those critiquing the work prior to submission—that is, the advisor, project team members, or peers. After all, a substantial amount of the work occurs after the content of the manuscript has been established: the editing. The student should plan on the editing process constituting about 70% of the total time it takes to write a manuscript (Heyman & Cronin, 2005).

> *Insufficient time for creative thinking and analysis and synthesis of the literature ... can lead to fragmented thoughts that are difficult to follow.*

Another point worth mentioning relates to the need to properly cite sources. The student must have a clear understanding of how to reference another author's work, both parenthetically and in the reference section. Many schools of nursing in the university setting follow the *Publication Manual of the American Psychological Association* (APA) for communicating scholarly work in written form. The student should be familiar with the APA format before beginning the writing process.

The student should also understand the difference between primary and secondary sources and the importance of avoiding plagiarism. Primary sources are work from the original author; it comes from the source. For example, when a researcher conducts a study and then publishes the results, the researcher is the primary source; he or she conducted and interpreted the research. Secondary sources, on the other hand, discuss work from primary sources, offering interpretation and discussion. The problem with using secondary source material stems from the fact that one author is analyzing, synthesizing, interpreting, and then discussing another author's work. If he or she interprets the results inaccurately and the student then cites the work from this secondary source, the information provided by the student is inaccurate as well. The takeaway message here is to cite primary sources whenever possible.

Plagiarism, simply defined, occurs when one person uses another person's or group's work, idea, or words as his or her own without citing the source ("Plagiarize," 2018). Some refer to this as literary theft. Certainly, this can occur inadvertently if the student is not familiar with the rules for citing sources or does not take the time to organize and document referenced material. To avoid plagiarism, the student should familiarize himself or herself with what constitutes plagiarism. For example, if the student used words from a journal article verbatim without using quotation marks and without citing the source, this would constitute plagiarism. Using quotation marks but failing to cite the source also is considered plagiarism because the source is not cited. Another example includes paraphrasing another person's work without citing the source.

> Plagiarism *occurs when one person uses another person or group's work, idea, or words without citing the source* ("Plagiarize," 2018).

Self-plagiarism is also considered as a form of plagiarism. The process of self-plagiarism involves "presenting one's own previously published work as if it were new" (APA, 2010, p. 170). Even though one may not be using another person's work, the concern centers on the potential of copyright infringement. According to APA (2010), "the core of the new document must constitute an original contribution to knowledge, and only the amount of previously published material necessary to understand that contribution should be included" (p. 16).

Remember, plagiarism occurs when one person uses another person's or group's work, idea, or words without giving credit to the source, and self-plagiarism occurs when one presents his or her own previously published work as if it were new. The only exception to this is if the information being used is considered common knowledge—that is, information the average person already knows. The student can avoid plagiarism by consistently documenting sources used to substantiate or inform his or her work. For students who wish to learn more about plagiarism, Indiana University offers an online plagiarism module that may be helpful (Frick et al., 2014). This resource is available at https://www.indiana .edu/~istd/plagiarism_test .html. See Chapter 15, Disseminating the Results, for a discussion of plagiarism detecting programs.

One final thought that the student should keep in mind: His or her writing style may not be refined at the beginning of the process, but over time, it should become clearer and the student should become a stronger writer (Heyman & Cronin, 2005; Shirey, 2013). Multiple approaches can be used to manage writing the proposal for a scholarly project. For example, some writers choose to follow a systematic approach to writing—that is, starting at the beginning with the completion of the abstract (allowing the writer to plan the manuscript content), followed by the introduction, background, literature review, and so on. Others choose to start in the middle of the manuscript. In this case, the focus is on capturing the key points on paper and then substantiating the work with the literature review, followed by the approach used, the intervention or proposed improvement process, analysis, implications for practice, and ending with the abstract. The DNP student will need to identify the process that works best for him or her.

▶ Writing the Proposal

The lessons from Stephen Covey (1989) are applicable when embarking on any significant project or major undertaking (such as writing a doctoral proposal): *to begin with the end in mind.* Simply stated, this means that the writer should plan ahead. First, review the college or university's requirements for the DNP project, which will vary from university to university. For example, some universities use a dissertation format, while others use an executive summary format or a quality improvement process format. Second, know what it is you want to write (your message), for whom (the audience), and why (ultimate goal).

The importance of a well-written proposal cannot be overstated. This document is essentially a vehicle by which the student *makes the case* for his or her project. He or she must express why his or her project is important, that it will be valued by society (the stakeholders), and that it can be done.

Begin with the end in mind. . .

Developing an Outline

Developing an outline is a great way to organize thoughts and to ensure that the key points of the manuscript are captured. However, to develop the outline, the student will need to know the expectations of the university regarding the doctoral proposal format. The student should schedule time to meet with his or her advisor or DNP project mentor to review how the manuscript should be organized; what the reviewers will be looking for; and what format should be used, including the required length, typeface, font size, word spacing, and margin size.

How to Approach the First Draft

Just start writing! It is helpful for writers, regardless of their preferred writing style, to write a rough draft as soon as possible (Happe, 2005). As the name implies, the rough draft is not the final draft. Therefore, focusing on every little detail is not the purpose of this stage in the writing process. The rough draft should be viewed as simply getting the ideas on paper; otherwise, the ability to write freely is lost (Happe, 2005). The student should allocate a certain amount of time each day or week to writing. This time should be spent *only* on those activities relevant to the proposal writing process. Do not allow other competing priorities to take precedence, even if that means sitting quietly gathering thoughts.

Once the first draft is complete, time can be spent perfecting the manuscript—adding references, checking the structure and content for accuracy, and ensuring that the message is clear and the flow is appropriate. Remember that the goal in writing the proposal is to transfer information from the writer to the reader in a manner that is easily understood. At this point, in addition to having an advisor or project faculty mentor review the manuscript, it is helpful to have the manuscript reviewed by a peer with experience in the content area to ensure that the presentation of the material is both accurate and easy to follow (Happe, 2005).

Writing Resources

As mentioned, most nursing programs and professional nursing journals use APA as the preferred editorial style guide. Further, many universities offer some type of writing support for students to help them with APA style and with general writing skills. These services may be offered either on campus, such as through an academic writing center or writing labs, or via online tutorials available through the university's library and/or electronic database. A few helpful writing tips are included at the end of this chapter.

▶ Components of the Proposal

Although the requirements for a doctoral proposal may vary from institution to institution, many include an informative title, an abstract or executive summary, an introduction, the background and significance, a statement of the problem and/or clinical question, the literature review, the organizational assessment (internal evidence) if appropriate, the project aim or purpose, and the theoretical or conceptual framework. This is typically followed by the methodology, including ethical considerations, a description of the setting and participants, the intervention or proposed improvement process, measures and instruments chosen to study the processes and/or outcome of the intervention, analysis, sustainability plan, and implication for practice. In an effort to address the broad and varying needs of DNP students, the following hypothetical pilot study is used to illustrate a comprehensive project proposal that evaluates a healthcare program and the potential to impact outcomes in a specific population. The student should follow his or her college or university's proposal requirements when developing the project proposal. The outline followed here builds on the components of the Standards for Quality Improvement Reporting Excellence (SQUIRE) guidelines, which were developed to assist those reporting quality improvement in health care (SQUIRE, 2015). Other resources that may be helpful when developing the project proposal include the Consolidated Standards of Reporting Trials (CONSORT), which are useful for improvement projects or effectiveness studies that use a randomized controlled trial design (CONSORT, n.d.), or the Strengthening the Reporting of Observational Studies in Epidemiology (STROBE) guidelines for projects that use observational or qualitative techniques (STROBE, 2009).

The Title

The title of the proposal is very important. It is the student's first opportunity to gain a reader's interest in his or her work. The title should briefly articulate what the project is about. Avoid using a long, descriptive title but make sure enough information is provided for the reader to understand the overall purpose of the proposal. To illustrate this, consider a hypothetical project that involves African American women who suffer caregiver stress when caring for sick family members at home. The proposed program is provided by a parish nurse who is able to positively affect stress levels through the introduction of stress reduction techniques using a caring approach. A title using this same information would be too wordy and may disengage the reader. A succinct title that includes the necessary information would be: *Introducing a Stress Reduction Program to African American Women Suffering from Caregiver Stress.*

The Abstract/Executive Summary

The abstract/executive summary should be concise, but should be sufficient to arouse the reader's interest. In other words, the abstract/executive summary should include a succinct summary of the proposal yet give enough information to be informative. Some find writing this section difficult because of the need to condense the main points of the manuscript into a few short sentences. It may be helpful for the student to review abstracts from peer-reviewed journals to get a sense of how published authors accomplish this task. The abstract typically includes the statement of the problem, a description of the purpose of the project, methods or approach, data analytical procedures, and implications for practice. An executive summary includes the background, summary of main points, conclusion, and recommendations. An example follows.

> **Problem Statement:** African American women caring for loved ones over time are experiencing high levels of caregiver stress that negatively impact their health, increase medical costs, and result in loss of work productivity.
>
> **Purpose:** Determine if a stress reduction program introduced by a parish nurse using a caring approach that focuses on the patient relationship is a cost-effective method to decrease stress scores, reduce the number of lost workdays, and increase self-rated health in African American women experiencing caregiver stress.
>
> **Methods:** A two-group pretest–posttest design will be used. Participants will be recruited from three community churches.
>
> **Inclusion Criteria:** English-speaking, African American women, between 20 and 60 years of age, with no comorbid conditions, who have provided caregiving services for a loved one ≥ 6 months, with a self-rated stress score ≥ 5, who are not practicing stress reduction techniques. The intervention includes an assessment and introduction of stress reduction strategies by the parish nurse that will be practiced by the participants over a period of 6 months. All participants will be asked to complete a self-rated stress level questionnaire, a survey of workdays over the past 6 months, and self-rated perception of health survey.
>
> **Analysis:** Paired sample t-tests will be used to evaluate whether the participants experienced reduction in stress levels, fewer lost workdays, and higher levels of perceived health after participating in the program. A cost analysis will be conducted to determine the sustainability of the program and potential to replicate the initiative throughout local parishes.

Implications for Practice: Reducing caregiver stress may lead to a decrease in stress-related health issues, fewer lost days of work, and an improvement in perception of health.

The Introduction

The introduction tells the reader why the topic is important; it sets the stage for what is to come. The student should spend time briefly describing the impetus to the project, the relevance of the topic, and the scope of the potential problem.

Background and Significance

In this section, the student should expand on the introduction. For example, for a quality improvement project, the student would describe how a dysfunction in a healthcare service delivery system adversely affects patients, staff, or the system as a whole, or prevents care from reaching its full potential (SQUIRE, 2015, p. 5). Regardless of the type of DNP project the student is embarking on, the student should seek to answer the following questions: Why is it important for this work to be completed? What are the problems that have been identified, and what are the implications? Why should the reader be interested in this project or topic? This section should give the reader an idea of what the local problem is and the characteristics of the organization in which it occurs; it is a lead-in to the problem statement.

Using the previous example of African American women experiencing caregiver stress, the student may want to begin by giving the statistics regarding the prevalence of caregiver stress among this group. The student may want to talk about the type of problems these women experience when caring for their loved ones, perhaps describing the family members who are receiving care and the type of care the women are providing. It may also be helpful to discuss the obstacles these women have to overcome to provide care for their family members; how providing this care is affecting their physical, psychological, or emotional health; the financial cost to individuals, families, and society of providing this care; and what is likely to occur if this care is not provided (implications).

The Problem Statement

The statement of the problem should be concise but clearly articulate the breadth and depth of the problem, why it is a concern, and why it should be evaluated (i.e., the nature and the severity of the specific problem). Given that the introduction, background, and significance sections provided the background for the problem (the lead-in), the student should spend time justifying the need for embarking on this project. Substantiating the problem with factual information or personal opinion is helpful (Nolinske, 1996). Finally, the student may want to conclude this section with a statement indicating why this is a problem for society (based on what was stated previously) and that it should be evaluated. For example,

African American women are experiencing high levels of caregiver stress that negatively impact their health, increase medical costs, and result in loss of work productivity. This is a trend that has increased more than 30%

over the past 10 years and is not expected to change in the near future. If this trend is allowed to continue, the health status of these women is likely to continue to decline, and medical costs will increase, which will negatively impact individuals, families, and communities; therefore, this phenomenon should be evaluated.

The Clinical Question

The problem statement leads to the development of a clinical question that is relevant to practice (Velasquez & Bonham, 2015). The clinical question helps the student describe the phenomenon of interest, informs the reader about an issue, and clarifies previous research, or it can add to the body of knowledge already available (Nolinske, 1996). One clinical question for caregiver stress could be:

Do African American women who participate in stress reduction activities rate their level of self-rated health higher after participating in the program?

As mentioned in Chapter 6, Developing the DNP Project, the *PICO approach* is an effective method to use to develop a good clinical question. PICO stands for Population, Intervention, Comparison, and Outcomes. In the clinical question example, the population is African American women, the intervention is stress reduction activities, the comparison includes preintervention and postintervention self-rated health data, and the outcome is how women who participate in stress reduction activities rate their level of health.

The information presented here is specific to a pilot project; however, it is useful information that is applicable to many types of DNP projects. For example, the formation of a clinical question could be used to help guide the student who is embarking on a program evaluation project, a quality improvement project, or a project with a focus on contributing to health policy. Using the example above, a program evaluation question could be: *Is a stress reduction program for African American women in a parish setting beneficial, sustainable, and replicable?* More information regarding scholarly project methods is available in Chapter 7, Aligning Design, Method, and Evaluation with the Clinical Question.

The Literature Review

Exploring the current literature (available knowledge) is helpful because it gives the student an opportunity to see what has been done around his or her phenomenon of interest, to synthesize the information, and to come to a conclusion about what is available. A comprehensive literature review provides the evidence to defend a *logical argument* supporting the need for and value of the proposed scholarly project, such as:

- African American women are experiencing high levels of caregiver stress.
- Caregiver stress can result in health issues and loss of work productivity.
- Stress reduction techniques are not being used by this population.
- If stress reduction techniques are introduced by a parish nurse using a caring approach, women may practice the techniques.
- If stress reduction techniques are being used, stress levels may decrease.

■ If stress levels decrease, there may be a subsequent decrease in stress-related health issues, an improvement in perception of health, and a decrease in lost days of work.

The literature review is used to provide a logical and concise description of what is known about the problem, present external data that support the need for the project, and present data that support the project plan. The content of the literature review should come from peer-reviewed journals or other academic sources. The results of the search should then be discussed and appraised. The level of evidence should be identified when the student describes how the literature supports the proposed intervention (Velasquez & Bonham, 2015).

The literature review is not a summarized list of literature available on the phenomenon of interest. Again, the goal of a literature review is to obtain a representative sample of the literature that describes the concepts related to the phenomenon of interest, demonstrates the results of research applicable to the topic, and provides a preponderance of high-quality evidence to support the proposed intervention (Velasquez & Bonham, 2015). All perspectives regarding the topic should be presented, even if the perspective is not favorable. A good proposal represents all viewpoints described in the literature, including grey literature. According to GreyNet International (2018), grey literature includes the multiple document types produced on all levels of government, academics, business, and organization not controlled by commercial publishing (para. 2). Examples of organizations that may be a source for grey literature include the World Health Organization (WHO), National Committee for Quality Assurance, Healthcare Effectiveness Data and Information Set, the Patient Protection and Affordable Care Act (ACA), and Medicare Access and Children's Health Insurance Program (CHIP) Reauthorization Act. More information about grey literature and a description of the process used to conduct a literature search and to write a literature review is provided in Chapter 6.

The goal of a literature review is to obtain a representative sample of the literature that describes the concepts related to the phenomenon of interest, the results of research applicable to the topic, and to provide a preponderance of high-quality evidence to support the proposed intervention.

The following is the initial portion of a hypothetical literature review, with hypothetical references, using the caregiver stress phenomenon as an example.

Literature Review

African American women are more likely to experience caregiver stress than Hispanic, Asian, or Caucasian women of the same age and socioeconomic background (Jones, 2015; Peters, 2016; Smith, 2017). Many healthcare professionals caring for these women contend that this population is also developing hypertension, diabetes, and symptoms of chronic fatigue more frequently than women of Hispanic or Asian descent (Gunther, 2015; Sindler, 2014; Vanhouser, 2018).

Paterson and Swender (2015) found that more than 40% of African American women in the United States who are caring for loved ones on a regular basis (a minimum of 5 days per week) experience at least 4 lost workdays per month. Another study by Johnson (2016) that followed 598 women over a period of 3 consecutive years confirmed this finding, with an average of 5 (25%) lost workdays experienced per month.

The literature suggests that this population is not utilizing stress reduction strategies on a regular basis (Bender, 2017; Ebstein, 2015; Marks, 2016; Paul, 2018). However, there is substantial evidence to support the use of stress reduction techniques in this population to improve health and/or reduce lost workdays (Lorden, 2016; Macon, 2017; Porrett, 2018).

The Organizational Assessment (Local Context)

The organizational assessment is used to obtain internal evidence regarding the local problem. All projects may not require an organizational assessment (for example, a project with a population health focus or policy analysis); however, when indicated, the assessment of the organization is used to describe the organizational culture and "physical and sociocultural makeup of the local environment . . . and the interpretation of these factors ("sense-making") by the healthcare delivery professionals, patients, and caregivers that can affect the effectiveness and generalizability of intervention(s)" (SQUIRE, 2015, p. 4). The culture of the organization influences the people, practices, and ultimately the organization's readiness for change (Velasquez & Bonham, 2015). A comprehensive organizational assessment should also include the identification of facilitators and barriers to the change initiative (including stakeholders) and other organizational specific factors (such as cost, policies, and alignment with the strategic plan) that can be used to determine project feasibility. More information regarding organizational assessment is provided in Chapter 6.

The Purpose of the Project

The project aim or purpose should be limited to one or two key areas that are clearly articulated. It should describe what the project will involve and what it will accomplish. Those reading your proposal should have a clear understanding of what the proposal is about just from reading the project aim or purpose.

Using the previous example, the purpose may be:

> This project attempts to determine if a stress reduction program introduced by a parish nurse using a caring approach that focuses on the patient relationship is a cost-effective method to decrease stress scores and the number of lost workdays and increase self-rated health in African American women experiencing caregiver stress.

The Conceptual and Theoretical Framework

The conceptual and theoretical framework for the DNP project includes "informal or formal frameworks, models, concepts, and/or theories used to explain the problem, any reasons or assumptions that were used to develop the intervention(s), and reasons why the intervention(s) was expected to work" (SQUIRE, 2015, p. 2).

A conceptual framework is similar to a map. The conceptual framework can be used to connect all the important aspects of the project. DNP students are expected to utilize a conceptual framework to guide the study as outlined in DNP *Essential* I: Scientific Underpinnings for Practice. As mentioned in Chapter 6, one example of a conceptual framework is the Donabedian model, which focuses on three main categories: structure, process, and outcome (Donabedian, 1988). Using this framework, the student is able to identify all the concepts that affect the project structure (the setting in which the project will be implemented and who will be involved in the project), the process (what will be done and how it will be delivered), and, finally, the outcome (what will be measured, reviewed, or assessed). Using the previous example, a project could be developed and implemented in a community setting, such as community churches within the inner city.

The intervention could include a presentation given by one parish nurse introducing stress reduction techniques to the target population that will be practiced over a 6-month period. The variables measured could include preintervention and postintervention levels of perceived stress, self-rated health, number of days of work missed over the same period, and use of stress management techniques, which would be assessed postintervention. A postintervention cost analysis could be used to determine program sustainability and the potential to spread the program to other local parishes (see **TABLE 12-1**).

A theoretical framework, on the other hand, helps guide and inform the project. For example, Jean Watson's theory of human caring focuses on human caring processes and experiences and makes the assumption that effective caring will promote health and individual or family growth (Watson, 2012). Therefore, using this theory as a guide, the student could illustrate how the parish registered nurse, using a caring approach, establishes a relationship with the patient and guides the patient through a stress reduction intervention to help her learn how to reduce stress levels.

TABLE 12-1 Project Conceptual Framework

Structure	Process	Outcome
St. Charles Church, St. Michael's Parish, and St. Bartholomew Church of Christ	Group intervention—concentrating on stress reduction techniques	Perceived stress Self-rated health
The expertise of the parish registered nurse—how the utilization of this care provider affects outcomes	The nurse–patient relationship—may help the participant integrate the stress reduction strategies	Use of stress management techniques
Inclusion criterion for participant selection	Inclusion criteria used to identify appropriate participants	Days of missed work Cost analysis

▶ Project Design

The project design will be determined based on the type of project being implemented. Any proposed project should have a project design plan, which includes anything from a quality improvement project to a pilot study, and the design should be discussed in detail. For example, a pilot study could use either an *experimental design* (used to show cause and effect, such as an intervention that manipulates the variables) or a *nonexperimental design* (data are collected based on observation, without manipulating the variables), whereas a project improvement project may use rapid improvement cycles (Plan-Do-Study-Act cycle) or Six Sigma to affect a change. The DNP student should consult with his or her advisor or partner with an experienced mentor to help guide him or her through the process.

The Methodology

This section is used to describe how the project will be done, connecting it to the project purpose. The project plan is described in detail, including ethical aspects in implementing the improvement, human subjects considerations and a description of the participants (if applicable), the setting, the tools/instruments used to evaluate the phenomenon of interest, the data collection or process improvement/intervention (if an intervention is included), and how the work will be evaluated. The methodology section provides an opportunity for the DNP student to describe how the clinical question will be answered.

This section may also include a financial analysis, which may be needed to demonstrate the feasibility and cost effectiveness of a project, as well as the potential impact. Because there is an increasing need for, and focus on, both clinically effective and cost-effective care, a cost analysis is important to consider. The student should make a list of what would be included in the total costs of implementing the project if someone was to replicate it. These costs should include direct costs (those costs that are easily assigned to the project, for example, salary/wages of those individuals implementing the project, project supplies, and subject costs) and indirect costs (those costs that are used for more than the project alone, for example, utilities, office supplies, and postage). An example of a project budget is provided in Chapter 13, The DNP Project Toolbox.

> *Because there is an increasing need for and focus on both clinically effective and cost-effective care, a cost analysis is important to consider.*

Ethical Consideration

Before implementing a DNP project, the student needs to consider ethical aspects related to implementing and studying the impact of the project. For example, how will potential ethical aspects be addressed? This may include a formal ethics review and potential conflict(s) of interest (SQUIRE, 2015 p. 2). Authorization from the institutional review board (IRB) should be included in the proposal. It is vital that the ethical concerns related to the safety of the participants be addressed. In this section, the DNP student should describe how much information the participants will receive regarding the project's purpose, whether they will need to sign a consent form, whether a stipend for participation will be provided, and a detailed plan of how the student will maintain participant confidentiality. See Chapter 10, Creating and Developing the Project Plan, for more information regarding the IRB process.

The Setting

In this section, the student has the opportunity to describe the environment where the project will take place. This provides a clear picture of the setting for those who may want to replicate the project in the future.

The caregiver stress scenario setting could be described as follows:

Data will be collected in three local community churches serving Wayne County in Southeast Michigan. The population within these three churches consists of primarily African American families with a mean age of 46.2 years. More than 800 families worship at these three churches; of that number, approximately 25% have one or more family members in need of caregiver support.

The Participants

When the project includes participants, it is important to discuss how the participants will be chosen, the actual description of the participants, as well as the total number of participants that will be included in the project. Accurate description of the sample population is useful to the reader because it helps him or her understand the composition of the sample and the degree to which the results of the project may or may not be generalized to other settings. For example, in a quality improvement project that focuses on organizational process or policy change, participants may also include providers, staff, and patient charts to assess and measure quality metric improvement.

The process for choosing participants can be accomplished using any number of sampling procedures, such as a convenience sample or a randomized sample. The description of this process becomes especially important when the project involves a pilot study. Finally, the actual description of the participants should include attributes such as gender, age, racial or ethnic group, marital status, socioeconomic status, and level of education.

The DNP student should also discuss the inclusion and exclusion criteria that will be used to identify participants. For example, the project described earlier may include only English-speaking African American female participants who are between the ages of 21 and 60 years, have no comorbid conditions, have provided ongoing caregiving services for a loved one for least 6 months, have a self-rated stress score of 5 or higher, and are not practicing any stress reduction techniques. Therefore, all males would be excluded, as would females who are not African American, African American females younger than 21 or older than 60, those who do not speak English, those who have comorbid conditions, and those who are not providing caregiving services, who have not provided caregiving services for at least 6 months, or who have a stress score lower than 5.

When conducting a pilot study, the student should also confirm that an appropriate sample size is obtained to ensure the validity of the project. A number of methods are available to assist in determining an adequate sample size. As mentioned, the DNP student should ensure that he or she is working with an experienced mentor who can guide him or her through this process.

The Intervention

When the DNP project includes an intervention, this section will be used to describe the process step by step, from start to finish. It includes the rationale for the intervention, a broad overview of the description of the intervention, and an operational plan. For quality improvement projects, this section should include the intervention inputs, internal activities, and outputs (in the form of a logic model, for example), and how these components are expected to produce changes in a system's performance (SQUIRE, 2015). The intervention will be guided by the conceptual and theoretical framework of the project. Again, the purpose of this section is to describe what will be done (including the collection of data and the purpose), how it will be done (the approach or process that is appropriate for the project design), where it will occur, who will be responsible for implementing the process (including background and credentials), how many people are involved in the process, and the expected timeline. Think of this section as a plan that can be used to train the members of the project team.

Next are a few points to consider. When using a questionnaire, remember to identify the response rate that will be considered acceptable (count on an average fall-off rate of 10–20%). When describing the procedure or intervention, remember to use future tense (because the project has not yet been completed) and to clearly describe the project variables. It is also helpful to consider what will be done to increase the response rate and how nonresponders will be tracked (Saunderlin, 1994).

In the caregiver stress scenario, the following may be included:

> An educational program will be implemented to impact the stress levels of the participants, reduce lost workdays, and improve perception of health. Participants will be recruited from three Southeast Michigan community churches located in Wayne County. A letter will be sent to all parishioners describing the program and the inclusion criteria. A telephone number and email address will be included for those who are interested; individuals who meet the initial inclusion criteria will be asked to meet with the parish nurse individually. These individuals will be given a stress level questionnaire to determine continued eligibility. One bachelor's-prepared registered nurse (parish nurse) will provide the intervention across the three sites.
>
> Each participant with a stress score of 5 or higher will be provided with a comprehensive description of the program, including the program purpose; what to expect as a participant, including potential risks; and the project lead's contact information if she has questions or concerns. Those who desire to participate will be asked to sign an informed consent.
>
> Each participant will be directed to return to the parish on a predetermined day for a 1-hour appointment, at which time she will receive an individual assessment with the parish nurse, a survey that evaluates the

participant's work history over the past 6 months, and a perception-of-health survey. The participants will be asked to return to the parish 1 week later for a 1-hour group educational intervention with the parish nurse that includes an introduction to comprehensive evidence-based stress reduction strategies (progressive muscle relaxation, guided imagery, mindfulness, and diaphragmatic breathing) and a teach-back opportunity to verify understanding.

Participants will be asked to follow up with the parish nurse every 2 weeks for 6 months via telephone, email, or in person to assess barriers to implementation, answer questions, and provide support. All participants will receive the parish nurse contact information for follow-up as needed between visits. A caring approach will be used by the parish nurse during all interactions to foster the development of a relationship with each participant. The parish nurse will contact any participant who does not attend the group intervention via telephone 1 week after the event and attempt a one-time makeup session.

After the completion of the 6-month intervention period, the participants will be asked to meet with the parish nurse one final time in person to complete the stress level questionnaire, the perception-of-health survey, the participant's use of mental stress management techniques questionnaire, and a work history survey for the prior 6-month period. In the event that a participant does not complete the postintervention session, the parish nurse will make one attempt via telephone and email to reschedule the session.

Measures/Tools/Instruments

This section should include a description of the measurement strategies and tools and/or instruments that will be used to evaluate the phenomenon of interest (when applicable). The conceptual framework should delineate the dependent variables and/or outcomes to be measured, as well as the strategy used. The instruments chosen to measure the outcome should be consistent with the project purpose/clinical question and population of interest (Velasquez & Bonham, 2015). In the example of a quality improvement project to affect an organizational process or policy change, the measures may include provider/staff pre- and post-testing of knowledge gained following an educational session and/or quality metrics data change pre- and postintervention.

This would include any questionnaires given to the participants, evaluation forms, or any other tools used to measure the variables of interest. Great care should be taken to identify an established tool that has been validated and is reliable. A description of the tool should be included in the project proposal, as well as a description of the validity and reliability of the tool. This last point is particularly noteworthy; validity of an instrument is important because it describes how well the instrument

The DNP student will want to choose a tool that captures the essence of the phenomenon and produces consistent, stable results over time.

(questionnaire, evaluation, or survey) will measure what it is *intended* to measure. In the caregiver stress scenario, the DNP student would want to choose an instrument that accurately captures the essence of *stress*. On the other hand, the *reliability* of the instrument is important because it describes how well the instrument consistently produces the same results on repeated tests. Simply stated, the DNP student will want to choose an instrument that captures the essence of the phenomenon and produces consistent, stable results over time.

The reliability of an instrument also includes interrater and/or intrarater reliability. Interrater reliability refers to consistency of measurements from rater to rater, whereas intrarater reliability specifically involves the reliability of measurements obtained from a single rater. For instance, in the caregiver stress scenario, if several raters will be used to administer a perceived stress questionnaire, the student will want to ensure that the questionnaires are implemented consistently by all raters—that is, that all raters use the same questionnaire, that the instructions for completing the questionnaire are the same from group to group, that each rater scores the questionnaire using the same scale, and so forth. This speaks to the value of having a well-defined data collection plan in which the steps involved in implementing the project, especially measuring the variables of interest, are described in detail.

Many data collection tools are referred to in the literature. The Medical Outcomes Trust (MOT) identify eight review criteria that can be used when evaluating an instrument: reliability, validity, sensitivity, interpretability, burden, alternative forms of administration, cultural adaptations, and language adaptations (Velasquez & Bonham, 2015). A simple search of the literature for the tool in question should produce at least one tool that would be appropriate for the project. In some instances, however, the student will need to develop his or her own tool to accurately measure the variables of interest. In this case, the student should note how it will be developed and any evidence that supports its development. Remember that the DNP student will need to work with his or her advisor or project faculty mentor to ensure that the reliability and validity of tools used in the project are maintained. Finally, a copy of the tools that the student plans on using in the project should be provided in the appendix.

Analysis

This section of the proposal focuses on how the student plans to evaluate the results of the project and/or analyze the data. The evaluation plan identifies the criteria that will be used to evaluate what worked and what may not have worked in the project and serves as a mechanism to help the student determine needed next steps or recommendations (i.e., what needs to occur after completion of the project). The project evaluation plan or approach may include key individuals who will be involved in the process, the overall goals of the project and/or the outcomes-based performance measures that will be used to assess change, the description of how the goal will be evaluated, and the reason for using the chosen evaluation method.

For projects involving a pilot study, for example, the level of statistical significance must be stated, the test used for analysis described, and the statistical software identified. It is imperative that an appropriate test be chosen to measure the variable of interest, which is also influenced by the clinical question. Again, describing the rationale for using specific analytical methods is beneficial. It is also wise to consult with a statistician at this point in the project, because he or she has the expertise to ensure that the appropriate test(s) is/are selected for analyzing the clinical question.

Following are just a few points to consider. Descriptive results, such as the number of men and women in the study, should be included to describe the population. When statistics are used to predict an outcome, or to determine differences or a relationship, the student should plan on reporting the results using conventional terminology (see **TABLE 12-2**). Some clinical questions, on the other hand, may require methods of analysis other than traditional statistics. For example, program evaluation projects may include budget analysis and data related to potential for program replication.

The analysis section, in essence, organizes the data in a way that answers the clinical question; in other words, it addresses the problem statement (Saunderlin, 1994). An effective analysis section presents a *summary* of how the results will be interpreted in logical succession.

Sustainability Plan

The DNP student should also include a sustainability plan in the project proposal. According to the Institute for Healthcare Improvement (IHI) (2015), sustainability refers to locking in the progress made by an improvement initiative, and spread [replication] occurs when best practices and knowledge about successful interventions

TABLE 12-2 Sample of Statistical Terminology

Test	Purpose	Statistical Symbol	Expression
p value	Tells you how likely you are to get the same results if the null hypothesis is true; the significance.	p	Report the significance (0.01 or 0.05 are typically used). $p \leq 0.05$
t statistic	Determines if there is a statistically significant difference in mean values between two groups.	t	Report degrees of freedom (df), the t value, and p value. $t(30) = 5.29$ $p = 0.000$
Pearson's product–moment correlation	Measures two variables at the interval or ratio level to determine if there is a relationship.	r	Report the df (always $N - 2$), the r value, and p value. $r(55) = 0.49, p < 0.01$
Chi square	Used to analyze nominal and ordinal data to determine if there are any differences.	χ^2	Report df and sample size in parentheses, the chi square value, and the p value. $\chi^2(1, N = 80) = 0.89$, $p = 0.25$

are actively disseminated to every available care setting. Sustainability speaks to the potential for the project to endure over time. This means the DNP student will need to define what is needed to assure project sustainability, but also what sustainability means for the project, the organization, and perhaps even nursing. A few factors specific to sustainability include:

1. Obtaining input and buy-in for continued project support from the organization and key decision makers
2. Defining critical long- and short-term policy strategies needed to assure sustainability
3. Acquiring resources—human, financial, and in-kind
4. Defining the process for ongoing documentation and organization of the project —continued evaluation, criteria grids, budgets, and more (National Center for Chronic Disease Prevention and Health Promotion, n.d.)

Through facilitation of the project, the DNP student can demonstrate the value of a DNP-prepared nurse in leading change initiatives, such as improved outcomes that are sustainable.

Implication for Practice

Before writing this section, think about how the results of the project may impact practice, patient outcomes, and so forth. Describe how the project will provide new insight into the existing knowledge where there is currently a gap regarding the phenomenon of interest or regarding the clinical significance and cost-effectiveness implications of the project. For the DNP student, it is particularly important to include information regarding the clinical significance when describing the implications of the project. Clinical significance refers to whether or not the intervention has an impact on everyday life, etc. In other words, what does it mean for the patient population that you are trying to impact or the clinical environment? How important is it clinically? Sometimes interventions can have statistical significance, but are not practical for the clinical environment and therefore are not clinically important.

The DNP student should also address the cost effectiveness of the project whenever possible. In today's healthcare environment all costs are scrutinized. As a result, most administrators will assess projects to determine if there is a potential for a return on investment before authorizing project implementation. To this point, it is wise to also include information on how you plan on sustaining and spreading improvements, as this will invariably impact return on investment. Finally, it is also appropriate to discuss the potential for subsequent clinical inquiry, how the project could influence current programs, or perhaps even healthcare policy.

▶ Citing References

Only the material referenced in the body of the proposal should be cited in the reference section. As mentioned previously, APA style of writing is used by many schools of nursing in universities across the United States. Other styles include the *American Medical Association (AMA) Manual of Style*, which is often used to present scientific data in biomedical journals (AMA, 2018). The *Recommendations for the Conduct,*

Reporting, Editing and Publication of Scholarly Work in Medical Journals (ICMJE Recommendations) submitted to biomedical journals is yet another example; this style focuses on both ethical and technical aspects of publishing (International Committee of Medical Journal Editors [ICMJE], 2018). Again, the DNP student should consult with his or her advisor or project faculty mentor to determine the appropriate style manual. Refer to the reference section of this chapter for an example of APA-formatted references. Other styles are available in the Helpful Resources section of this chapter.

> *Only the material referenced in the body of the proposal should be cited in the reference section.*

▶ Appendices

When additional information is needed to support the presented work, but is too cumbersome to include in the body of the work (e.g., a tool used to evaluate outcomes), the information can be presented in the appendix section. In other words, appendices are used for reference to additional documentation necessary to complete the project. The type of documents included in the appendices section will vary based on the project. The following materials may be appropriate for this section (note that it is best to confirm the requirements with an advisor or committee chair prior to submitting the final product):

- Participant invitation letter
- Conceptual/theoretical framework (if not included in the body of the proposal)
- Instruments/tools used to measure variables
- Informed consent form
- Participant instructions
- Letters to stakeholders
- Transcripts of interviews
- Budget
- Needs assessment report
- SWOT analysis report

A proposal template is provided as a reference at the end of this chapter (see the appendix). As mentioned, the requirements for the doctoral proposal will vary from institution to institution. Therefore, the student should check with his or her advisor or project faculty mentor for specific information regarding the proposal requirements.

▶ Writing Tips

The following writing tips from Venolia (2001) may help the DNP student when writing the DNP proposal.

1. Use a comma to:
   a. Separate independent clauses that are joined by coordinating conjunctions—*and, but, or, for, yet,* and *so.*

b. Separate three or more items in a series—*popcorn, peanuts, and pretzels.*

c. Between consecutive adjectives that modify the same noun—*an inexpensive, worthwhile program.*

d. Where needed for clarity—*whatever you decide to do, do it right* (Venolia, 2001).

2. Use a semicolon or period preceding the conjunctive adverb, not a comma—*The dean will be late for the recognition ceremony; however, she does plan to attend.* Also use a semicolon to join two independent clauses that are not joined by a conjunction—*The dean will not attend the recognition ceremony; she will be missed.*

3. Avoid misplaced modifiers (may alter the intended meaning)—*She told him that she wanted to move to a new location frequently.*

a. Right: *She frequently told him that she wanted to move to a new location.*

4. Avoid dangling modifiers—*Hidden in the armoire, Aunt Suzy found her missing sweater.*

a. Right: *Aunt Suzy found her missing sweater hidden in the armoire.*

5. Tricky words

a. *Affect* is most often used as a verb (to influence)—*The physician hopes to affect the patient's decision.*
And *effect* as a noun (consequence)—*The effect of the policy change was to reduce falls on the unit.*

b. Use *that* to introduce restrictive or defining clauses—*The sweater that needs to be washed is on my bed.* In this case, the sweater is one of several and thus must be further identified. And use *which* to introduce nonrestrictive clauses—*The sweater, which needs to be washed, is on my bed.* In this case, there is only one sweater that needs to be washed (*which* adds further meaning and could be dropped from the sentence without changing the meaning). Tip: A *which* clause should be separated with a comma.

c. Who or Whom? The best guide is to substitute a personal pronoun for who or whom. If he, she, or they fits, use *who*; if him, her, or them fits, use *whom*—*The woman who entered the store* (*she* entered the store). *To whom shall I send the check?* (I shall send the check to *him, her,* or *them*).

6. Write in active voice. In the active voice, the subject acts (*Kathy passed the medications for the unit*) instead of being acted upon (*the medications for the unit were passed by Kathy*).
Tip: Write in active voice unless the thing acted upon is more important than the person performing the action—*the game was canceled.*

7. Plural vs. singular nouns or pronouns. Check that there is agreement between the pronoun and the antecedent. For example, "Each patient took their medication . . ." is incorrect because one patient cannot be a "they" (Venolia, 2001). Right: "Each patient took his or her medication . . ."

8. Literature review vs. annotated bibliography

a. A literature review is both a *product* and a *process*. The process involves collecting and reading the relevant literature, coming to some understanding (comprehension) based on what has been read, making connections/applying what is learned to your project, analyzing it (to determine how it fits together), evaluating the strengths and weaknesses of your findings, then coming to a conclusion (what you think the scientific literature says about the topic; for example, you may identify a gap in the literature). The literature review as a product is a written *synthesis* of your findings.

b. Annotated bibliography—a list of sources used to research a topic with notes that describe and/or evaluate your findings.

9. Avoid writing in first person (i.e., using pronouns "I" or "me").

10. Add structure to your work by using subheadings and transitional phrases. Introduce new topics or ideas with a transitional statement (to connect separate thoughts or ideas together for the reader).

11. The body of the work should be written in a logically succession (do not skip around) and there should be a connection between the introduction, body of the work, and the conclusion.

12. Remember: The author/researcher studied a phenomenon . . . not the article or journal.

APA Format

1. Include a running head (maximum of 50 characters, spaces, and punctuation) in the upper left-hand side of the first page (the words "running head" are on the first page only) and a page number in the upper right-hand side of every page.

   To create a header using Microsoft Office Word, click on the "Insert" tab → choose "Header" → check "Different first page" box → click on "Page number" → choose option for the page number at the top of the page, flush right → to the left of the page number type the words "Running head:" followed by your title in UPPERCASE → then press the tab key until the title is flush left. On the next page click on the header section and type your title next to the page number (in UPPERCASE), then press the tab key until the title is flush left.

2. Title page: The title should be a maximum of 12 words, centered in the upper half of the page, followed by your name (omit title/degree), then your affiliation (university, organization, etc.).

3. Times New Roman 12-point typeface is the APA typeface preference, although other serif typefaces with 12-point font are also acceptable.

4. Use at least 1-inch margins all around (top, bottom, left, and right) on standard-sized paper (8.5 × 11 inches) and double space between lines. Margins should only be left justified.

5. Abstract: This is a concise summary of your manuscript. It should be approximately 150 to 250 words. Do not indent the paragraph.

6. Introduction: starts on page 3 of a manuscript. Do not use "Introduction" as a heading; the title of the manuscript is used (centered) instead.

7. In text quotations:

   a. By two authors: Research by Williams and Jones (2014) supports . . . The latest research indicates . . . (Williams & Jones, 2014)

   b. By three to five authors: (Williams, Jones, Sun, Berry, & Harlow, 2014). In subsequent citations (Williams et al., 2014)

    c.   Six or more authors: (Williams et al., 2014)

    d.   Two or more works in the same paragraph: (Williams et al., 2014; Wolker & Peamont, 2012)

8.   References page: the heading "References" should be centered at the top of the page; double-space reference entries; the first line of every entry should be flush left then all lines that follow are indented. To use "hanging" indent feature in Microsoft Office Word, click on the "Page Layout" tab, then click on "Paragraph" option and use the down arrow to select "Hanging" in the indentation section "Special" box.

9.   All entries in the references should be ordered alphabetically by the author's surnames (last name followed by initials, i.e., Moran, K. J.). If you have a source that is anonymous, then the title of the work is used (instead of the author's surname).

10.   The author name should be inverted (last name first, then initials: "Williams, J. Q.")

11.   Only the first word of a title and subtitle are capitalized. Or, if a colon is used in the title then the first word after a colon is capitalized. The same is true following a dash in a title. Of course, all proper nouns should be capitalized. When hyphenated compound words are in the title do not capitalize the second word.

12.   *Block quotations* (any quotation of 40 words or more) do not use quotation marks to enclose the block. Block quotes are indented one-half inch on the left margin for the whole quote, but not on the right margin. Here's an example:

With regard to plagiarism, the *Publication Manual of the American Psychological Association* (APA, 2010) makes the following statement:

> Quotation marks should be used to indicate the exact work of another. Each time you paraphrase another author (i.e., summarize a passage or rearrange the order of a sentence and change some of the words), you will need to credit the source in the text. . . . The key element of this principle is that authors do not present the work of another as if it were their own work. This can extend to ideas as well as written words. (pp. 15–16)

▶ Summary

To ensure one has a successful writing experience, the student should review the university requirements for the proposal before beginning to write, seek clarification and support from faculty as needed, and ask for feedback on their work from mentors and peers throughout the writing process.

Key Messages

- The doctoral proposal represents the student's intellectual ability, knowledge in the subject area, and contributions to nursing.
- Proposal format may vary by institution. Check with your institution to determine the format you should use.

- When writing a project proposal, insufficient time for creative thinking and analysis and synthesis of the literature can lead to fragmented thoughts that are difficult to follow.
- When starting the proposal writing process, begin with the end in mind.
- The student can avoid plagiarism by consistently documenting sources used to substantiate or inform his or her work.
- Only the material referenced in the body of the proposal should be cited in the reference section.

Action Plan—Next Steps

1. Evaluate your writing skill set.
2. Check with your advisor or project faculty mentor regarding the institutional proposal format requirements.
3. Develop an outline.
4. Choose an appropriate project title.
5. Start writing!
6. Seek feedback from colleagues early in the writing process.

References

American Medical Association (AMA) (2018). *American Medical Association (AMA) manual of style*. Retrieved from http://www.amamanualofstyle.com/

American Psychological Association (APA). (2010). *Publication Manual of the American Psychological Association* (6th ed.). Washington, DC: Author.

Consolidated Standards of Reporting Trials (CONSORT) (2010). *CONSORT statement*. Retrieved from http://www.consort-statement.org/

Covey, S. R. (1989). *The 7 habits of highly effective people: Powerful lessons in personal change*. New York, NY: Simon & Schuster.

Dols, J. D., Hernandez, C., & Miles, H. (2017, February). The DNP project: Quandaries for nursing scholars. *Nursing Outlook, 65*(1), 84–93. Retrieved from http://dx.doi.org/10.1016/j.outlook.2016.07.009

Donabedian A. (1988). The quality of care: How can it be assessed? *Journal of the American Medical Association, 260*, 1743–1748.

Fauchald, S. K., & Bastian, H. (2015). Utilizing an interdisciplinary approach to increase student writing abilities in doctor of nurse practice programs. *Journal of Professional Nursing, 31*(1), 64–70. Retrieved from http://dx.doi.org/10.1016/j.profnurs.2014.05.004. © 2015 Elsevier Inc. All rights reserved.

Frick, T. W., Boling, E., Barrett, A., Dagli, C., Myers, R., & Albayrak-Karahan, M., . . . Matsumura, N. (2014). *How to recognize plagiarism: Tutorial and tests*. Bloomington, IN: Department of Instructional Systems Technology, School of Education, Indiana University. Retrieved from https://www.indiana.edu/~istd/

Giddens, J. F., & Lobo, M. (2008). Analyzing graduate student trends in written paper evaluation. *Journal of Nursing Education, 47*(10), 480–483.

GreyNet International. (2018). Retrieved from http://www.greynet.org/

Happe, B. (2005). Disseminating nursing knowledge: A guide to writing for publication. *International Journal of Psychiatric Nursing Research, 10*(3), 1147–1155.

Heyman, B., & Cronin, P. (2005). Writing for publication: Adapting academic work into articles. *British Journal of Nursing, 14*(7), 400–403.

Institute for Healthcare Improvement (IHI). (2015). *How-to-guide: Sustainability and spread*. Retrieved from http://www.ihi.org/resources/Pages/Tools/HowtoGuideSustainabilitySpread.aspx

International Committee of Medical Journal Editors (ICMJE) (2018). *Recommendations for the conduct, reporting, editing and publication of scholarly work in medical journals (ICMJE Recommendations)*. Retrieved from http://www.icmje.org/about-icmje/faqs/icmje-recommendations/

Leddy, C. (2011). Advice from the master of the writing craft. *The Writer, 124*(6), 36–38.

Lee, N. J. (2010). Preparing for thesis and viva: Some practicalities. *Nurse Researcher, 17*(3), 52–59.

Moos, D. D., & Hawkins, P. (2009). Barriers and strategies to the revision process from an editor's perspective. *Nursing Forum, 44*(2), 79–92.

Morse, G. G. (2009). Faculty application of the American Psychological Association style. *Journal of Nursing Education, 48*(10), 542–551.

National Center for Chronic Disease and Health Promotion (n.d.). A sustainability planning guide for healthy communities. Atlanta, GA: Centers for Disease Control and Prevention. Retrieved from https://www.cdc.gov/nccdphp/dch/programs/healthycommunitiesprogram/pdf/sustainability_guide.pdf

Nolinske, T. (1996). Writing a research proposal. *Journal of Prosthetics and Orthotics, 8*(4), 132–137.

Plagiarize. (2018). *Merriam-Webster*. Retrieved from http://www.merriam-webster.com/dictionary/plagiarize

Saunderlin, G. (1994). Writing a research proposal: The critical first step for successful clinical research. *Gastroenterology Nursing, 17*(2), 48–56.

Shirey, M. R. (2013). Building scholarly writing capacity in a doctor of nursing practice program. *Journal of Professional Nursing, (29)*, 137–147,

Standards for Quality Improvement Reporting Excellence (SQUIRE) 2.0 (2015). *Revised standards for quality improvement reporting excellence.* Retrieved from http://squire-statement.org/index.cfm?fuseaction=document.viewDocument&documentid=1&documentFormatId=1&vDocLinkOrigin=1&CFID=33187921&CFTOKEN=601f5bf702fd3c6d-A613A60E-1C23-C8EB-801327165B903DC1

Strengthening the Reporting of Observational Studies in Epidemiology (STROBE). (2009). *STROBE statement.* Retrieved from https://www.strobe-statement.org/index.php?id=strobe-home

Velasquez, D. & Bonham, E. (2015). The clinical practice project: Planning to publish. *Journal of the American Association of Nurse Practitioners, 27,* 420–425. doi: 10.1002/2327-6924.12226

Venolia, J. (2001). *Write right!* Berkeley, CA: Ten Speed Press.

Watson, J. (2012). *Caring science ten caritas processes.* Boulder, CO: Watson Caring Science Institute. Retrieved from https://www.watsoncaringscience.org/

Helpful Resources

American Psychological Association (APA) style guide available at http://www.apastyle.org/

BioMedical Editor available at http://www.biomedicaleditor.com/ama-style.html

CONSORT 2010 statement available at http://www.consort-statement.org/consort-2010

Indiana University plagiarism module available at https://www.indiana.edu/~academy/firstPrinciples/choice.html

International Committee of Medical Journal Editors (ICMJE) (uniform requirements for manuscripts) available at http://www.icmje.org/

Purdue Online Writing Lab (OWL) available at http://owl.english.purdue.edu/owl/section/2/10/

SQUIRE guideline available at http://www.squire-statement.org/

STROBE statement available at https://www.strobe-statement.org/index.php?id=strobe-home

Appendix

Running head: SHORTENED TITLE ALL UPPERCASE   1

[Project Title – Upper and lowercase no more than 12 words]

[Student First Name Middle Initial(s) Last Name]

[Name of University]

[Date]

Abstract/Executive Summary

The abstract is a brief summary of the proposal. Review the university requirements for specific instructions related to the format—for example, word count, margins, and font size. The abstract generally does not exceed one page, whereas the executive summary may be several pages in length. Although the requirements for the content may vary from institution to institution, most require the problem statement, a project purpose, overall project design with description of the sample and the proposed methods, analysis procedures, and implications for practice.

Table of Contents

(Check with university to determine if a table of contents is required.)

List of Tables

Table 1. The table title belongs here

List of Figures

Figure 1. The figure title belongs here

1. INTRODUCTION

The introduction tells the reader why this topic is important; it sets the stage for what is to come. Even though a heading is provided in this example to illustrate placement, because a manuscript always begins with an *introduction*, the title *introduction* is not used in the actual proposal.

Background/Significance

In this section, the student should expand on the introduction. Why is it important for this work to be completed? What are the problems that have been identified, and what are the implications? Why should the reader be interested in this project or topic?

Problem Statement/Clinical Question

The statement of the problem should be concise but clearly articulate the breadth and depth of the problem, why it is a concern, and why it should be evaluated. The clinical question helps the student describe the phenomenon of interest, informs the reader about an issue, and clarifies previous research, or it can add to the body of knowledge already available (Nolinske, 1996).

Review of the Literature

The literature review is used to present the data that support the need for the DNP project, such as a gap in knowledge or flaws within the current literature. A comprehensive literature review provides the evidence to defend a *logical argument* supporting the need for and the value of the proposed scholarly project.

Organizational Assessment

The organizational assessment describes the internal evidence regarding the local problem. All projects may not require an organizational assessment; however, when indicated, the assessment of the organization is used to describe the organizational culture and "physical and sociocultural makeup of the local environment. . . . and the interpretation of these factors ("sense-making") by the healthcare delivery professionals, patients, and caregivers that can affect the effectiveness and generalizability of intervention(s)" (SQUIRE, 2015, p. 4).

Purpose of the Project

The project aim or purpose should be limited to one or two key areas that are clearly articulated. It should describe what the project will involve and what it will accomplish.

2. CONCEPTUAL AND THEORETICAL FRAMEWORK

A conceptual framework is similar to a map; it can be used to connect all the important aspects of the project. A theoretical framework helps inform the project.

3. METHODOLOGY

This section is used to describe how the project will be done, connecting it to the project purpose and describing how the clinical question will be answered. The project design will be determined based on the type of project being implemented. Any proposed project should have a project design *plan*. The project plan describes the ethical aspects in implementing the improvement, human subjects considerations, and a description of the participants (if applicable), the setting, the tools/instruments used to evaluate the phenomenon of interest, the data collection or process improvement/intervention (if an intervention is included), and how the work will be evaluated.

Setting

Describe the environment where the project will take place. This provides a clear picture of the setting for those who may want to replicate the project in the future.

Participants

When describing the project participants, it is important to discuss how they will be chosen, give a description of the participants, as well as indicate the total number of anticipated participants.

The Intervention and Data Collection

When the DNP project includes an intervention, this section is used to describe the process step by step, from start to finish. It includes the rationale for the intervention, a broad overview of the description of the intervention, and an operational plan.

The purpose of this section is to describe what will be done (including the collection of data and the purpose), how it will be done (the approach or process that is appropriate for the project design), who will be responsible for implementing the process (including background and credentials), how many people are involved in the process, and the expected timeline. Think of this section as a plan that can be used to train the members of the project team.

Measures/Instruments/Tools

In this section, describe the tools and measures that will be used to evaluate the phenomenon of interest (if applicable).

4. ANALYSIS

This section of the proposal focuses on how the student plans to evaluate the results of the project and/or analyze the data. The evaluation plan identifies the criteria that will be used to evaluate what worked and what may not have worked in the project and may help the student determine the next steps or recommendations (i.e., what needs to occur after completion of the project). The project evaluation plan or approach may include key individuals who will be involved in the process, the overall goals of the project and/or the outcomes-based performance measures that will be used to assess change, the description of how the goal will be evaluated, and the reason for using the chosen evaluation method. An effective data analysis section presents a *summary* of how the results will be interpreted in logical succession.

5. SUSTAINABILITY PLAN

The sustainability plan should define what is needed and what will be done to assure the project endures over time.

6. IMPLICATIONS FOR PRACTICE

The implications section should describe how the results of the project may impact practice, patient outcomes, and so forth. The student should describe how the project will provide new insight into the existing knowledge where there is currently a gap regarding the phenomenon of interest or regarding the clinical and cost-effectiveness implications of the project. It is also appropriate to discuss the potential for subsequent clinical inquiry, how the project could influence current programs, or perhaps even healthcare policy.

REFERENCES

The following are a few examples of reference types available using APA style guide, Sixth Edition; refer to APA section 7.01–7.11. The student can also refer to http://www.apastyle.org/.

References in APA format should start on a new page, the word *References* is centered at the top of the page using uppercase and lowercase letters. The references section is double spaced and should begin with a hanging indent (as illustrated in this section).

Journal example:

Author, A., Author, B., & Author, C. (2012). Title of article. *Title of Periodical in Italics, xx*(x), xxx–xxx. doi:xx.xxxxxxxx (Please note: the volume number *is* italicized, but the issue [in parentheses] is not; the page numbers are not prefaced with pp. or p. The student should list only the page numbers; the student should include the digital object identifier [doi] if there is one assigned.)

Journal from online source (without doi) example:

Author, A., Author, B., & Author, C. (2012). Title of article. *Title of Periodical in Italics, xx*(x), xxx–xxx. Retrieved from http://www.xxx.xxxx

Special issue or section of a journal example:

Author, A. A., & Author, B. B. (Eds.). (2012). Title of article [Special issue or Special section]. *Title of Periodical in Italics, xx*(x), xxx–xxx.

Magazine article example:

Author, A. A., Author, B. B., & Author, C. C. (2012, Month). Title of article. *Title of Periodical in Italics, xx*(x), xxx–xxx.

Book example:

Author, A. A. (2012). *Title of the book.* City of publication, STATE abbreviation: Publisher. Editor, A. A. (Ed.). (2012). *Title of the book.*

Online book example:

Author, A. A. (2012). *Title of book.* Retrieved from http://www.xxxxx.xxxx

Chapter in a book example:

Author, A. A., & Author, B. B. (2012). Title of chapter. In A. Editor, B. Editor, & C. Editor (Eds.), *Title of book* (pp. xxx–xxx). City of publication, STATE abbreviation: Publisher. (Please note: In this example, pp. does precede the page numbers for the chapter.)

APPENDIX A: THE TITLE OF APPENDIX GOES HERE

When additional information is needed to support the presented work but is too cumbersome to include in the body of the work (e.g., a tool used to evaluate outcomes), the information can be presented in the appendix section. The type of documents included in the appendices section will vary based on the project.

When only one appendix is included in the manuscript, it should be labeled *Appendix*. If more than one appendix is included, they are labeled with letters rather than numbers (i.e., Appendix A, Appendix B, Appendix C) in the order they appear in the manuscript. Each appendix should also have a title, and each should begin on a separate page (**TABLE 12-3**).

TABLE 12-3 A Clear and Concise Table Title Goes Here*		
Heading 1	**Heading 2**	**Heading 3**
The data that will be illustrated below each heading belong here.	Use headings and labels that the reader will understand.	A table key may help provide clarity.
The information within a table must be able to stand alone.	Check with the university to verify format requirements.	Be sure to arrange the data in the table logically.

*Tables describe data using columns and rows.
Source for data used to create table should be included here if appropriate.

Figure Example

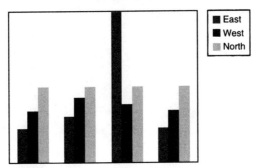

FIGURE 12-1 A clear and concise figure title goes here.
Source for figure should be included here if appropriate.

Figures are used for visual presentation of data and may include charts, graphs, photographs, illustrations, maps, and so on (see **FIGURE 12-1**). A caption should follow the figure title that explains what the figure illustrates. A legend should be included to explain the information in the figure.

CHAPTER 13

The DNP Project Toolbox

Katherine Moran, Rosanne Burson, and Dianne Conrad

CHAPTER OVERVIEW

Multiple tools are available to help the doctor of nursing practice (DNP) student develop a plan for the project, ensure seamless implementation, and drive efficient project management. The goal of this chapter is to introduce the student to a sample of available tools to use throughout the DNP project development and implementation cycle.

CHAPTER OBJECTIVES

After completing this chapter, the learner will be able to:

1. Identify one assessment tool that may be useful for the DNP project.
2. Select a tool to use for project management.
3. Describe a tool used for budget management.
4. Identify two tools appropriate for process improvement.
5. Explain how scheduling tools may be used within the DNP project.
6. List three examples of tools used for project evaluation.
7. Identify information technology tools that can assist with management of the DNP project.

▶ Utilizing the Toolbox

The toolbox is designed to help the student identify the tools that will be most beneficial during the project development and implementation phases and that will ultimately help ensure a successful outcome. A description of each tool and/or intended purpose is provided, followed by an example and/or tool template.

1. Assessment Tools

Assessment tools include those items that help the student organize thoughts and work through conceptual ideas, as well as in the decision-making process. The following tools can be used early in the project planning phase.

Organizational Assessment Tools

Evaluating the organization in which the project will take place is a helpful exercise in project planning. Identifying the organization's strengths, weaknesses, resources, and other attributes can help in planning and implementing a project smoothly and successfully. **TABLE 13-1** lists resources for choosing an appropriate organizational assessment aid discussed in Chapter 8, Interprofessional and Intraprofessional Collaboration in the DNP Project.

Self-Assessment Tool–Competency Assessment for Practicum Design

This tool is used to assess the student's current skill set prior to the onset of the practicum. Completing this self-assessment based on the DNP *Essentials* (AACN, 2006) helps the student develop a practicum plan that strengthens core competencies. It can also be used as a tracking tool throughout the DNP curriculum to

TABLE 13-1 Organizational Assessment Tools		
Tool	**Description**	**Resource**
Free Management Library	Website with tools for evaluating and improving organizations	https://managementhelp .org/aboutfml /diagnostics.htm https://managementhelp .org/organizations/index .htm
Reflect & Learn Frameworks	Organizational assessment frameworks, including: ■ Universalia Institutional and Organizational Assessment Model (IOA Model) ■ A Causal Model of Organizational Performance & Change (Burke & Litwin Model) ■ The Seven-S Model ■ The Marvin Weisbord Six-Box Model (Weisbord's Model) ■ Open Systems Model	http://www.reflectlearn .org/discover/frameworks

Tool	Description	Resource
Reflect & Learn Self-Assessment Tools	Over 60 tools for various types of organizational self-assessment: ■ By type of organization (profit, non-profit, donors/grantmakers, governmental agencies/organizations) ■ By area of the Universalia IOA Model (organizational capacity, external environment, organizational motivation, organizational performance)	http://reflectlearn .org/discover /self-assessment-tools
Canadian International Developmental Agency	Organizational Assessment Guide presents a framework for conducting assessments and guidelines for shaping execution	http://documents .reflectlearn.org /Offline%20Docs%20 for%20Your%20 Introductory%20 Guide%20to%20OA /OA%20Guide-E.pdf
American Medical Association	Communication Climate Assessment Toolkit (C-CAT)	http://www.ucdenver .edu/academics/colleges /medicalschool/centers /BioethicsHumanities /C-CAT/Pages/C-CAT.aspx

show progression in the attainment of competencies related to the DNP *Essentials* (AACN, 2006) (**Appendix A**). See Chapter 11, Driving the Practicum to Impact the DNP Project, for more information on completing the tool.

2. Tools to Connect Relationships and Organize Thoughts

The following tools can help as the DNP student brings multiple ideas and data together to formulate a problem statement.

Concept Map

A concept map is used to show relationships or connections among words, ideas, or a general notion (concept) (see **FIGURE 13-1**). Using the concept of health as an example, one can quickly see that health encompasses more than the absence of disease; it involves physical, social, spiritual, and mental health. The concept map provides a means for the student to graph and organize knowledge in a way that promotes logical thinking and thus helps the student better understand ideas from a larger whole. Concept mapping is also a helpful tool in nursing to promote critical thinking (Schmehl, n.d.). A concept map template is provided in **Appendix B**.

FIGURE 13-1 Concept map.

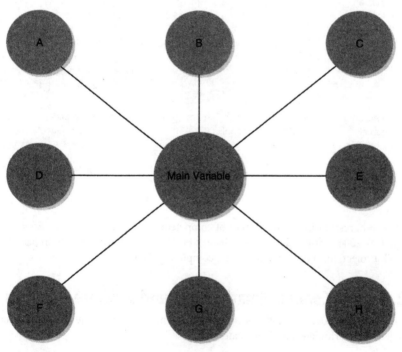

FIGURE 13-2 Mind map.

Mind Mapping

Mind mapping is a technique used to organize data in an attempt to develop or visualize ideas, solve problems, or even make a decision. This tool is often used as a brainstorming approach to show connections between ideas. In **FIGURE 13-2**, multiple like variables are linked to the central or main variable to show possible associations.

3. Tools to Help Define the Problem

The student will want to summarize assessment data to get a comprehensive view of the true components of the problem. The following tools will assist in gathering the data accurately and simply.

Check Sheet

The check sheet is used to gather data about a process. The user typically places a check mark on the sheet to indicate observation of a specific point in a process. A check sheet can be customized to meet the specific needs of a project (see **FIGURE 13-3**).

Fishbone Diagram

The fishbone diagram is also known as the *cause and effect* diagram or the *Ishikawa diagram*, and is used to identify potential causes of a problem or to help the team members when they are having difficulty coming to a conclusion (see **FIGURE 13-4**). To use a fishbone diagram, the team must first agree on a problem statement, which is captured on the horizontal center line running through the diagram. The team

☐ **Checkpoint One**	☐ **Checkpoint Two**	☐ **Checkpoint Three**
☐ Step/Item 1	☐ Step/Item 1	☐ Step/Item 1
☐ Step/Item 2	☐ Step/Item 2	☐ Step/Item 2
☐ Step/Item 3	☐ Step/Item 3	☐ Step/Item 3
☐ Step/Item 4	☐ Step/Item 4	☐ Step/Item 4
☐ Step/Item 5	☐ Step/Item 5	☐ Step/Item 5
☐ Step/Item 6	☐ Step/Item 6	☐ Step/Item 6

FIGURE 13-3 Check sheet.

Reproduced with permission from QI Macros. http://www.qimacros.com

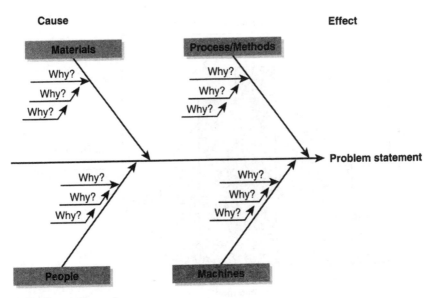

FIGURE 13-4 Fishbone diagram.

Reproduced with permission from QI Macros. http://www.qimacros.com

then begins to brainstorm ideas about the cause of the problem. These ideas are captured on vertical lines running into the center (problem) line. As more and more ideas are added to the figure, it begins to take on the appearance of an arrow, or fishbone (hence the name). If it is difficult for the team to generate ideas, headings can be used to facilitate the process (e.g., materials, process/methods). As the team continues to drill down, subcategories that further describe the problem are generated.

Another use for tools is to present data, including assessment or evaluation data, in a powerful and efficient manner. Basic graphs, such as bar graphs, will highlight differences between groups or categories. Other examples include radar or spider charts, frequency histograms, line graphs, pie charts, and run charts. A few specific examples follow.

Histogram

A histogram is a bar graph that is used to illustrate the frequency distribution of a phenomenon. It is a rough estimate of the probability distribution of the given variable. For example, **FIGURE 13-5** illustrates the frequency distribution of patient arrivals in the emergency department over a period of time. "A histogram can evaluate the capability of a process to meet specifications using variable data like time, money, weight" (Arthur, 2011, p. 11). In the example in Figure 13-5, time is used as the variable.

Scatter Plot

The scatter plot is a tool used to display the distribution of two variables to show relationship. In **FIGURE 13-6**, one can see that as speed increases, fuel consumption

FIGURE 13-5 Histogram.

FIGURE 13-6 Scatter plot.
Reproduced with permission from QI Macros. http://www.qimacros.com.

increases as well. Use a scatter plot when there is a believed relationship between two variables.

4. Project Management Tools

As mentioned in Chapter 10, Creating and Developing the Project Plan, project management involves planning, organizing, acquiring, managing, leading, and controlling resources to achieve the overall project goal(s). Clearly, multiple tools may be needed to manage a project effectively. The following tools will assist in determining alternate solutions to problems and will help identify the appropriate plan for implementing change. Finally, a project plan template is provided in **Appendix C**.

Action Plan

The project action (implementation) plan, in essence, articulates how to achieve the project goals. It controls the execution of the project plan and delineates the details of project implementation by addressing *who, what, where, when, why,* and *how* (see **TABLE 13-2**).

Balanced Scorecard

The balanced scorecard is a value-added management process that aligns the organizational mission and/or vision to project/business activities and other nonfinancial performance measures to help improve communication, monitor performance, and give managers a balanced view of the organization's performance (Balanced Scorecard Institute, 2012; see **FIGURE 13-7**). The balanced scorecard incorporates a variety of perspectives, including financial, customer, and internal business process perspectives (McLaughlin & Hays, 2008).

To be successful, companies need to measure and monitor metrics that align with the business vision and strategy. Examples of measures that matter include:

1. Financial—profit
2. Customer satisfaction
3. Employee satisfaction
4. Product quality
5. Cost to produce the product
6. Growth

TABLE 13-2 Action Plan						
Type	**What**	**How**	**Who**	**When**	**Where**	**Why**
Strategy						
People Organization						
Process						
Technology						

Reproduced with permission from QI Macros. http://www.qimacros.com

These items are examples of key performance indicators (KPIs) and can be used to define values for measuring and monitoring achievement toward goals.

Process Flowchart

The flowchart is used to map a process showing all the steps involved (see **FIGURE 13-8**). This can be a very high-level chart or it can be a visual graphic depicting a very simple

FIGURE 13-7 Balanced scorecard.

Reproduced with permission from QI Macros. http://www.qimacros.com

process. These flowcharts can also be used to streamline a process by identifying opportunities for improvement.

5. Process Improvement Tools

Lean Methodology

Lean is a process management methodology based on the Toyota Production System. The aim of Lean is to improve efficiency through the use of tools by removing waste, such as:

- Overproduction—making too much
- Transportation—moving resources—that is, people, material, and information
- Motion—unnecessary movement
- Correction—refers to a product/information that needs to be fixed

Step

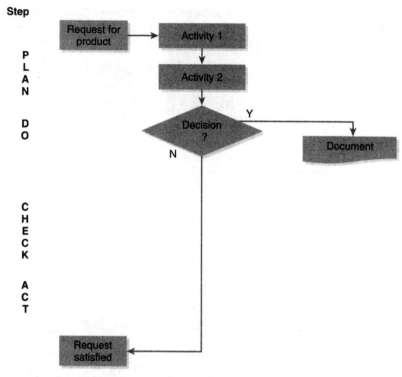

FIGURE 13-8 Process flowchart.
Reproduced with permission from QI Macros. http://www.qimacros.com.

- Overprocessing—anything that is done to the product/information that does not add value
- Inventory—product/information that is waiting to be used
- Waiting—people waiting for product/information to arrive
- Unused employee ideas and talent—people's ideas or talents not being used (Pinnacle Enterprise Group, 2012, para. 1)

Lean methodology involves various tools that help the project manager assess the project flow at a very detailed level, with a goal of removing complex processes that are associated with higher costs.

Six Sigma

This methodology or management system was developed in 1986 as a method to reduce variability in manufacturing at Motorola. Today, Six Sigma methods are used in a variety of arenas ranging from manufacturing, to government, to healthcare organizations (Chapman, 2011). The term is used to evaluate quality, based on a scale that aims to achieve no more than 3.4 defects per one million opportunities (DPMO). The focus of this methodology is improving quality and reducing errors and variation (McLaughlin & Hays, 2008). "A good Six Sigma implementation plan will identify what activities to implement, how to do them, who will do them, when they will be started and completed, and how they will be measured" (Arthur, 2011, p. 44).

DMAIC Process

The DMAIC process, which stands for define, measure, analyze, improve, and control, is a Six Sigma problem-solving method that uses the five stages of quality improvement:

1. *Define* the opportunity for improvement, the project goals, and the key stakeholders.
   Tools that may be used: project charter, project status report, issue log, process flowchart, and work breakdown structure
2. *Measure* performance; the current state of the process. Determine what to measure and collect the data.
   Tools that may be used: Pareto chart, process flowchart
3. *Analyze* the data to identify opportunities, improve the process, or fix the problem.
   Tools that may be used: Pareto chart, fishbone diagram, histogram, scatter plot, statistical analysis, and hypothesis testing
4. *Improve* the process by making the needed changes based on analysis.
   Tools that may be used: brainstorming, failure modes and effects analysis (FMEA)
5. *Control* the outcome by making sure the changes are set in the process by developing and initiating a monitoring plan.
   Tool that may be used: control plan

6. Budget Tools

Budget tools help estimate how much a project will cost based on the project activities, as well as monitor the costs during project implementation. Generally, project budgetary tools include revenues (if applicable) and expenditures (costs) as outlined in the project plan.

Project Budget

The project budget includes both direct and indirect costs. Direct costs include items such as equipment and supplies. Indirect costs are those associated with the day-to-day operation of an organization—for example, electricity and heat. A budget template is provided in **Appendix D**.

Cost–Benefit Analysis (CBA)

As the name implies, a cost–benefit analysis is used to determine the costs and/or benefits associated with implementing a change (see **TABLE 13-3**). To conduct a cost–benefit analysis, all the costs (e.g., resources used) associated with the change (countermeasure) are listed, followed by all the potential benefits (e.g., time savings). Both columns are totaled, and then the costs are subtracted from the benefits. Decision-making tools help the student identify which potential change is most cost effective. Table 13-3 details a few sites that can assist in completing a CBA.

TABLE 13-3 Cost–Benefit Analysis Tools

Tool	Description	Resource
Mind Tools Limited Cost-Benefit Analysis (CBA)	Discussion, process, and examples provided	https://www.mindtools.com/pages/article/newTED_08.htm
Smartsheet CBA Template	Free CBA template	https://www.smartsheet.com/free-cost-benefit-analysis-templates

Reproduced with permission from QI Macros. http://www.qimacros.com

TABLE 13-4 Risk Assessment Matrix

Risk Description	Business Impact	Probability of Occurrence	Priority
	(1, 3, 5)	(1, 3, 5)	
			0
			0
			0
			0
			0
			0
			0
			0
	1-low, 5-high		

Reproduced with permission from QI Macros. http://www.qimacros.com

7. Risk Assessment Tools

As mentioned in Chapter 10, a risk assessment (see **TABLE 13-4**) is suggested to identify and evaluate the potential impact of project risks. Conducting a risk assessment helps the student prioritize these risks and determine which may require a mitigation plan.

Force Field Analysis

The force field analysis is a decision-making tool used to identify all the potential forces driving and restraining a proposed change. Using the template in **TABLE 13-5**, the student would identify all the potential forces that will help him or her implement a project in the *driving forces* section, then fill in all the potential forces that would work against or impede the implementation of the project in the *restraining forces* section.

In the *action to be taken* section, the student should list the actions that could be taken to strengthen the driving forces, as well as those that can be taken to weaken the restraining forces, thereby improving the chance of success. This tool is useful because it helps the student identify the potential for successfully implementing a project.

8. Disseminating the Plan—Communication Tools

Project Charter

The purpose of this document is to formally recognize the existence of a project. It is a valuable tool to use when securing commitment for project implementation

TABLE 13-5 Force Field Analysis			
	Forces		
Countermeasures Proposed Solutions	**Driving Forces (For)**	**Restraining Forces (Against)**	**Action to Be Taken**

within an organization. Even if the charter is not required by the institution, it is a useful tool to ensure that all aspects of the project, including potential constraints, are addressed. The project charter typically includes:

- Project title and high-level description
- Project lead/manager
- The overview/rationale—explains the problem being solved by completing the project (business case)
- Project scope—the features and functions of the project
- Risks—if the project is not done
- Stakeholders
- Project goals, objectives, and deliverables (metrics)
- High-level timeline
- Project risks/constraints
- Anticipated resources—team members, equipment, and so on
- Preliminary budget
- Project approval—signature required

A sample of a project charter is provided in **Appendix E.**

Communication Plan

As mentioned in Chapter 10, the purpose of the communication plan is to describe how communication will occur during the project. This plan includes how and when information will be communicated, who communicates the message, and what is communicated. A sample of a communication plan is provided in **Appendix F.**

Project Meeting Agenda/Minutes

When conducting a project meeting, having an agenda will help ensure that key points are addressed, efficiency is improved, and that the meeting is kept on schedule. Following the meeting, the team will need a synopsis of the discussion points, the assigned action items, the members responsible for the action items, and the timeline for completion. The meeting agenda and minutes can be combined into one succinct form to meet the needs of both. An example of a meeting agenda/minutes form is provided in **Appendix G.**

Project Milestones

As mentioned in Chapter 10, project milestones are important events or key deliverables that are completed during the life cycle of the project (see **TABLE 13-6**). A table can easily be used to describe and track the estimated time of completion for each milestone.

Project Status Report

Communication is the key to successful project management. The project status report helps maintain communication during the project implementation phase. The project manager or lead uses the report to communicate the status of the project against the project plan on a regular basis to the key stakeholders. The content of the report varies from project to project based on the project size and so on. The

TABLE 13-6 Project Milestones		
Milestones	**Description**	**Estimated Completion Date**

TABLE 13-7 Issues Log						
Issue Number	**Description of Issue**	**Date Reported**	**Assigned To**	**Status**	**Date Resolved**	**Resolution**

typical report will include information on the project milestone overview and status, issue summary, risks summary, and metrics. An example of a project status report is provided in **Appendix H**.

Issues Log

An issues log is simply a record of all the issues or problems that arise during a project that require some type of resolution. This record helps the student keep track of and effectively manage these issues during project implementation (see **TABLE 13-7**).

9. Scheduling Tools

Scheduling tools can be used to assign duties to team members so they know what they are expected to accomplish and by when (deadline). However, scheduling tools can also be used to plot out all the activities and resources required to complete a project. The following tools can be used to help the DNP student manage project resources and activities so the project goals are accomplished on time!

Project Time Worksheet

The project time worksheet is used to track project team members' time on the project. The example in **TABLE 13-8** identifies each team member, the date and hours worked, and the total hours that each team member and the team as a whole worked over a given period of time.

Project Schedule

This document is used to estimate the time and effort required to complete the project. In some cases, it is used to hold people accountable (see **TABLE 13-9**). However, it is important to note that the focus should be only on those activities that are important for achieving the overall project goal.

Project Timeline

The project timeline is a visual representation of tasks to be completed related to calendar dates (see **FIGURE 13-9**). It helps organize the project and establish deadline

TABLE 13-8 Project Time Worksheet					
Period Start					
Team Member	**Date and Hours Worked**	**Date and Hours Worked**	**Date and Hours Worked**	**Date and Hours Worked**	**Total Hours**
Project Lead					
Team Member A					
Team Member B					
Team Member C					
Team Total					

TABLE 13-9 Project Schedule

Project Schedule for . . .

Tasks	Who	Hours	Start	End	1/1	1/8	1/15	1/22	1/29	2/5	2/12	2/19	2/26	3/5
Planning Phase		84.0	1/2	1/11										
Task 1		45.0	1/2	1/5										
Task 2		15.0	1/5	1/8										
		24.0	1/8	1/11										

FIGURE 13-9 Project timeline.

FIGURE 13-10 Work breakdown structure.

Reproduced with permission from QI Macros. http://www.qimacros.com.

dates for each task. When setting up a project timeline, it is often helpful to begin with the deadline for completion of the project and work backward to the present to establish the framework for realistic completion of the tasks.

Work Breakdown Structure

The work breakdown structure is also included in the *project scope*. This document helps identify how the objectives and goals of the project will be met. The work breakdown structure lists the tasks (or milestones) that must be completed to meet an objective and the resources that will be needed to accomplish the task (McLaughlin & Hays, 2008). In the example in **FIGURE 13-10**, the work breakdown structure is provided for building a bicycle.

10. Evaluation Tools

A wide variety of evaluation tools are available for use, and they can be used for a variety of reasons. For example, evaluation tools can be used to help the student problem solve, brainstorm ideas, determine risk, answer basic questions about a program, or even determine effectiveness of an action, intervention, or project. Many of the previous assessment tools can and should be used as part of the evaluation to compare pre- and post-intervention data.

11. Information Technology Tools

Melissa Stec, DNP, APRN, CNM, FACNM, FAAN

There is evidence that technology-enhanced teaching and learning improves student outcomes (Beetham & Sharpe, 2013; New Media Consortium, 2012); however, a significant barrier to realizing technology's promise is the educational community's ability or willingness to capitalize on this opportunity. Adopting and integrating emerging technologies throughout teaching and learning culture relies on the successful diffusion of the innovations, and diffusion depends on acceptance of change (Rogers, 2003). As nursing is an interactive, kinesthetic profession that requires the use of both technological and visual expertise, it is believed that parallels between these attributes and use of technology will directly contribute to the preparation, success, and excellence of its students and their abilities to transform health care.

The infusion of technology in education has broad implications for DNP students. Tablet devices are providing students with a creation tool that allows for small-scale, application-based learning rather than the more traditionally directed software-based project tools that are often cumbersome and difficult to negotiate (Walters & Baum, 2011). Several opportunities are available for students to use informatics tools throughout the DNP project process. The informatics toolbox has provided a robust resource for students to consider when engaging in project development, implementation, and evaluation. **TABLE 13-10** outlines tools that work to enhance the project process and ensure a streamlined, comprehensive output that accomplishes the student's goals.

TABLE 13-11 features applications for Windows, iOS, and Android operating systems along with approximate costs.

TABLE 13-10 Informatics Tools to Enhance the DNP Project Process		
Function	**Application**	**Description**
Annotation	iAnnotate Skitch	Used to read, markup, and share files in various file types; improves productivity.
Sharing	Flipboard Box	Share information with others with secure file space or with interactive magazines.
Logic Models	iThoughts Mindmap PureFlow	Create multidirectional flow charts and logic maps that can be color coded, easily edited, and exported in multiple file formats.
Portfolios	Evernote Box Google Drive	Allow users to write, present, collect, and use information in one place.

(continues)

TABLE 13-10 Informatics Tools to Enhance the DNP Project Process *(continued)*

Function	Application	Description
Posters and Presentations	PowerPoint Keynote Google Slides Nearpod Explain Everything Presentation Maker	Create interactive posters and presentations with graphics, data, and voice-over components; used to create both static and dynamic presentations on a variety of platforms.
Project Planning and Budget	Microsoft Project Planning Pro Plus	Produce complex project plans that include GANTT charts, resource usage tracking, budgets, risk management tools, and multitasking gestures.
Risk Management	Risk Registrar	Used for organization risk assessment and as a repository for all identified risks of a project or business plan.
White Boards	Collaborate LiveBoard	Use electronic white space to write, draw, and collaborate; can be captured and used later.

TABLE 13-11 Informatics Tools: Functions and Operating Systems

	Tablet Applications		
Functions	**Windows**	**iOS**	**Android**
Annotation	Skitch (NC) PDF markup	iAnnotate ($$)	iAnnotate ($$)
Information Sharing	Flipboard (NC), web based, all devices		
Logic Models	Ithoughts HD ($$)	PureFlow ($)	iMindMap HD (NC)
Portfolios	Evernote (NC, $$$), web based, all devices Box (NC), web based, all devices Google Drive (NC), web based, all devices		
Posters	PowerPoint (NC, $$$)	Keynote (NC)	Google Slides (NC)
Presentations	Nearpod ($$)	Explain Everything ($$)	Presentation Maker (NC)

	Tablet Applications		
Functions	**Windows**	**iOS**	**Android**
Project Planning and Budget	Microsoft Project (NC) Planning Pro Plus ($)	Planning Pro ($$$)	Planning Pro ($$$)
Risk Management	Risk Registrar (NC)	Risk Register + ($)	Not available
Sharing	Box (NC), web based, all devices Good drive, Google Docs (NC), web based, all devices		
White Boards	Collaborate (NC)	Explain Everything ($)	LiveBoard (NC)

Key: NC, no charge; $, $0–$5; $$, $5–$10; $$$, $10–$20.

TABLE 13-12 Device-Agnostic Tools for Faculty and Students

Purpose	Tool
Information Sharing and Portfolios	Flipboard Box Dropbox Google Drive, Docs, and Sheets Evernote Seesaw
Presentations	Nearpod Prezi Picktochart
Video Discussion	Flipgrid
Notetaking	Simplenote
Collaboration	Zoom Skype
Project Management	Basecamp

See **TABLE 13-12** for technology tools that are device agnostic, meaning that they can be used on any device, and are gaining popularity in education. Device-agnostic platforms are often web based and provide flexibility to students and faculty when working on projects.

The following excerpt from Dr. Maria Maloney highlights the value of using technology to enhance the learning experience (**EXEMPLAR 13-1**).

EXEMPLAR 13-1 Using Technology Tools to Assist in the DNP Project Process

Maria Maloney, DNP, APRN, CPNP

To assist in the DNP project process, I used many applications available on an iPad. Thanks to the portability of the iPad, I could work on my project anytime, anywhere! All of my coursework, including readings, assignments, and discussion boards, are conveniently available on the iTunesU app. Additionally, I used the Evernote application to compile and organize all my completed coursework, including papers, videos, and presentations. The Evernote application allows the creation of many folders that can be used for different courses, and professors and peers can be invited to see your folder, ensuring easy transmission of coursework. Planning Pro allowed me to create an interactive project timeline and incorporate needed resources and budget on a per step basis. One of my favorite applications for the DNP program is Keynote. I have made all my presentations, study guides, and even labels for printing in this application. Lastly, Explain Everything is an application that allows you to add voiceover to presentations made in Keynote. Even if your program does not require an iPad as mine did, I would recommend iPad use for DNP students as it allows your coursework to be available at your fingertips for even the busiest of students.

▶ Summary

A vast amount of resources are available to assist the DNP student in the planning and implementation phase of the DNP project. This chapter provided only a sample of the potential tools available for use; a wealth of additional information is available via the Web and project management textbooks. The student should check with an advisor or his or her DNP project team to identify those resources that may be available through the university at no or reduced cost.

References

American Association of Colleges of Nursing (AACN). (2006). *The essentials of doctoral education for advanced nursing practice.* Retrieved from http://www.aacnnursing.org/Portals/42/Publications/DNPEssentials.pdf

Balanced Scorecard Institute. (n.d.). *Balanced scorecard basics.* Retrieved from http://www.balancedscorecard.org/BSCResources/AbouttheBalancedScorecard/tabid/55/Default.aspx

Beetham, H., & Sharpe, R. (2013). *Rethinking pedagogy for a digital age.* New York, NY: Routledge Publishing.

Chapman, A. (2011). *Six Sigma definitions, history, overview. Businessballs.* Retrieved from http://www.businessballs.com/sixsigma.htm

McLaughlin, D. B., & Hays, J. M. (2008). *Healthcare operations management.* Chicago, IL: Health Administration Press.

New Media Consortium (NMC). (2012). *Horizon report – 2012 higher education edition.* Retrieved from http://www.nmc.org/pdf/2012-horizon-report-HE.pdf

Pinnacle Enterprise Group. (2012). *Lean and Six Sigma.* Retrieved from http://www.pinnacleeg.com/shp-lean-and-six-sigma.php/page/services/service/lean-and- six-sigma

QI Macros. (2012). *The shortcut to lean Six Sigma results!* Retrieved from http://www.qimacros.com

Rogers, E. (2003). *Diffusion of innovations.* New York, NY: Free Press.

Schmehl, P. (n.d.). *Concept mapping.* Retrieved from: http://www.nursingconceptmapping.com/

Walters, E., & Baum, M. (2011). Point/counterpoint: Will the iPad revolutionize education? *Learning and Leading with Technology, 38*(7), 6–7.

Appendix A: Competency Assessment for Practicum Design

Essential I: Scientific Underpinnings for Practice Competencies	DNP Student Competency Rating (1–5)	Needed for Project	Needed for Practicum
1. Integrate nursing science with knowledge from ethics and from the biophysical, psychosocial, analytical, and organizational sciences as the basis for the highest level of nursing practice.			

2. Use science-based theories and concepts to:
  a. Determine the nature and significance of health and healthcare delivery phenomena.
  b. Describe the actions and advanced strategies to enhance, alleviate, and ameliorate health and healthcare delivery phenomena as appropriate.
  c. Evaluate outcomes.
  d. Develop and evaluate new practice approaches based on nursing theories and theories from other disciplines.			

Essential II: Organizational and Systems Leadership for Quality Improvement and Systems Thinking Competencies	DNP Student Competency Rating (1–5)	Needed for Project	Needed for Practicum
1. Develop and evaluate care delivery approaches that meet current and future needs of patient populations based on scientific findings in nursing and other clinical sciences, as well as organizational, political, and economic sciences.			
2. Ensure accountability for quality of health care and patient safety for populations with whom they work. a. Use advanced communication skills/processes to lead quality improvement and patient safety initiatives in healthcare systems. b. Employ principles of business, finance, economics, and health policy to develop and implement effective plans for practice-level and/or system-wide practice initiatives that will improve the quality of care delivery. c. Develop and/or monitor budgets for practice initiatives. d. Analyze the cost effectiveness of practice initiatives accounting for risk and improvement of healthcare outcomes. e. Have demonstrated sensitivity to diverse organizational cultures and populations, including patients and providers.			
3. Develop and/or evaluate effective strategies for managing the ethical dilemmas inherent in patient care, the healthcare organization, and research.			

Essential III: Clinical Scholarship and Analytical Methods for Evidence-Based Practice Competencies	DNP Student Competency Rating (1–5)	Needed for Project	Needed for Practicum
1. Use analytical methods to critically appraise existing literature and other evidence to determine and implement the best evidence for practice.			
2. Design and implement processes to evaluate outcomes of practice, practice patterns, and systems of care within a practice setting, healthcare organization, or community against national benchmarks to determine variances in practice outcomes and population trends.			
3. Design, direct, and evaluate quality improvement methodologies to promote safe, timely, effective, efficient, equitable, and patient-centered care.			
4. Apply relevant findings to develop practice guidelines and improve practice and the practice environment.			
5. Use information technology and research methods appropriately to: a. Collect appropriate and accurate data to generate evidence for nursing practice, inform/guide database designs that generate meaningful evidence for nursing practice, analyze data for practice, and design evidence-based interventions. b. Predict and analyze outcomes, examine patterns of behavior and outcomes, and identify gaps in evidence for practice.			

(continues)

Essential III: Clinical Scholarship and Analytical Methods for Evidence-Based Practice Competencies	DNP Student Competency Rating (1–5)	Needed for Project	Needed for Practicum
6. Function as a practice specialist/consultant in collaborative knowledge-generating research.			
7. Disseminate findings from evidence-based practice and research to improve healthcare outcomes.			

Essential IV: Information Systems/Technology and Patient Care Technology for the Improvement and Transformation of Healthcare Competencies	DNP Student Competency Rating (1–5)	Needed for Project	Needed for Practicum
1. Design, select, use, and evaluate programs that evaluate and monitor outcomes of care, care systems, and quality improvement, including consumer use of healthcare information systems.			
2. Analyze and communicate critical elements necessary to the selection, use, and evaluation of healthcare information systems and patient care technology.			
3. Demonstrate the conceptual ability and technical skills to develop and execute an evaluation plan involving data extraction from practice information systems and databases.			

(continues)

Essential IV: Information Systems/ Technology and Patient Care Technology for the Improvement and Transformation of Healthcare Competencies	DNP Student Competency Rating (1–5)	Needed for Project	Needed for Practicum
4. Provide leadership in evaluation and resolution of ethical and legal issues within healthcare systems relating to the use of information, information technology, communication networks, and patient care technology.			
5. Evaluate consumer health information sources for accuracy, timeliness, and appropriateness.			

Essential V: Healthcare Policy for Advocacy in Health Care Competencies	DNP Student Competency Rating (1–5)	Needed for Project	Needed for Practicum
1. Critically analyze health policy proposals, health policies, and related issues from the perspective of consumers, nursing, other health professions, and other stakeholders in policy and public information.			
2. Demonstrate leadership in development and implementation of institutional, local, state, federal, and/or international health policy.			
3. Influence policymakers through active participation on committees, boards, or task forces at the institutional, local, state, regional, national, and/or international levels to improve healthcare delivery and outcomes.			
4. Educate others, including policymakers at all levels, regarding nursing, health policy, and patient care outcomes.			

(continues)

Essential V: Healthcare Policy for Advocacy in Health Care Competencies	DNP Student Competency Rating (1–5)	Needed for Project	Needed for Practicum
5. Advocate for the nursing profession within the policy and healthcare communities.			
6. Develop, evaluate, and provide leadership for healthcare policy that shapes healthcare financing, regulation, and delivery.			
7. Advocate for social justice, equity, and ethical policies within all healthcare arenas.			

Essential VI: Interprofessional Collaboration for Improving Patient and Population Health Outcomes Competencies	DNP Student Competency Rating (1–5)	Needed for Project	Needed for Practicum
1. Employ effective communication and collaborative skills in the development and implementation of practice models, peer review, practice guidelines, health policy, standards of care, and/or other scholarly products.			
2. Lead interprofessional teams in the analysis of complex practice and organizational issues.			
3. Employ consultative and leadership skills with intraprofessional and interprofessional teams to create change in health care and complex healthcare delivery systems.			

Essential VII: Clinical Prevention and Population Health for Improving the Nation's Health Competencies	DNP Student Competency Rating (1–5)	Needed for Project	Needed for Practicum
1. Analyze epidemiological, biostatistical, environmental, and other appropriate scientific data related to individual, aggregate, and population health.			
2. Synthesize concepts, including psychosocial dimensions and cultural diversity, related to clinical prevention and population health in developing, implementing, and evaluating interventions to address health promotion/disease prevention efforts, improve health status/access patterns, and/or address gaps in care of individuals, aggregates, or populations.			
3. Evaluate care delivery models and/or strategies using concepts related to community, environmental and occupational health, and cultural and socioeconomic dimensions of health.			

Essential VIII: Advanced Nursing Practice Competencies	DNP Student Competency Rating (1–5)	Needed for Project	Needed for Practicum
1. Conduct a comprehensive and systematic assessment of health and illness parameters in complex situations, incorporating diverse and culturally sensitive approaches.			
2. Design, implement, and evaluate therapeutic interventions based on nursing science and other sciences.			
3. Develop and sustain therapeutic relationships and partnerships with patients (individual, family, or group) and other professionals to facilitate optimal care and patient outcomes.			

(continues)

Essential VIII: Advanced Nursing Practice Competencies	DNP Student Competency Rating (1–5)	Needed for Project	Needed for Practicum
4. Demonstrate advanced levels of clinical judgment, systems thinking, and accountability in designing, delivering, and evaluating evidence-based care to improve patient outcomes.			
5. Guide, mentor, and support other nurses to achieve excellence in nursing practice.			
6. Educate and guide individuals and groups through complex health and situational transitions.			
7. Use conceptual and analytical skills in evaluating the links among practice, organizational, populations, fiscal, and policy issues.			

Key:

Assessment	Explanation (based on Benner's *From Novice to Expert* [1984])
1–5	Student self-rated competency

- 5 = **Expert**: Highly competent or expert demonstration of the competency.
- 4 = **Proficient**: Understands a situation as a whole, but not yet an expert with the competency.
- 3 = **Competent**: Does not yet have enough experience to recognize a situation in terms of an overall picture, but has an understanding of the competency.
- 2 = **Advanced Beginners**: Able to demonstrate marginally acceptable performance of the competency.
- 1 = **Novice**: No experience with the competency expected to perform.

*	Competencies needed for the scholarly project.
**	Identified professional growth need for the project.
^	Additional identified professional growth need.

Modified from American Association of Colleges of Nursing (AACN). (2006). *The essentials of doctoral education for advanced nursing practice.* Retrieved from http://www.aacnnursing.org/Portals/42/Publications/DNPEssentials.pdf
Benner, P. (1984). *From novice to expert: Excellence and power in clinical nursing practice.* Menlo Park, CA: Addison-Wesley.

Appendix B: Concept Map Template

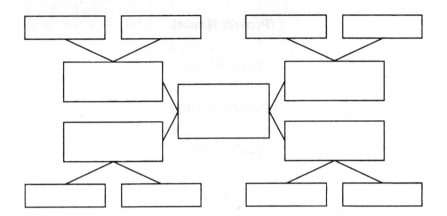

Appendix C: Template for Project Plan

(Project Name)

Project Plan

(Student Name)

(University)

(Date)

Table of Contents

This plan was adapted from the Centers for Disease Control (n.d.), North Carolina Enterprise (2004), and Project Management Docs (n.d.).

Appendix D: Sample Budget

Program Expenses		
Salaries/Wages[a]		
Itemize human resource costs in this section (i.e., administrative support, practitioner, etc.).		
	Monthly	**Total**
		$
•	$	$
•	$	$
•	$	$
Total Salary Costs		$
Startup Costs		
Itemize startup costs in this section (i.e., copies, charts, display board, etc.).		
•		$
•		$
•		$
Total Startup Costs		$
Capital Costs		
Hardware		$
Equipment		$
Other		$
Total Capital Costs		$

Operational Costs		
Itemize operational costs in this section (i.e., electricity, heat, etc.).		
•		$
•		$
•		$
Total Project Expenses		$
Program Revenue[b]		
Revenue Generation		
Itemize potential revenue in this section.		
•		$
•		$
•		$
		$
Total Project Revenue		$
Program Benefit/Loss		
Total Revenue		$
Less Expenses		$
Total Program Benefit/Loss		$

[a] Include either actual wages paid (if available) or median full-time salary for the same position in the United States. An additional 30% may be added to wages to cover benefits.

[b] For example, revenue attained through billable evaluation and management codes, teaching codes, and so on.

Adapted from Moran, K., Burson, R., Critchett, J., & Olla, P. (2011). Exploring the cost and clinical outcomes of integrating the registered nurse certified diabetes educator in the patient centered medical home. *The Diabetes Educator, 37*(6), 780–793.

Appendix E: DNP Project Charter

Project Name:

Project Lead:

Date:

Project Overview (Including background)

Project Scope

Risks (If the project is not done)

1.
2.
3.
4.

Stakeholders

1.
2.
3.
4.

Project Team (List team members and roles each will play.)

1.
2.
3.
4.

Desired Outcomes (Overall goals)

1.
2.
3.
4.

Objectives (Must be achieved to complete the project)

1.
2.
3.
4.

Project Deliverables (Those tasks that must be achieved to meet the objectives/complete the project)

<u>Metric</u>   <u>Target</u>

1.

2.

3.

4.

Project Timeline

Project Phase	Milestone	Estimated Month of Completion[a]					
		Jan	Feb	Mar	Apr	May	June
Initiation	Project charter approved	→					
Planning	Project planning meeting	——→					
	Project plan completed	————→					
	Communication plan completed						
	IRB approved						
	Hardware and software approved						
Implementation	Training completed						
	Equipment approved						
Monitoring	Mid-project evaluation complete						
Closing	Project completion meeting						

[a]An arrow (→) is used to indicate the month the activity is estimated to be completed.

Project Risks/Constraints and Mitigation Plan (Any event that could have a negative impact on the project objectives and what will be done to address it proactively)

          Risks   **Mitigation**

1.

2.

3.

4.

5.

Assumptions (Factors that are assumed—for example, access to the setting, access to participants where applicable, and use of equipment)

1.

2.

3.

4.

5.

Project Resources (Staffing, equipment, etc.)

1.

2.

3.

4.

5.

Preliminary Budget		
One-Time Costs	**Project**	**Ongoing**
Staff	$	$
Professional services	$	$
Other	$	$
Total One-Time Costs	**$**	**$**
Capital Costs	**Project**	**Ongoing**
Hardware	$	$
Equipment	$	$
Other	$	$
Total Capital Costs	**$**	**$**
Ongoing Costs	**Project**	**Ongoing**
Software license fees	$	$
Maintenance fees	$	$
Other	$	$
Total Ongoing Costs	**$**	**$**
Signatures:		
Advisor/Chair		[date]
DNP Student		[date]

Adapted from Stanford University Information Technology Services. (2008). *IT services project charter*. Retrieved from http://web.stanford.edu/dept/its/projects/service_management_toolkit/

Appendix F: DNP Communication Plan

1. Introduction
In this section, briefly describe the project and communication goals.

2. Contact List

Team Member Name	Role	Work Number	Cell Number	Email Address

3. Reports

Document (Description)	Name of Recipients	Method for Distribution (email, etc.)	Who Is Responsible for the Distribution?	Frequency of Distribution

4. Project Meetings

Meeting	Purpose	Participants	Meeting Leader	Meeting Frequency

Adapted from North Carolina Enterprise. (2004). *Project management plan template*; Institute of Electrical and Electronics Engineers (IEEE). (1988). 1058.1-1987 IEEE standard for software project management plans.

Appendix G: DNP Project Meeting

| Date: |
| Location: |
| Facilitator: |
| Attendees: |

Please review before the meeting:

AGENDA ITEMS

Discussion Topic
✓
✓
✓
✓
✓
✓
✓
✓
✓
✓

ACTION ITEMS

Description:	Assigned to:	Due date:
✓		
✓		
✓		

Appendix H: Project Status Report

Name:

Date:

Completed Activities

Activity/Date of Completion
-
-

Activities in Progress

Activity/Estimated Date of Completion
-
-
-

Issues
-

Planned Activities

Planned Activity/Estimated Date of Completion
-
-
-
-

Risks
-
-

Modified from Centers for Disease Control and Prevention (n.d.). *Status reporting*. CDC Document Library. Retrieved from http://www2.cdc.gov/cdcup/library/matrix/default.htm

CHAPTER 14

Project Implementation

Katherine Moran and Rosanne Burson

CHAPTER OVERVIEW

The implementation phase occurs only after extensive development, planning, and communication. This chapter highlights aspects of the implementation phase that the doctor of nursing practice (DNP) student must consider to reach his or her intended goals.

CHAPTER OBJECTIVES

After completing this chapter, the learner will be able to:

1. Identify components of implementation success.
2. Discuss the importance of project implementation planning.
3. List the key factors associated with operationalizing the project plan.
4. Define the most valuable characteristics of an effective leader.
5. Describe the project implementation close-out phase.

▶ The Implementation Process

When it is finally time to implement the DNP project, the student will undoubtedly feel a sense of relief, excitement for what is yet to come, and possibly a little trepidation. Progressing to this point in the DNP program takes a lot of commitment and perseverance. It is likely that many months of planning have already been invested in conceptualizing the project. The phenomenon of interest has been identified, various project types have been explored, appropriate identification of measurable outcomes has occurred (see Chapter 7, Aligning Design, Method, and Evaluation with the Clinical Question), and finally a decision has been made and the project plan is developed. Now it is time for the next step—operationalizing the plan. This is the action phase of the project plan.

How Leadership Influences Project Implementation

Operationalizing the plan is the action phase of the project plan.

Most people would agree that the project leader/manager influences or at least has an impact on the overall project success, especially where project implementation is concerned. Right or wrong, good results or outcomes tend to be associated with good leaders. However, there is more to the story than meets the eye. Successful project management involves the coordination of project activities, team member needs, team needs, stakeholder needs, and organizational needs. The goal is to reach a balance with these competing priorities (see **FIGURE 14-1**).

There is a plethora of information in the literature on the topic of what it takes to be an effective leader. **TABLE 14-1** outlines a few of the characteristics associated with

Project activities

Team member, team, stakeholder, and organizational needs

FIGURE 14-1 Balancing priorities.

TABLE 14-1 Characteristics of an Effective Leader

Personal	Skills	Qualities
Charismatic	Leads by example	Enthusiastic
Confident	Persuasive	Assertive
Humble	Communicates effectively	Knowledgeable
Selfless	Manages multiple priorities	Flexible
Visionary	Motivational	Respectful
Caring	Active listener	Emotional intelligence
Positive attitude	Fiscally responsible	Imaginative
People oriented	Decisive	Driven to succeed

effective leadership. A good leader is able to draw on his or her skill set and use the appropriate skills, at the appropriate time, to keep the project in balance. The skills used are based on the needs of the moment. For example, when there is an urgent matter that needs resolution, the leader will be assertive, confident, and decisive.

The skills or competencies the DNP student will need to demonstrate to be a successful project leader are incorporated in *Essential* II—Organizational and Systems Leadership for Quality Improvement and Systems Thinking (American Association of Colleges of Nursing [AACN], 2006). See Chapter 8, Interprofessional and Intraprofessional Collaboration in the DNP Project, for the National Center for Healthcare Leadership (2017)–defined leadership competencies for medicine, nursing, and administration. The project leader must have an understanding of his or her skill set as a leader and the behaviors that correspond to project implementation factors. A few critical leadership abilities include setting goals and objectives, project planning, team building, decision making, consulting with stakeholders, project ownership, problem solving, communicating, being enthusiastic, and motivating others.

A high degree of emotional competence is required to become a successful project leader (see Chapter 11, Driving the Practicum to Impact the DNP Project). Emotional competence behavior includes self-awareness, compassion, passionate optimism, mindfulness, personal humility, appreciation of ambiguity and paradox, appreciation of knowledge, willpower, resilience, and impulse control (Porter-O'Grady & Malloch, 2015). Self-awareness includes understanding self and others' unique perceptions and preferred styles of interaction. It also incorporates the ability to be comfortable with ambiguity and unclear paths, to be open to other viewpoints and new information. Compassionate leaders combine an understanding of the context of situations with the policies of an organization. In other words, a leader looks at the personal side of the equation, as well as what is best for the organization, to deliver a solution. Passionate optimism involves maintaining a positive mindset and resilience, even with the promise of disappointments. Mindfulness refers to being aware of recurring situations, how other members of the team responded, then being able to interpret these situations and use what is learned to guide future behavior. Finally, impulse control is the ability to temper negative feelings while sharing feelings (Porter-O'Grady & Malloch, 2015). Chism (2019) discusses the aspects of emotional competence specifically in the DNP-prepared nurse as an important leadership competency.

Project implementation is also the time during which the DNP student will demonstrate the characteristics and behaviors of all the DNP *Essentials* (AACN, 2006). Those involved with the project will have an opportunity to view the competencies of the DNP-prepared nurse. This is the time to begin marketing yourself and your degree. Chism (2019) states that DNP-prepared nurses ". . . may develop a brand to share what unique talents, skills and knowledge they bring to their career environment" (p. 302). The DNP student should focus on articulating what a DNP degree *is* as well as the *strengths* the DNP-prepared nurse brings to the organization. This can be accomplished using an "elevator speech" (Chism, 2019). Be prepared to present a 1-minute, 3-minute, and 5-minute version of your elevator speech. There will be opportunities, often when least expected, to market the DNP degree and the skills that DNP-prepared nurses bring to the table.

The DNP student should develop business acumen, as this is also important to successful project implementation. According to Reilly and Reilly (2009), business acumen "is keenness and quickness in understanding and dealing with a business situation in a manner that is likely to lead to a good outcome" (p. 10). Examples of characteristics of an individual with business acumen include:

- Has an acute perception of the dimensions of business issues.
- Can make sense out of complexity and an uncertain future.
- Is mindful of the implications of a choice for all the affected parties.
- Is decisive.
- Is flexible if further change is warranted in the future (Reilly & Reilly, 2009, p. 10).

Individuals with these characteristics are able to recognize the changing environment, can "think ahead" to identify and circumvent potential barriers, and are able to orchestrate project implementation efficiently. Having good judgement and being able to make quick decisions is essential.

Along with business acumen, the DNP student should develop his or her financial acumen. Being able to understand and decode the relationship among numbers, people, process, and technology is important when implementing a project in any healthcare environment today (Theodotou, 2018). Financial acumen certainly includes financial skills, but also skills in business quality and global skills. According to Theodotou (2018), possessing financial skills means that one has a good understanding of core financial literacy concepts, and can manage budgets, forecasting, and reporting requirements. Business quality skills include the ability to manage costs; focus on process quality, standards, and metrics; and effectively manage resources. Global skills are essential to effectively analyze local, regional, and global trends and risk, and to develop a sustainability strategy to assure project success now and in the future.

While some DNP students may possess many of these skills, others will not. If further business acumen development is needed, the student should discuss this with his or her project mentor. Often, opportunities are available for the student to design a practicum experience with a business mentor to improve his or her competency in this area (see Chapter 11).

▶ What Constitutes Project Success?

Whether a project is considered a success is largely dependent on the perception of the key stakeholders, including the student, university, organization where the project is implemented, and patients (when applicable). In Chapter 10, Creating and Developing the Project Plan, it was noted that if the project goals are met on schedule and within the budget, and there is a high level of satisfaction regarding the outcome, then the project will likely be considered a success. This makes sense, but what are the factors that are associated with successful projects? How can these factors be leveraged to improve outcomes?

▶ Factors to Consider During Project Implementation

Pinto and Slevin (1987) are well versed in project implementation and have been recognized for their interpretation of factors associated with successful project implementation. According to Pinto and Slevin (1987), the following factors are involved in project implementation:

- Top management support, mission, and schedule
- The client, personnel, and technical skills
- Monitoring, feedback, and communication
- Troubleshooting
- Client acceptance

Project Planning

Management Support, Mission, and Schedule

As mentioned in Chapter 10, an important aspect of successful project implementation is a carefully considered plan. From this perspective, the most important piece of advice the doctoral student should consider when developing the DNP project is to *plan ahead*. The student really needs to take the time to carefully consider what he or she wants to achieve in the project and build a solid business case that will garner top management support. First, be clear regarding what the overall goal is; what is it that you want to achieve (i.e., the expected benefits), and then develop objectives that will lead to the desired outcome. These objectives need to be measurable (so that you know if you achieved the goal). When developing the project objectives, think about the "critical success factors" and/or project deliverables that will be needed to assure project success (Haughey, 2018). The project deliverables should be relevant to the project, of course, but they should also be of interest to the stakeholders. From the organization's perspective, deliverables that relate to improving healthcare quality, the patient experience, and efficiency; reducing costs; and so on, are always important to keep in mind. Next, consider the time that will be needed to complete the project, and then *add time* to the schedule to account for unexpected delays. In other words, expect the unexpected.

> *The most important piece of advice the doctoral student should consider when developing the DNP project is to plan ahead.*

There is an old carpenter saying, "measure twice, cut once," which essentially means that a person has only one shot at cutting the piece of wood, so he or she should take the time to get it right the first time. In other words, it pays to do the legwork up front. As mentioned in Chapter 6, Developing the DNP Project, Pareto's principle is applicable to planning the DNP project; approximately 80% of the project is planning and 20% is implementation.

The first three factors of project implementation relate to the planning phase (Pinto & Slevin, 1987). These factors were addressed in Chapter 10 in more detail. However, the key messages here are to first make sure there is top management support for the project before even considering implementation. Without management support, the resources needed for the project are in jeopardy (see **FIGURE 14-2**).

As mentioned, presenting a solid business case for the project is critical. The DNP student can strengthen the business case by taking the time to complete an organization needs assessment. Using the information gleaned from the organizational assessment, the student should determine if what is needed within the organization can

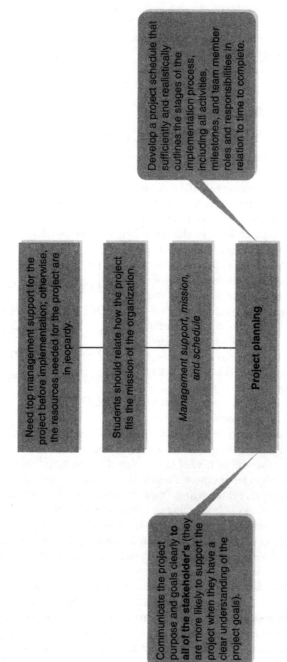

FIGURE 14-2 Project planning.

be achieved through the planned project, and if the project aligns with the organization's mission, priorities, and strategic plan. The student will also want to assess whether the organization has the capacity and is ready for the change, and if the project needs modification to fit the setting and/or target group (see Chapter 6).

Key stakeholders are more likely to support the project when they have a clear understanding of the project goals, and stakeholder support is critical.

Equally important is the need to communicate the project purpose and goals clearly to all of the stakeholders. Key stakeholders are more likely to support the project when they have a clear understanding of the project goals, including how the goals are aligned with the mission and vision of the organization; stakeholder support is critical. Taking the time to assess the organization will help the student build a solid business case that will garner top management support.

A white paper, a 5–7 page document that is targeted at the organization, may be helpful in communicating the recommended project to the stakeholders. The purpose of a white paper is to provide useful, practical, and educational content that helps stakeholders understand an issue, solve a problem, and/or make a decision regarding a project (Graham, 2013). The organizational needs assessment informs the following elements of the white paper:

- Purpose
- Significance
- Current practice
- New evidence
- Intervention
- Considerations
- Recommendations (Graham, 2013)

Finally, the doctoral student should develop a project schedule that sufficiently and realistically outlines the various stages of the implementation process, including all activities, milestones, and team member roles and responsibilities in relation to the time needed for completion. The project schedule will be a useful document to help the student manage and meet the project deadlines. See Chapter 13, The DNP Project Toolbox, for an example of a project schedule. The next seven factors in the outline really involve operationalization of the project plan. This is the action phase of the project implementation process (Pinto & Slevin, 1987) (see **FIGURE 14-3**).

Operationalizing the Project Plan

The Client, Personnel, and Technical Skills

The next two factors to consider in the operationalization phase of project implementation relate to human resources. These include the client (defined as anyone who has an interest in the result of the project) and personnel recruitment, selection, and training (Pinto & Slevin, 1987). First, consider the client's needs. The student needs to make sure that the end users (i.e., key stakeholders or those who will be affected by the outcome of the project) are consulted during this process to help

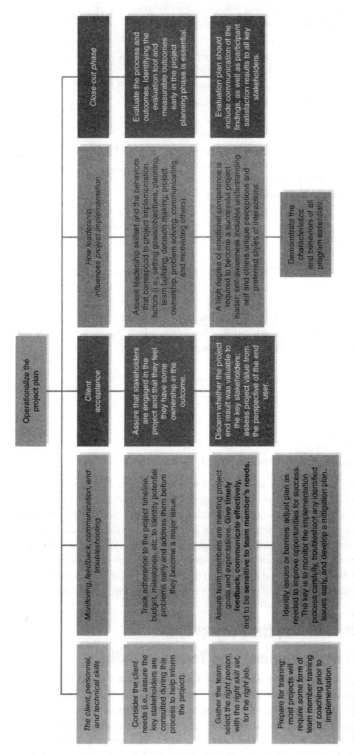

FIGURE 14-3 Operationalize the project plan.

inform the project. See Chapter 6 for more information on identifying key stake-holders. Next, the student needs to gather the team. What is most important to note about the team is the need to select the *right person* with the *right skill set* for the *right job*. Certainly, the team includes the student's project faculty mentor and practice mentor, but the team may also include additional members whose primary responsibilities are implementing various aspects of the project. For example, certainly it is important to have the technology available to support the project, but it is also important that team members possess the ability to use technology to successfully meet the project goals and objectives.

In addition to having the right skill mix, team members also need to be committed to the project. When commitment is lacking on the part of any team member, the project outcome can be negatively impacted. Once the team is gathered, it is time to prepare for training. As mentioned earlier, most projects will require some form of team member training or coaching prior to implementation. During this process, the training plan is considered and discussion regarding the need to work as a team to meet project goals is stressed. See Chapter 10 for more information on training the team.

Monitoring, Feedback, and Communication

Project monitoring and feedback are facilitated via a monitoring plan, which often involves further project refinement and/or adjustments to the plan. This includes tracking adherence to the project timeline, budget, and milestones. The goal is to identify any potential problems early in the implementation phase and to address them before they become major issues. For example, one problem that is sometimes encountered during project implementation is "scope creep," that is, the project grows in size. This can lead to a project running over budget or even not completing on time (Haughey, 2018). Having a well-defined project scope that all key stakeholders agree to is important; then you need to stick to it.

> *The goal is to identify any potential problems early in the implementation phase and to address them before they become major issues.*

The monitoring process involves problem solving, decision making, and managing any project changes and/or risks, but, part of the monitoring process also involves making sure that team members are meeting project goals and expectations, while encouraging them to continue to meet objectives. This is important because an essential piece of monitoring and communication is motivation. Prabhakar (2008) states, "One of the biggest ways to motivate people and to convince them of the potential for successful outcomes is to communicate effectively" (p. 6). Therefore, when monitoring team members' productivity, it is important to give timely feedback, communicate effectively, and to be sensitive to individual team members' needs. In addition, as stressed by Pinto and Slevin (1987), it is critical to communicate effectively with key stakeholders, such as the organization where the project is being implemented.

Finally, the identification of issues and barriers is also part of the monitoring process. As mentioned in Chapter 11, barriers may be identified prior to or during implementation. To keep the project on track, the DNP student should consider the following common barriers to project implementation (Flick, 2009):

1. Lack of clarity—when the project team or stakeholders do not understand the project goals and objectives and/or their respective roles and responsibilities.

2. Project requirements have not been defined—also a contributing factor to lack of clarity; make sure all of the stakeholders agree on the project requirements.

3. Resources are not adequate to meet project goals—a comprehensive project plan must include all of the resources needed to implement the project, including resources that may be needed to sustain the change once the project is completed.

4. Lack of stakeholder support—ongoing effective communication can help mitigate this barrier.

5. Biases (the stakeholders' and yours)—make sure you can deliver what you promise. Stakeholders may have had past experiences where outcomes were "overpromised and underdelivered." This can set a negative tone before the project begins; again, effective communication is the key.

6. Technology gap—as mentioned, it is important to have technology available to support the project, but it is also important that team members possess the ability to use technology to successfully meet the project goals and objectives. The DNP student will also want to consider whether a technology gap exists from the perspective of the stakeholders; especially if the project is technology based.

7. Resistance to change—as most projects involve interaction with other people, it is wise for the DNP student to assess the potential for resistance to change and consider ways to overcoming resistance when developing the project plan. One way to overcome resistance is to make sure all stakeholders understand the benefits of the project. A white paper may be a useful tool in communicating succinctly to stakeholders.

8. Lack of time—this is a critical factor that can be mitigated with a realistic timeline.

9. Not invented here—this barrier relates to DNP students who attempt to implement a project in an organization where they do not have an established relationship. If this is the case, it is helpful for the student to choose a practice mentor who can open organizational doors and be a champion for the project early on.

10. Political barriers—organizational culture, strategic priorities, and so on are examples of political barriers that are important to consider. Again, a thoughtful project plan prevents most problems.

For the most part, successful project implementation begins and ends with effective communication as well as having a well-developed plan to address and hopefully overcome barriers. Prabhakar (2008) notes that it may be necessary to adjust the plan to improve opportunities for success and cites the following 10 key factors that can be used to improve project performance during implementation:

1. Bypass an obstacle.
2. Cause people to stretch.
3. Focus on the goal.

4. Follow a standardized process.
5. Learn from the past.
6. Maintain ongoing communications.
7. Document the work being done.
8. Reuse previous work.
9. Seek buy-in from all involved.
10. Seek simplicity, not complexity, in goal and path (p. 6).

Following these recommendations will ensure a path to project success that will be identified in the close-out phase. Further, the identification and eventual overcoming of the barriers may actually strengthen the commitment of the key stakeholders and improve the final product.

Troubleshooting

It is virtually impossible to predict every potential problem that could come up during project implementation. The key is to monitor the implementation process carefully, troubleshoot any identified issues early, and develop a mitigation plan. Here is where the value of the student's problem-solving skills will be recognized, as he or she works with the team to develop a strategy to overcome barriers. Monitoring and troubleshooting could be necessary in the areas of the planning process, the budget, personnel issues, or identification of participants, to name a few. See Chapter 13, The Scholarly Project Toolbox, for information regarding the tools available for the student to use in the troubleshooting/problem-solving process.

> *The key to successful project implementation is to monitor the process carefully, troubleshoot any identified issues early, and develop a mitigation plan.*

Client Acceptance

At this stage in the process, the student will find out if the project end result was valuable to the key stakeholders. In most cases, the student will already have a good idea of how the project has been received. However, in some cases, even though the project was completed on time, stayed within its budget, and the student had communicated effectively and managed the project as expected, the end user of the project *may or may not* find the end result valuable. The best way to prevent an unexpected outcome is to include key stakeholders early in the process (Pinto & Slevin, 1987). The student should ensure that stakeholders are engaged in the project and that they feel they have some ownership in the outcome. As mentioned previously, stakeholder support is critical, even at the end of the project.

> *Stakeholder support is critical, even at the end of the project.*

Close-out Phase

Once the implementation phase is complete, the close-out phase begins. The close-out phase includes an evaluation of the process and the outcomes. Clearly delineating the evaluation tool that will be used in the project and identifying the measurable outcomes early in the project planning phase are essential. Certainly by now one can recognize how important it is to plan appropriately for each phase of the project. Choosing an evaluation method that is appropriate for the project and its purpose is necessary to effectively evaluate the final outcome of the project. Hickey and Brosnan (2017) state that, "the form of an evaluation is based on its intended purpose and use" (p. xi). Areas of evaluation include:

1. Economic
2. Organization and system
3. Healthcare informatics and patient care technology
4. Patient care standard guidelines and protocols
5. Populations
6. Conceptual models (Hickey & Brosnan, 2017)

Other components of the evaluation plan should include communication of the findings, as well as participant satisfaction results, to all key stakeholders. "Lessons learned, barriers that were overcome during the implementation phase, and strategies used to overcome the barriers could further inform the project" (Beene, 2012, p. 83) and should be included in the final report.

At this point in the project implementation phase, it is important to acknowledge the team and other supporters for a job well done and to show appreciation for all efforts. Also acknowledge your own accomplishment and take time to reflect on the experience and satisfaction of completing the project.

In the following excerpt, Dr. Mary Walczyk shares her DNP project implementation experience in a post-anesthesia care unit setting (see **EXEMPLAR 14-1**).

EXEMPLAR 14-1 Implementation of a "One Team" Approach to PACU Handoff

Mary Walczyk, DNP, CRNA

My DNP project was to develop, implement, and evaluate a *"one team"* approach when transferring total joint arthroplasty patients from the operating room (OR) to the post-anesthesia care unit (PACU). Variations and inconsistencies in information transfer, the lack of standardization, and the fact that only one member of the OR team provides the transfer of information confirmed the need for a change in practice and subsequently drove this project. My goal was to create an efficient and effective way to transfer the postsurgical patient from the OR to the PACU grounded in the themes of standardization and multidisciplinary collaboration. The standardized structure through the use of a protocol and checklists provides the conveyance of detailed, pertinent, and meaningful communication between providers. The multidisciplinary approach involving the OR nurse, surgical provider, and anesthesia provider collaboratively brings all key providers involved in the care of the surgical patient together as *one* for the PACU handoff.

As I reflect back on my DNP project, several themes come to mind that lead to a successful implementation phase: strong leadership skills to drive the DNP project; a robust literature search; and an in-depth strengths, weaknesses, opportunities, and threats (SWOT) analysis. As a future DNP-prepared certified registered nurse anesthetist (CRNA), this quality improvement project focused on the elements of leadership, the art of interprofessional collaboration, and the processes needed for implementation of *change* in a healthcare organization. Lessons learned during the implementation stage highlighted that leadership styles are not static, but rather dynamic, as you need to adapt to each situation. An effective leader adapts to different situations by taking on different roles such as leading and directing in some situations or inquiring and seeking out advice in other situations. However, one static attribute one must possess as the leader of a DNP project is accountability and the need to gain trust and confidence in administrators as well as from the staff.

As I started the implementation phase of my DNP project, I needed to demonstrate leadership in my project. At the numerous meetings with the director of the operating room, director of anesthesia, and chief of orthopedic surgery, I needed to quickly instill confidence and trust to gain their support in this quality improvement project. The earning of trust and confidence from the departmental leaders and staff was the result of a well-organized evidence-based presentation and proposal and empirical driven strategies for success. The interprofessional dimension of this project, and the importance of collaboration among the departments of nursing, orthopedic surgical providers including physician assistants, and anesthesia providers, was paramount for successful implementation. My leadership style morphed from "the leader" of the project with the departmental administrators, to more of a leader "inquiring and seeking out advice" with the staff from the various disciplines. It was essential to listen to the staff and brainstorm with them in order to get collective buy-in, as this was evident in the development of the provider-specific checklists. Allowing staff to assume ownership in the project was crucial as this truly promoted engagement and collaborative decision making.

The extensive literature review guided my path from proposal development to implementation. Combing through the vast studies, key strategic themes on staff engagement and staff education emerged, and these strategies were integrated into my proposal. As one incorporates strategies for success into the project, keep in mind that refinement may be needed for the implementation plan. For example, my plan was for the interprofessional team to meet to discuss the needed items for each of the checklists; however, it was realized very early on that these meetings would directly impact staff productivity. I followed the main theme of the strategy, which was staff engagement and representation of stakeholders, and made a few changes to my implementation plan. I developed draft checklists for each of the disciplines (OR nurse, surgical provider, and anesthesia provider) based on an extensive review of the literature, and then met individually with members of the interprofessional team and staff to revise the checklists based on their clinical expertise and experiences. This slight modification to the empirical driven strategy on engagement was a way to break down the staff's culture of complacency, move away from the status quo, and make a change in their practice.

The empirical literature demonstrated that staff education was a crucial step in the implementation phase of this project. It was my intent to provide a formal PowerPoint presentation addressing current research studies and the success stories of other hospitals to the operating room nurses and surgical and anesthesia providers. However, the dynamic perioperative setting and time restraints did not allow for formal meetings. To complete the important step of staff education efficiently, I was creative in providing several informal meetings to the various stakeholders. The venue of a 6:00 a.m. meeting at Starbucks was used for the anesthesia residents, as were huddles with the operating room staff at the start of their 7:00 a.m. shift. The venue may have changed, but the content mirrored the anticipated formal presentations.

As I look back, performing the SWOT analysis was a crucial and essential step to this quality improvement initiative and strategic planning as it provided a global analysis of the organization's macro and microsystem. Through this process, the strengths and weaknesses were identified at the microsystem level as well as potential

(continues)

EXEMPLAR 14-1 Implementation of a "One Team" Approach to
PACU Handoff

barriers to implementation. Performing an organizational assessment allowed for the identification of supportive leadership, which is key to drive the idea from conception to implementation to sustainability. However, be prepared as your implementation path based on your SWOT analysis may have some bumps and twists. Mine certainly did, as some of the departmental leaders that were identified as strengths to the project and whose approval was procured were no longer with the organization. This directly impacted and delayed the implementation phase of my project. This is where the skill set of *intuition* plays a pivotal role, as you must be thinking ahead and most importantly deciding the right time to initiate a change. I waited several weeks, until the new departmental leaders were acclimated to their roles, before approaching them with this quality improvement project. To be honest, it was agonizing to wait; however, it was a needed step for a seamless implementation.

You are the driver of your DNP project. These words are paramount to the success of your project's implementation phase. It is through your attributes as a leader, diving into the empirical literature, and knowing the organization at a macro- and microsystem level that contribute to the success. The journey from conception to implementation of my DNP project is the deliverable that exemplifies how a DNP student can be a system leader making innovative changes in clinical practice.

▶ Summary

Understanding implementation science and applying this knowledge to the project implementation process ensures success when engaging in the challenging arena of healthcare organizations. The DNP-prepared nurse uses many aspects of the DNP *Essentials* (AACN, 2006) to produce change that is measurable, meaningful, and sustainable.

Impact

- Project implementation is the time during which the DNP student will demonstrate the characteristics and behaviors of all the DNP *Essentials* (AACN, 2006), and, the value of the DNP-prepared nurse.
- An effective project implementation plan that is supported by top management and other key stakeholders is key to a successful project outcome.

Key Messages

- Include key stakeholders early in the planning and implementation process.
- Gather an effective team by selecting the *right person* with the *right skill set* for the *right job*.
- Identify any potential problems early in the implementation phase and address them before they become major issues.
- When monitoring team members' productivity, it is important to give timely feedback, communicate effectively, and be sensitive to individual team members' needs.

- Successful project management involves the coordination of project activities, team member needs, team needs, stakeholder needs, and organizational needs.
- A good leader is able to draw on his or her skill set and utilize the appropriate skills, at the appropriate time, to keep the project in balance.
- Emotional competence in the DNP is an important leadership competency.
- The close-out phase includes an evaluation of the process and the outcome.
- After the project is completed, it is important to acknowledge the team and other supporters for a job well done.

Action Plan—Next Steps

1. Plan ahead to implement your project.
2. Implement the project using leadership skills.
3. Monitor the progress of the project through implementation.
4. Close out the project by reporting the planned outcomes and lessons learned.
5. Plan an elevator speech.

References

American Association of Colleges of Nursing (AACN). (2006). *The essentials of doctoral education for advanced nursing practice.* Retrieved from http://www.aacnnursing.org/Portals/42/Publications/DNPEssentials.pdf

Beene, M. S. (2012). Implementing a project. In J. L. Harris, L. Roussel, S. E. Walters, & C. Dearman (Eds.), *Project planning and management* (pp. 79–92). Burlington, MA: Jones & Bartlett Learning.

Chism, L. A. (2019). *The doctor of nursing practice: A guidebook for role development and professional issues* (4th ed.). Burlington, MA: Jones & Bartlett Learning.

Flick, S. (2009). *How to reduce barriers to project implementation.* Bizmanualz. Retrieved from http://www.bizmanualz.com/blog/top-ten-obstacles-to-project-implementation.html

Graham, G. (2013). *White papers for dummies.* Hoboken, NJ: John Wiley & Sons, Inc.

Haughey, D. (2018). *Eight key factors to ensuring project success.* Project Smart. Retrieved from http://www.projectsmart.com/articles/eight-key-factors-to-ensuring-project-success.php

Hickey, J. V., & Brosnan, C. A. (2017). *Evaluation of health care quality in advanced practice nursing.* New York, NY: Springer Publishing Company.

National Center for Healthcare Leadership (NCHL). (2017). *National Center for Healthcare Leadership competency model summary.* Retrieved from http://www.nchl.org/static.asp?path=2852,3238;/

Pinto, J. K., & Slevin, D. P. (1987). Critical success factors in effective project implementation. *Institute of Electrical and Electronics Engineers Transactions on Engineering Management, EM-34(1).* Retrieved from https://www.researchgate.net/publication/267559698_20_Critical_Success_Factors_in_Effective_Project_implementation

Porter-O'Grady, T., & Malloch, K. (2015). *Quantum leadership: Building better partnerships for sustainable health* (4th ed.). Burlington, MA: Jones & Bartlett Learning.

Prabhakar, G. P. (2008). What is project success: A literature review. *International Journal of Business and Management, 3(9),* 3–10.

Reilly, R. R., & Reilly, G. P. (2009). *Building business acumen: What it is, why it's important and how to get it.* Retrieved from https://acumenlearning.com/media/1402/reilly-building_business_acumen-hrwest1209.pdf

Theodotou, M. (2018). *3 financial acumen skills that you don't want to ignore.* American Management Association. Retrieved from http://www.amanet.org/training/articles/3-financial-acumen-skills-you-dont-want-to-ignore.aspx

SECTION III

Doctor of Nursing Practice Outcomes

CHAPTER 15

Disseminating the Results

Rosanne Burson

CHAPTER OVERVIEW

Some of the first items the doctor of nursing practice (DNP) student should consider as he or she is preparing for the project are the required deliverables within the specific DNP program. Keep the end in mind. What are the requirements for graduation in relation to disseminating the results of the DNP project? Some type of dissemination will be required, although there is variability across programs. The requirements typically include a public presentation, a defense of the project, and a written manuscript for the college or university. A journal article may also be a requirement. Finally, there should be dissemination of the project outcomes as an executive summary or a written report within the organization that supported the project (American Association of Colleges of Nursing [AACN], 2015). Each of these formats will require very different approaches; they need to be considered early to avoid unnecessary rework. This chapter will review the various options that can be developed as part of disseminating the results of the DNP project.

CHAPTER OBJECTIVES

After completing this chapter, the learner will be able to:

1. Identify the available options for disseminating the results of the DNP project.
2. Discuss recommendations for effective public presentations.
3. Review pointers for manuscript submissions.
4. Verbalize the importance of communicating and disseminating the results of the DNP project.

▶ What are the Deliverables?

Dissemination of the findings from evidence-based practice and research to improve health outcomes is described in DNP *Essential* III, Clinical Scholarship and Analytical Methods for Evidence-Based Practice (AACN, 2006). The use of evidence to improve practice or patient outcomes is highlighted by deliverables prior to graduation in a DNP program. A deliverable is a term used in project management to describe a tangible or intangible object produced as a result of the project that is intended to be delivered to a customer (Cutting, 2008). As mentioned in Chapter 2, Defining the Doctor of Nursing Practice: Current Trends, some recommended deliverables (AACN, 2015) include:

- Publishing in a peer-reviewed print or online journal
- Poster and podium presentations
- Presentation of a written or verbal executive summary to stakeholders and/or the practice site/organization leadership
- Development of a webinar presentation or video
- Submission and publication to a non-refereed lay publication
- Oral presentation to the public at large
- Development and presentation of a digital poster, grand rounds presentation, and/or a PowerPoint presentation

It is critical that the DNP student has an understanding of the expected time frame from completion of the final deliverables to graduation. For example, when must the project be completed to be eligible for graduation? When must all deliverables be accepted by the project team and graduate or nursing school to be ready for graduation? Can deliverables, such as a final presentation, be completed after this date? The DNP program may require that the full project team or faculty mentor sign off on all written work, or that the work be submitted to the college or university and/or a journal at a defined deadline prior to graduation, while allowing the presentation to occur at project completion.

> *It is critical that the DNP student has an understanding of the expected time frame from completion of the final deliverables to graduation.*

▶ Public Presentations

Public presentation of the DNP project may be a graduation requirement, so be sure to have a thorough understanding of the requirements for your specific DNP program. The public presentation may occur as a *proposal* prior to the implementation of the project or as a *presentation* after the completion of the project. The overall look of the presentation changes on the basis of its timing (before or after the project is implemented).

A presentation that occurs prior to the project is often considered a verbal defense of the project. A verbal defense includes:

- Introduction
- Background to the problem
- Literature review
- Clinical question

- Project plan (may include budget)
- Methodology
- Projected sample requirements
- Tools for evaluation
- Expected implementation process
- Time for questions and comments from the audience

See Chapter 12, The Proposal, for details in preparing the proposal. Sometimes the defense occurs in front of the project team only, and team members can add suggestions, ask questions, and finally approve the defense. The proposal may also be a public defense. In this format, there is often a public declaration of the presentation, with an invitation from the college or university to interested audiences to attend. The audience asks questions and may make additional comments. Audience members may consist of nursing faculty from the university or other universities, faculty from outside the school of nursing, graduate program faculty, deans from various colleges within the university, students from various programs, interested persons from healthcare organizations, or other interested parties.

A presentation that occurs after the project is completed has the purpose of disseminating results, so it will also include project results; an interpretation of the results; and sustainability, recommendations, and implications for practice. Forums used for disseminating results include conferences sponsored by the university, or podium and poster presentations outside the university in various local, regional, or national venues, including within the organization where the project was implemented.

Regardless of the timing or the place, there are a few items to consider in relation to the development of the presentation. The DNP student should understand:

- The purpose of the presentation (defense of the proposal vs. dissemination of results)
- The makeup of the audience attending the presentation
- When the presentation should occur during the education process
- How much time is allowed for the presentation
- The required format of the presentation

The student will work with his or her DNP project team to negotiate a date for the defense. Several meetings with the DNP project faculty mentor, or project team, can be expected as the student fine tunes his or her writing and develops all of the components of the project. The evaluation of the final DNP project is the responsibility of the faculty (AACN, 2015); hence, the faculty mentor will confirm with the project team that the student is indeed ready to defend.

In preparing the presentation, it is important to know the time allotted and the presentation format. A typical time allotment is 30 minutes, with an additional 30 minutes for questions. It can be challenging to focus on the high points of all the work that has been done in this brief time frame. A PowerPoint format can assist the presenter in staying focused on the points that must be considered and presented.

PowerPoint Pointers

In preparing a PowerPoint presentation, there are a few standard expectations to consider.

1. Express appreciation to the agencies, the project team members, and others who have been instrumental to the project.
2. Identify grant support or other funding sources, if any.

3. Cite references on your slides and list references at the end.
4. Use graphs and charts to make a point.
5. Use 32-point font or larger.
6. Do not crowd slides with too much information.
7. Follow the topic items to keep the presentation on track.
8. Practice, so that you stay in the time frame available.

Remember that although competency in developing a slide set is important, the PowerPoint presentation is just a tool to assist the presenter in providing information to the group. The way the presenter stands and his or her tone of voice, eye contact, and professional attire contribute to the entire package (Lim, 2012). The depth of knowledge regarding the topic, supported by the literature, as well as the creativity of the innovation and attention to the detail of the project plan, will enhance the presentation far beyond the features of PowerPoint.

> *The depth of knowledge regarding the topic ... will enhance the presentation far beyond the features of PowerPoint.*

Podium Presentations and Posters

Another mechanism for disseminating the results of the DNP project includes podium presentations and posters. Typically, more poster presentations are scheduled at a conference venue than podium presentations in order to provide more opportunities to disseminate creative work (Berg & Hicks, 2017).

For either format, the presenter must submit an abstract to the conference review committee and have it accepted. Aligning the abstract with objectives of the conference will improve opportunities for successful submission and acceptance. In addition, the author should carefully follow submission guidelines that are described by the conference planners. The process of preparing for either method is summarized as follows:

1. Identify which meeting would be most appropriate for the presentation.
2. Read/evaluate abstract submission guidelines regarding the format, word limits, space constraints, and deadline.
3. Most abstracts are submitted online, where one will cut and paste or upload the final version.
4. Be concise in your message, which should be carefully thought out.
5. The title should represent the content.
6. Project abstracts will contain five sections:
   - Background/Problem: Introduction to the topic and what is currently known.
   - Objective: The aim or purpose of the project.
   - Methods/Approach: How one addressed the purpose.
   - Results/Outcomes: Pertinent results presented in text or table/figure.
   - Conclusions/Implications: Focus on the response to the objective and how it fits in with future practice. (Berg & Hicks, 2017; Boullata & Mancuso, 2007)

There are a few key recommendations to consider for the podium presentation. First, one must have a good understanding of the time allotted for the presentation. Always consider the audience and the purpose of the presentation in developing the poster for a short presentation of 10 to 15 minutes. The following points by Weber and Cobaugh (2008) are recommended:

1. Present concisely and be specific to the audience.
2. Share the most important objectives and results.
3. Relegate background information to one or two points.
4. Use graphic presentation of results.
5. Avoid "busy" tables that take too long for the audience to absorb.
6. Always take the time to discuss the limitations of the study.
7. Request faculty and/or peer review prior to the presentation, both of the slide set and the actual presentation.

A poster is a presentation that provides a visual means of communicating information and should be visually appealing while transferring knowledge and stimulating discussion (Berg & Hicks, 2017; Boullata & Mancuso, 2007). For poster presentations, the visual aspect is critical for success and is prepared with two areas in mind: content and display.

For poster content, use the same title as the abstract. Material should be organized, concise, and free of spelling or grammar errors. When considering the display, it is recommended to use the "10-10 rule." Keep in mind what a participant can look at in 10 seconds from 10 feet away (Boullata & Mancuso, 2007). Color, layout, and well-placed graphs can be instrumental in attracting participants to the poster. Other conference specifications to consider include:

1. Poster format and size—freestanding or attached to a wall or corkboard or digital image projection.
2. Location of the posters—conference room, hall, or lobby.
3. Number of posters/presenters, number of conference attendees.
4. Bring copies of abstracts, contact information, push pins, and business cards.
5. Know dates that the poster must be delivered. (Berg & Hicks, 2017; Christenbery & Latham, 2013)

There are multiple poster templates available online, as well as companies that will produce a poster at a reasonable charge. Consider the type of material for the poster. If one is traveling a distance and may use the poster several times, consider a cloth poster that can be rolled up in the suitcase. Some conferences are moving to electronic posters to provide more space. Bring a backup digital file of your poster to the conference in case of technical difficulties. Be sure that poster submissions meet all requirements of the specific conference that is being attended, especially in relation to formatting criteria, which can include PowerPoints, website live demonstration, and other web-focused media (Christenbery & Latham, 2013).

Podium and poster presentations are important, because they are great ways to

Keep in mind what a participant reviewing a poster may look at in 10 seconds from 10 feet away.

disseminate information in areas of practice. These types of presentations can be a precursor to a journal article or a follow-up to the article. Another feature is that podium and poster presentations are a connection to other potential opportunities that can occur only through networking.

Podium and poster presentations are a connection to other opportunities that can occur only through networking.

For example, one of the authors of this book was invited to be a guest lecturer at a DNP program to present poster material to a leadership class because of a conversation with a professor who attended a poster session at a national conference. Including your contact information in a handout and/or having business cards available are great tools for networking with those interested in your topic. Finally, presentations are another aspect of scholarship that can be used for promotion and tenure evaluation for individuals working in academia.

▶ Portfolios

A portfolio may be an expected deliverable within the DNP program, although it is not considered a DNP project (AACN, 2015). "Portfolio evaluation is an efficient and effective strategy to objectively demonstrate the accomplishment of program objectives using students' perceptions of their academic experience" (Kear & Bear, 2007, p. 109). The practice portfolio is described in the AACN DNP *Essentials* document (2006). It is recommended that the portfolio documents, the final practice synthesis and scholarship, include the impact or effect on practice. Examples of representation in the portfolio include pilot studies, program evaluation, quality improvement (QI), evaluation of a new practice model, consulting projects, integrated research reviews, and manuscripts submitted for publication. Reflections may be a portion of the portfolio that exemplify synthesis of the DNP *Essentials*.

Once again, it behooves the DNP student to be aware of this requirement early in the program. Knowledge of the required documents for the portfolio helps the DNP student to begin preparation throughout the educational process and saves tremendous time in rediscovering the needed documents at a later time.

▶ Executive Summary

The executive summary is another written method of dissemination that may be used to present the project outcomes within the organization where the project was implemented. The executive summary is an efficient and impactful tool to support dissemination of the results of the work within the organization and supports next step sustainability as well.

This document is typically one to two pages and is a great tool to have available with an oral presentation. The format of the document will include:

- Description of the current status and why change is needed
- Presentation of the project details and how it aligns with the organization's goals, objectives, mission, vision, and values

- Market analysis findings
- Implementation process
- Evaluation metrics
- Project outcomes as related to metrics:
  - Clinical
  - Financial
  - Satisfaction
  - Other as identified in the evaluation plan
- Sustainability
- Implications

▶ Written Manuscript

Understanding the written requirements of the college or university will be important for graduation as well. Written manuscripts will have requirements related to format and submission. Often there is a required date that the manuscript must be submitted by to be ready for graduation—this may be several weeks prior to actual graduation, so planning is essential. Be sure to get a list of the submission requirements. Manuscript submission requirements may include specific formatting such as that of the American Psychological Association (APA), as well as how the manuscript should be submitted, such as hard copy or bound.

For some programs, a requirement for graduation is submission of an article for publication, which integrates well with the purpose of the DNP to disseminate evidence-based practice. Even if it's not a requirement for graduation, DNP students and graduates need to have a commitment to publishing. Disseminating results provides others with information that is needed for evidence-based practice and success for other writers to build upon. Scholarly dissemination is an important aspect of developing future scholarship, becoming a part of a network of scholars (Carlson, Staffelino, & Murphy, 2017), and substantiating the rigor of doctoral level work. Replication of best practices in varied clinical environments closes the gap between research and implementation in practice, thus building practice knowledge.

Scholarly dissemination is an important aspect of developing future scholarship, becoming a part of a network of scholars, and substantiating the rigor of doctoral level work.

▶ Journal Submissions

Reasons to write for publication include:

1. Dissemination of evidence
2. Sharing initiatives and innovation with others
3. Keeping nurses updated

4. Communicating research findings
5. Developing the science base of nursing
6. Directing the future of the profession
7. Communicating the importance of clinical practice findings to build evidence (Oermann & Hays, 2016)

Too often, the journal submission is the last item on the list separating the DNP student from graduation, if this is a requirement of the college or university. If this submission is considered in the planning phase, it will be done well and there will be an improved opportunity for successful publication of an article on the DNP project. However, there are many considerations in transitioning the manuscript of a project to a suitable article for publication.

> *Too often, the journal submission is the last item on the list separating the DNP student from graduation.*

▶ Process for Journal Submissions

Understanding the process for peer-reviewed journal submissions is essential for the prospective author. When an article is submitted, the editor will review it to determine if it aligns with the aims of the journal and/or interests of the readership. The editor will send out a call for a panel of reviewers with expertise that matches the manuscript, such as expertise on the topic and/or the manuscript design. Sometimes obtaining a reviewer may be a challenge. Reviewers are very busy; even once assigned, it may take some additional time to complete the review.

Peer reviewers have an allotted time period to complete the review, which is typically 2 to 3 weeks. The reviewers will send back comments, as well as an opinion of acceptance/not acceptance or acceptance with revisions. The editor then compares the comments, reads the article in more depth, and makes a decision. The editor will write a summary letter, collating the comments from the reviewers.

The minimum time for turnaround is 6 to 8 weeks; however, it could take 3 months or longer, depending on the journal. It behooves the author to speak with colleagues who are experienced with publishing to identify those journals that may be more responsive. Some journals have been known to hold onto articles for 1 to 2 years after acceptance. So, tapping into the "writing grapevine" prior to submission is in the author's best interest. Another tactic is emailing the editorial office to find out the percentage of articles chosen for publication, how long the review process is, and how long after acceptance articles are generally published. This information can be obtained prior to a query letter and put in a file for future review prior to actual submission to the journal. Another area to explore is the journal's use of unsolicited manuscripts. Some journals only publish solicited articles, others publish a combination.

Not many articles are accepted as written. The article may be accepted with minor revisions, the article may be sent back to the writer asking him or her to revise and resubmit the manuscript, or the article may be rejected. Authors are encouraged to revise their manuscript when revisions are requested, because both the writer and the journal have already invested significant time in the endeavor. When revising the manuscript, the author should respond and detail what has been incorporated into the revision. However, if the writer does not agree with the recommendations, he or she needs to document why he or she disagrees. Once the editor receives the revised manuscript, he or she may send the article back out to one or two reviewers. Keep in mind, the author may even need to revise the manuscript again. The article may be rejected even later in the process if the author and reviewers cannot agree on revisions.

There are many journals and many opportunities to submit a well-written manuscript. The author must be thoughtful and spend the time to research the best fit for the article, including the possibility of journals outside of nursing.

▶ Tips for Successful Journal Submission

Recognizing that students sometimes struggle when preparing a manuscript for submission to a peer-reviewed journal, this section will review tips for journal submission.

Understanding the process and gaining important pointers for manuscript submission will assist the author in producing a polished paper and provide a smoother journey to publication. Each of these recommendations will be explored further in this chapter.

1. Choose the journal carefully based on its mission, readership, and types of articles.
2. Match the manuscript to the journal.
3. Follow all author guidelines for:
   - Manuscript style and format
   - Abstract guidelines
   - Development of tables, figures, and graphs
4. Expect recommendations from reviewers and be willing to resubmit.
5. If needed, develop writing skills by using writing resources.

Choose the Journal Carefully Based on Its Mission, Readership, and Types of Articles

A place to begin the search for an appropriate journal is to peruse journals that were included in the literature review for the project and scan journals that have published articles on topics that are related to the DNP project.

A helpful tool to use when considering potential journals for an article is the Journal/Author Name Estimator (Jane): http://jane.biosemantics.org/. This tool allows the author to submit an abstract, and then, based on the information received, provides the author with a list of journals that have accepted similar topics. The author can then access the recommended journals to review the types of articles that have been published.

The *impact factor*, often abbreviated *IF*, is a measure of the frequency that articles from the journal are cited, which reflects the journal's importance. The University of Virginia Health System website gives a step-by-step direction on how to identify the IF of journals of interest: www.hsl.virginia.edu/services/howdoi/hdi-jcr.cfm.

Most journals outline specific requirements for a manuscript in their particular publication. The author should look at the mission and/or vision statement of the journal, the type of topics in the journal's call for papers, and the journal's reader audience, all of which will identify the level of content that is required. Questions to ask include: Does the journal publish articles like the manuscript in hand? For example, is this a research article or a case study? Does the journal target the population the author would like to reach?

Select four to five journals based on the type of journal, the articles in the journal, and its readership and audience, and then write with those journals in mind. Remember, the submitted manuscript must be consistent with *the journal's mission*. Focus on the journal's *target audience* by reviewing recent issues of the journal to identify topics of interest and depth of content. Another aspect of the journal review is getting a sense of *timing*. In other words, what else has been published in this journal and other journals? How does this manuscript add to the body of nursing knowledge? The editor is not just trying to fill space, but is highlighting an issue that is of interest to the audience and is important for building nursing's body of knowledge. It is plausible that the student's article could be considered a follow-up to some of those articles; however, the topic should not be overdone (i.e., there are too many recent similar articles). The author may not know what is in the pipeline, but a review of recent articles in the journal may give perspective on what topics have already been published. A query letter may also give the author insight into what the journal is looking for in unsolicited articles and if the proposed manuscript would be a match for the readership. To appeal to the audience, the topic should be well developed and the manuscript should have good readability.

Match the Manuscript to the Journal

The university requirement for the DNP project may differ from manuscript format. For example, if the article was originally developed for an academic setting, it must be rewritten to fit the journal. As the author aligns with specific journals, consider what he or she wants to present to the world. Does the project have a clinical or quality focus, or does it fit into a specialty journal? Is the topic appropriate for the chosen journal? For instance, if the article is more about the process than the disease state, consider a journal focused on quality.

In preparing the manuscript for a specific journal, write the article specifically for that journal. The *title is critical*—does it say what the article is about? In other words, the portrayal of content in the title is important. Other questions to ask include:

- Is the article consistent with the journal?
- Is the topic timely and innovative, or is it a twist on an older topic?
- Is the article unique?
- Is there consideration of the journal article categories such as case study, feature articles, or briefs?

As planning for the project submission occurs, think about how unique it is relative to the literature. It must be an innovative project that has not been done, or done with a new twist.

Follow All Author Guidelines

It is important to follow all of the recommended author guidelines for:

- Manuscript style and format
- Abstract guidelines
- Development of tables, figures, and graphs

When choosing a journal for submission, be sure to follow the author guidelines explicitly in relation to format, font, citations, and length of article. It is important to write to match the journal, which includes the length of paragraphs, headings, and depth of content. The final product should look like a paper that would fit in that journal. For instance, do not include a model in the article unless the paper is about a model. It may be helpful to review the table of contents of the journal to assist in this process.

Most journals will have guidelines for various types of submission. The author should identify the specific type of article that he or she plans to submit and follow those specific guidelines. Here is an example of the requirements within a specific journal: authors.jblearning.com.

Expect Recommendations from Reviewers and Be Willing to Resubmit

Many authors have had their work rejected or had to undertake a major revision at some point in time. The writer should expect direction or clarification and give him- or herself permission to grieve—this is a normal process related to the sense of ownership of an article. One should also expect good feedback and recommendations from the reviewers. Take all of the input and move forward. The writer should appreciate the opportunity for improvement and make the requested revisions and resubmit the manuscript.

Understand Why the Manuscript Was Turned Down

Take a deep breath and objectively consider the comments from the editor and the reviewers. If the comments indicate that the manuscript is well written but is not a match for the journal, the writer needs to resubmit to an appropriate journal. If there are content or writing recommendations, the author should take the feedback and make changes to strengthen the article before submitting it to another journal. Also, time and resources from the journal have gone into the author's article review, so be sure to follow through and resubmit the manuscript if changes are required. For instance, an author may not follow the previously discussed recommendation of using a specific reference style like the American Medical Association (AMA) or American Psychological Association (APA) format. Or, perhaps the topic was not innovative or the new practice initiative was limited by a brief intervention period with unsustainable outcomes. Sometimes articles have errors in references, which raises a flag about the content. Or, references may be incomplete, incorrect, or too old. It is recommended that others, such as a faculty mentor or other faculty, read the paper before submitting. Another suggestion is to get an editor to assist with writing.

The next step is to take the reviewer comments, incorporate the relevant ones, and send the manuscript to the next journal on the list. Less than one-half of authors resubmit. Be persistent in making revisions and keep submitting the article. There are 500 nursing and healthcare journals with plenty of opportunity! However, after four rejections, the author may need to reframe the topic. Consider the recommendation and add a twist. Perhaps not enough preliminary work was done. It is also important to think about the project design. Most DNP projects are not appropriate for research-oriented journals. However, journals focusing on quality improvement, innovation, or evidence-based practice may be a great fit.

Develop Writing Skills

It is important for students, faculty, and advisors to recognize the need to rework the article for publication versus an academic manuscript. Keep in mind, the editor is evaluating the author's writing skills from the first contact. There are specific clues that the editor keys into from the writer. For example, how does the query letter read in relation to composing a sentence? Does the DNP student's skill and content level match other manuscripts in the journal? Did the author pay close attention to methodology and design; this will also be assessed very carefully by the reviewers. It may be helpful to read articles in other journals to see how others are developing and presenting case studies, for example. Alternatively, consider a literature search on how to write for publication. *Nurse Author Editor* (www.nurseauthoreditor.com) offers articles and tips on writing (e.g., present sections in the manuscript that are based on research guidelines if the manuscript is a research article or performance improvement guidelines for QI manuscripts).

Finally, find a mentor for authorship. This should be someone who understands what mentorship entails. The mentor does not have to be geographically located near the writer—mentoring can occur via the Internet. If the writer does not have a mentor in mind, consider academic connections or contacting professional nursing organizations that have journals. Often colleges and universities have writing centers or other mentoring support. Some have resources to match new authors with senior writers or may even have a formal mentoring program. It may be helpful to offer to be a reviewer to learn about clear writing and publishing; writing skills improve the more one writes.

When manuscripts are accepted for publication, they may be offered online prior to being published in print. The appendix to this chapter includes a sample of a published article by Elizabeth Duffy and co-authors Cheryl Rogers, Leah Shever, and Marilyn Hockenberry. See Chapter 8, The Project Team, for a discussion regarding authorship of submitted manuscripts.

Online Manuscript Submission

Most journals will have an online submission process. Be sure to follow the directions explicitly. Typically, the article will be submitted in separate documents that include the title page, abstract, body of the manuscript with references, and tables and figures. The directions will include whether the manuscript should be sent in PDF or another format. Each of these components may have word limits. Using a tool like Microsoft Word's *word count* feature can ensure that the submitted piece is well within the specified limits. There may be a letter to the editor submission area as well, where the author highlights why this is an important article to consider. Finally, make sure to plan for enough time to upload the submission accurately.

Other Journal Considerations

Another area to consider prior to journal submission is using a plagiarism program like SafeAssign (www.blackboard.com/safeassign/index.html). There are many plagiarism programs available for use. For example, journals may first submit the manuscript through a program like iThenticate (www.ithenticate.com/). If the results are unfavorable, the manuscript may be rejected before the editor does an initial review. Even when references are cited correctly, a percentage over a predetermined level suggests that the article is not original material. For example, too many direct quotes will increase the percentage level. The writer should strive for a result less than 15% using SafeAssign.

▶ Summary

In summary, an important aspect of journal submission is communicating the writer's experience or findings to contribute to the body of knowledge within nursing and health care. Collectively, the value of DNP-prepared nurses' work will be discussed in the final chapter (Chapter 16, The Rest of the Story—Evaluating the Doctor of Nursing Practice).

In addition, there is great personal value in submitting for publication. This includes development of the author's own knowledge, personal satisfaction, sharing with a wider audience, and the potential benefits of promotion and tenure in a university setting for a faculty member (Oermann & Hays, 2016). When a manuscript presents timely and important content that is of interest to the journal's readership, and is in the appropriate style, the opportunity for publication becomes a reality!

The following excerpt by Dr. Diane Grimaldi describes her dissemination experiences with her DNP project (see **EXEMPLAR 15-1**).

EXEMPLAR 15-1 Association of Psychiatric History, Attendance of Postoperative Support Groups, and Outcomes Following Gastric Bypass Surgery: A Pilot Study

Diane Grimaldi DNP, PMHCNS, BC

I was interested in pursuing this field of inquiry because treating bariatric surgery patients is a clinical specialty for me. I had been providing full-spectrum psychiatric and psychopharmacologic services, both preoperatively and postoperatively, for this population for years prior to enrolling in my DNP program. A longstanding concern of mine has been the lack of standardized, evidence-based, psychological treatment protocols for patients undergoing bariatric surgical procedures.

A knowledge deficit regarding how to best meet the postoperative psychological needs of this population exists. Therefore, the aim of the project was to identify descriptors of long-term weight loss correlated with attendance of postoperative support groups following gastric bypass (GBP) surgery. Findings of this study revealed that approximately two-thirds of participants who underwent GBP screened positive for one or more Axis I diagnoses on the Psychiatric Diagnostic Screening Questionnaire

(continues)

EXEMPLAR 15-1 Association of Psychiatric History, Attendance of Postoperative Support Groups, and Outcomes Following Gastric Bypass Surgery: A Pilot Study

(PDSQ). Furthermore, higher numbers of comorbid psychiatric conditions were associated with less robust weight loss outcomes. It became clear that a more comprehensive understanding of the impact of a patient's psychiatric history on surgical outcomes might inform the development of evidence-based treatment protocols. Also, early identification of such conditions could reduce weight recidivism and improve outcomes.

The dissemination of project findings is an essential part of the process of sharing knowledge, translating outcomes, and deciphering implications in a local context for clinical application in a meaningful way. As abstract submissions for dissemination was a requirement for successful completion of the DNP program I attended, I took advantage of several opportunities to present the outcomes of my project in various venues. For example, a university-sponsored symposium for nursing faculty and students, including DNPs, enabled me to present a poster at the university and Lowell community toward the end of my program. I was also able to present my poster at the New England Chapter of the American Psychiatric Nurse's Association conference. During this conference I also presented a concurrent session, entitled *Psychosocial Issues Following Bariatric Surgery*, where I incorporated an executive summary of my project.

Results of my project were also disseminated to clinical and community audiences. Shortly after graduation, I was asked to present the project to a multidisciplinary group of staff members at a local psychiatric hospital and again at an informational session for people who were contemplating bariatric surgery as a possible treatment intervention. These different venues provided me with the opportunity to diversify the presentation of data and project outcomes in a way that addressed the interests of these audiences most effectively.

I also disseminated my work in a professional journal. To increase the likelihood of acceptance by a professional journal, I first identified my target audience, and then I searched for journals that were likely to reach that audience. The intention was to publish the manuscript in a journal that was read by healthcare professionals from different disciplines who provide treatment for bariatric surgery patients. I chose the *Bariatric Surgical Practice and Patient Care* journal because the journal met the criteria of having a multidisciplinary editorial staff, contributors, and readership. Acceptance of publication with minor revisions was achieved within 2 months of submission. Publication of the project in this peer-reviewed journal was accomplished 4 months after graduation.

Since the completion of this study and my doctoral program nearly 4 years ago, my primary clinical role as a practitioner with a private psychotherapy and psychopharmacology practice has not changed. The most significant impact of the DNP credential for me personally is that it solidified my status as a clinical expert in the field of obesity treatment and psychosocial issues associated with the bariatric surgery population. As a result, I have been invited to speak to multidisciplinary groups of clinicians and bariatric surgery candidates preoperatively and postoperatively on a regular basis. I have had the opportunity to consult with a significantly increased number of local bariatric surgeons and weight management programs. Establishing relationships with other clinicians in this field, coupled with high visibility from speaking to large groups on a regular basis, has resulted in many new referral sources for both individual and group treatment. Given that my reasons for pursuing the DNP were largely existential in nature, the outcome, though subtle as compared with some of my colleagues whose clinical roles changed far more dramatically, has been personally fulfilling.

Impact

- An important aspect of DNP scholarship is the dissemination of work that is being done in practice.
- Work that is appropriately disseminated strengthens practice-based evidence.
- It is through dissemination that the value of practice knowledge and the impact of the practice doctorate in nursing is understood.

Key Messages

- The DNP student should understand all of the college or university requirements for disseminating the results of the DNP project and the importance of including organizational stakeholders.
- The results of the DNP project may be disseminated in verbal presentations, such as an oral defense, or podium or poster presentations.
- The results of the DNP project may be disseminated in written documents that are submitted to the university or as a manuscript submitted to an appropriate journal.
- Consider the executive summary format to disseminate project outcomes to the organization where the project was implemented.
- Follow all specific guidelines for verbal or written dissemination.
- Plan for the time it takes to develop and submit the results of the DNP project.
- Consider manuscript submission to a journal, even when it is not a graduation requirement.

Action Plan—Next Steps

1. Know the requirements for communicating the results of the DNP project.
2. Plan how the results of the DNP project will be disseminated.
3. Develop a timeline to incorporate the planned communication.
4. Consider journal submission of a manuscript, even if it is not a requirement.
5. Review potential journals for the manuscript.
6. Write the manuscript with the journal in mind.
7. Happy writing!

References

American Association of Colleges of Nursing (AACN). (2006). *The essentials of doctoral education for advanced nursing practice.* Retrieved from https://www.aacnnursing.org/Portals/42/Publications/DNPEssentials.pdf

American Association of Colleges of Nursing (AACN). (2015). *The doctor of nursing practice: Current issues and clarifying recommendations.* Retrieved from https://www.aacnnursing.org/Portals/42/DNP/DNP-Implementation.pdf

Berg, J., & Hicks, R. (2017). Successful design and delivery of a professional poster. *Journal of the American Association of Nurse Practitioners, 29,* 461–469.

Boullata, J. I., & Mancuso, C. E. (2007). A "how-to" guide in preparing abstracts and poster presentations. *Nutrition in Clinical Practice, 22,* 641–646. doi: 10.1177/0115426507022006641

Carlson, E. A., Staffileno, B. A., & Murphy, M. P. (2017). Promoting DNP-PhD collaboration in doctoral education: Forming a DNP project team. *Journal of Professional Nursing,* doi: 10.1016/j.profnurs.2017.12.011

Christenberry, T. L., & Latham, T. G. (2013). Creating effective scholarly posters. *Journal of the American Association of Nurse Practitioners, 25,* 16–25.

Cutting, T. (2008). *Deliverable-based project schedules: Part 1.* Project-Management.com. Retrieved from http://www.pmhut.com/deliverable-based-project-schedules-part-1

Kear, M. E., & Bear, M. (2007). Using portfolio evaluation for program outcome assessment. *Journal of Nursing Education, 46*(3), 109–114.

Lim, F. A. (2012). Wake up to better PowerPoints. *Nursing 2012,* 47–48.

Oermann, M. H., & Hays, J. C. (2016). *Writing for publication in nursing* (3rd ed.). New York, NY: Springer Publishing Company.

Weber, R. J., & Cobaugh, D. J. (2008). Developing and executing an effective research plan. *American Journal of Health System Pharmacists, 65,* 2058–2065.

APPENDIX

Implementing a Daily Maintenance Care Bundle to Prevent Central Line-Associated Bloodstream Infections in Pediatric Oncology Patients

Journal of Pediatric Oncology Nursing
2015, Vol. 32(6) 394–400
© 2015 by Association of Pediatric
Hematology/Oncology Nurses
Reprints and permissions:
sagepub.com/journalsPermissions.nav
DOI: 10.1177/1043454214563756
jpo.sagepub.com

Elizabeth A. Duffy, DNP, RN, CPNP[1], Cheryl C. Rodgers, PhD, RN, CPNP, CPON[2], Leah L. Shever, PhD, RN[1], and Marilyn J. Hockenberry, PhD, RN, PNP-BC, FAAN[2]

Abstract

Eliminating central line-associated bloodstream infection (CLABSI) is a national priority. Central venous catheter (CVC) care bundles are composed of a series of interventions that, when used together, are effective in preventing CLABSI. A CVC daily maintenance care bundle includes procedural guidelines for hygiene, dressing changes, and access as well as specific timeframes. Failure to complete one of the components of the care bundle predisposes the patient to a bloodstream infection. A nurse-led multidisciplinary team implemented and, for 6 months, sustained a daily maintenance care bundle for pediatric oncology patients. This quality improvement project focused on nursing staffs' implementation of the daily maintenance care bundle and the sustainment of the intervention. The project used a pre–post program design to evaluate outcomes of CVC daily maintenance care bundle compliancy and CLABSI. A statistically significant increase between the pre- and post-assessments of the compliance was noted with the CVC daily maintenance care bundle. CLABSI infection rates decreased during the intervention. Strategies to implement practice change and promote sustainability are discussed.

Keywords

pediatric, oncology, CLABSI, care bundle, sustainability

1 The University of Michigan School of Nursing, Ann Arbor, MI, USA
2 Duke University School of Nursing, Durham, NC, USA

Corresponding Author:

Elizabeth A. Duffy, The University of Michigan School of Nursing, 400 North Ingalls, Room 2330, Ann Arbor, MI 48109, USA.
Email: eaduffy@umich.edu

Background

Central venous catheters (CVCs) are indwelling catheters that provide permanent or temporary stable venous access for both the acute and chronically ill patient. Approximately 80,000 central line–associated blood-stream infections (CLAB-SIs) occur each year in hospitals, and 30,000 of those results in death (Pronovost, Marsteller, & Goeschel, 2011). The cost of CLABSI to the United States health system is more than $2 billion annually, with an average cost per patient of $45,000 (Pronovost et al., 2011).

Children with cancer are disproportionately affected by CLABSI due to prolonged periods of immunosuppression that leaves them susceptible to infections. Pediatric oncology patients have CLABSI rates as high as 17.95% compared with children in the pediatric intensive care unit, whose reported rate is 3.71% (McMullen et al., 2013). More than 12 000 children are diagnosed with cancer each year in the United States (Center for Disease Control [CDC], 2010). The majority of these children will receive therapy that requires the use of a CVC, which may be in place for a number of years to administer intensive therapies including chemotherapy and various supportive intravenous (IV) products.

CVC Care Bundles

Prevention of CLABSI is an area of national concern; nurses assume frontline responsibility for safe, quality CVC care to minimize the risk of patients contacting life-threatening infections (Secola, Lewis, Pike, Needleman, & Doering, 2012). CLABSI can be reduced by 50% when evidence-based care around insertion and maintenance is provided through CVC bundles (Brungs & Render, 2006).

The Centers for Disease Control (CDC) CLABSI prevention guidelines provide the basis for both an insertion bundle and a CVC daily maintenance care bundle. The CVC maintenance-only focus was chosen for this project because evidence suggests that improved daily maintenance practices are significantly associated with decreased infection rates in the inpatient setting (Miller et al., 2010). The CVC daily maintenance care bundle includes seven best practices and specific timeframes associated with procedures for patient hygiene, dressing changes, access, and IV line care among patients with CVCs. Failure to complete one of the components of the care bundle predisposes the patient to a bloodstream infection. A CVC daily maintenance care bundle has been used to reduce CLABSI in pediatric intensive care units and neonatal intensive care units, and it has influenced CLABSI prevention strategies for pediatric stem cell transplant recipients and hospitalized pediatric oncology patients (Rinke et al., 2013).

In 2006, a major national initiative was conducted by the National Association of Children's Hospitals and Related Institutions (NACHRI) that focused on CLABSI among critically ill pediatric patients; this initiative reported a reduction in CLABSI from 6.3 infections per 1000 catheter days to 4.3 infections per 1000 catheter days (Jeffries et al., 2009; NACHRI, 2008). The NACHRI quality transformation effort demonstrated a decrease of CLABSI in pediatric oncology patients when nursing staff used the CVC daily maintenance care bundle. In 2008, our medical institution developed a multidisciplinary CLABSI work group and began to formally apply components of the NACHRI collaborative project in the care of pediatric oncology patients. Rigorous implementation of a pediatric hematology oncology-specific

CVC daily maintenance care bundle over a 3-year period significantly reduced the incidence of CLASBI from 2.92/1000 patient days at baseline to 1.6 CLABSI/1000 patient days—a 45% decrease (Choi et al., 2012). However, the CVC daily maintenance care bundle was not sustained over time, as evidenced by the variance of nursing practice in CVC care 12 months following the completion of the intervention.

The purpose of this quality improvement project was two-fold. The first was to re-implement a CVC daily maintenance care bundle among nursing staff, and consistently and accurately apply it to all hospitalized pediatric oncology patients with a CVC. The second was to incorporate proven sustainability efforts throughout the project to ensure the longevity of the CVC daily maintenance care bundle in future clinical practice. This article describes the re-implementation of a CVC daily maintenance care bundle, methods used to promote sustainability in clinical practice while also answering the following measures of implementation. Are the components of the CVC daily maintenance care bundle documented in the electronic medical record (EMR)? Are the documented components of the bundle in compliance with the CVC daily maintenance care bundle? Is there a decrease in the monthly CLABSI rates with the implementation of the CVC daily maintenance care bundle?

Conceptual Framework

Greenhalgh's (2004) model provides a framework for the diffusion, dissemination, implementation, and sustainability of health service innovations directed at improving health outcomes (White & Dudley-Brown, 2012). This model was used in the implementation of the project and provided the foundation to foster the sustainability of the intervention by focusing on individuals involved in direct patient care through a shared sense of priorities, needs, and potential solutions.

Method

The quality improvement project was reviewed by the institutional review board at Duke University and deemed exempt. The project used a pre–post program design comparing the rate of CLABSI over 6 months after implementation of the daily maintenance catheter care bundle to the rate of CLABSI from the previous 6 months. The setting was a 32-bed pediatric hematology, oncology, and bone marrow transplant unit located within a large tertiary medical institution. The unit sees approximately 100 new oncology diagnoses per year and more than 600 annual admissions to this unit. There are 68 nurses on the unit.

The first step in the project was to identify and interview nursing stakeholders regarding the multidisciplinary work group developed in 2008 and the current practice regarding CVC care bundles. In 2011, at the end of the multidisciplinary collaborative project the nursing staff's self-reported adherence to recommended maintenance bundle practices was generally high (>90%) in most domains (Choi et al., 2012). The pediatric nurse practitioner completed the interviews focusing on current CVC practice and the sustainment of the CVC daily maintenance care bundle following the completion of the project. One point of initial contestation among nursing staff was the importance of the standardization of the CVC daily maintenance care bundle. A few stakeholders believed that the patient should be able to choose the components of the dressing change and the decision to have a daily bath with chlorhexidine (CHG). One salient theme throughout the interview process was that nursing staff could not identify the components of the CVC daily maintenance care bundle. Subsequently, there was significant variance in nursing practice when performing dressing changes and promoting bathing practices. Interviews with stakeholders resulted in a consensus of the importance of reintroducing and sustaining the CVC daily maintenance care bundle to prevent CLABSI.

Assembling a Team

An innovation team was established with nursing leadership, nursing staff, and the infection control practitioner. The inclusion of a nursing leader that participated in the original collaborative project strengthened the team through her historical perspective and expertise in CLABSI prevention. A pediatric nurse practitioner facilitated the initial team discussions, documented agreed-on action items and time lines, and acted as a project manager for the implementation of the CVC daily maintenance care bundle. In addition, a physician champion, the medical director for the inpatient unit, agreed to participate in and support the team.

The innovation team met monthly to plan implementation strategies. One of the initial goals identified by the team was to have an infection rate of zero. The challenge of both reaching and maintaining a target rate of zero in pediatric oncology patients was recognized by all the team members. The end users (ie, the nursing staff) were deliberately involved in the development of processes that lead to sustainability. A group of nursing champions in collaboration with the innovation team determined the integration of the CVC maintenance care bundle into the health system education policies to decrease variance in nursing practice and strategies to engage other stakeholders. A multidisciplinary approach was applied to the dissemination of the innovation through the participation of a physician champion during the planning of the reimplementation and the inclusion of the pediatric oncology physician staff throughout the project.

Multidisciplinary Approach

The lead physician assembled a collaborative multidisciplinary team to analyze CLABSI in pediatric oncology patients 3 months into the re-implementation of the CVC daily maintenance care bundle. The multidisciplinary team met monthly to review the rate of CLABSI, discuss each individual patient that developed CLABSI, and used a root cause analysis to identify common factors in the care of those patients. Strategies to increase patient adherence to the CVC daily maintenance care bundle were discussed by each of the team members. The team meetings were led by the infection control practitioner and included members from the innovation team, nursing and physician leadership from the inpatient/outpatient pediatric oncology service, emergency department, pediatric surgery, and representatives from the phlebotomy department.

Standardizing Practice

The components of the CVC maintenance bundle include hand hygiene, dressing changes, daily bath or shower, use of institutionally approved injection caps, cleansing of access points, and line maintenance (**TABLE 1**). The nursing leadership and pediatric nurse practitioner developed a CVC dressing change competency,

TABLE 1 Central Venous Catheter Daily Maintenance Care Bundle.

Maintenance Care Bundle Task	Description
Hand hygiene	Proper hand cleansing before every catheter/tubing/dressing interaction
Dressing changed appropriately	Recommended intervals: 7 days for transparent dressing or 3 days for gauze Other indications: soiled, damp, loose, unknown date/time of last change Recommended practices: chlorhexidine gluconate skin antisepsis when dressing changed
Intravenous tubing changed appropriately	Recommended intervals: at ≥96 hours since last tubing change or 24 hours if blood/lipid exposure Other indications: medication hang-time expiration, unknown date/time of last change
Bathing or showering performed	Chlorhexidine (CHG) used for daily bath or shower Dressing and catheter covered during bath or shower Dressing changed immediately after bath or shower if dressing change due by date Caps/tape changed on unaccessed lumens after bath or shower
Central lines entered appropriately	Minimized entries through batching of medication administration and lab draws Maintained closed intravenous system (eg, pre-pierced ports/caps and bifuse extension sets) Cleansed access points with alcohol scrub prior to each line entry for 15 seconds

Adapted from Choi, S. W., Chang, L., Hanauer, D., Shaffer-Hartman, J., Teitelbaum, D., Lewis, I., . . . Niedner, M. F. (2012). Rapid reduction of central line infections in hospitalized pediatric oncology patients through simple quality improvement methods. *Pediatric Blood Cancer, 10*(1002), 1–8.

modified patient education materials to include one standard for a CVC dressing change based on patient age, and created one handout for nursing staff, parents, and patients delineating the components a CVC daily maintenance care bundle. The education materials were congruent with the institutional approved standard of care for CVC line maintenance. The staff education occurred 2 months prior to the implementation at an all nursing staff retreat in late May. A physician led the session with a case study of patient with CLABSI highlighting that this was a preventable infection that was almost fatal. The patient story generated an emotional response among nursing staff and facilitated buy-in to improve current nursing practice to prevent CLABSI.

The nursing staff education included a group demonstration of the compo-nents of the CVC daily maintenance care bundle, followed by small groups led by a member of the innovation team demonstrating a CVC dressing and a return demonstration by all staff. Education was provided to all staff through an initial in-service to decrease variance in practice in CVC care, with follow-up education occurring 1 and 6 months later.

A gap analysis of the pre-intervention chart audits at the start of the implemen-tation indicated an opportunity to increase adherence in the provision and docu-mentation of a daily bath or shower. Efforts were undertaken to address this gap in practice through targeted education for nursing staff, parents, and patients. The targeted education included posters placed throughout the inpatient unit with simple poignant phrases regarding the importance of a daily bath and prevention of CLABSI.

Three months after the education sessions the nursing staff and innovation team then rolled out the CVC daily maintenance care bundle to the bedside of all patients with a CVC. Nurses educated patients and families about the CVC daily maintenance care bundle. Oncology patients with a CVC were provided education during their inpatient admission regarding the components of the CVC daily main-tenance care. In addition, nursing staff began to include the time and completion of the daily bath or shower in their shift report. Posted on the patient census board in the nursing staff room were the preferred bath time and also a checklist to indicate when the bath was completed. These simple interventions were independently iden-tified and implemented by the nursing staff to increase adherence.

Evaluation

Data collection began in July 2013 and was completed in January 2014. The rate of CLABSI and documentation of the daily maintenance care bundle was assessed by electronic medical record (EMR) review. Pre-implementation data were collected in July 2013 and included a retrospective review of the average monthly rate of CLABSI from January 2013 to June 2013. Post-implementation data were collected monthly and included the average monthly rate of CLABSI from July 2013 to December 2013. CLABSI was defined as a confirmed bloodstream infection not secondary to an in-fection meeting the CDC/National Healthcare Safety Network criteria (CDC, 2010). The CVC must be placed at the time of or within 48 hours before the onset of the infection (CDC, 2010). The pediatric oncology infection control practitioner noted the inclusion criteria for a CLABSI based on the CDC standards and through a chart review determined if the primary site of infection was the CVC.

Assessment of the CVC daily maintenance care bundle included hand hygiene, dressing changed appropriately, IV tubing changed appropriately, daily bath or shower performed, and central lines entered appropriately (Table 1). The completion of components of the CVC daily maintenance care bundle was evaluated through a chart audit by the nursing staff using a standardized tool. Chart audits consisted of 35 randomly selected patients admitted in July 2013 to measure pre-intervention data and 45 randomly selected patients admitted in January 2014 to measure the adherence to the intervention. Specific questions that were evaluated in the chart review included the following: (1) Are the components of the bundle documented in EMR? (2) Are the documented components of the bundle in compliance with the daily maintenance care bundle? The four areas of the CVC daily maintenance care bundle captured in the EMR include date of the next dressing change, date of the next IV tubing change, date of the next cap change, and daily bath or shower. Each component of the bundle was individually evaluated.

Results

The sample for the CVC daily maintenance care bundle documentation included a total of 80 charts of patients admitted to the pediatric oncology unit who had a CVC at least one of the two assessment points. The pre-intervention chart audits included a convenience sample of 35 patients admitted to the pediatric oncology unit with a CVC. There was a greater than 90% compliance with timelines and accurate documentation regarding the date of the next dressing change, date of the next IV tubing change, and date of the next cap change. However, only 29.6% of the patients had a documented daily bath or shower. The post-intervention assessment included a convenience sample of 45 patients admitted to the pediatric oncology unit with a CVC and demonstrated a greater than 90% compliance with timelines and accurate documentation regarding the date of the next dressing change, date of the next IV tubing change, and date of the next cap change. Post-intervention demonstrated significantly higher compliance, 69.8%, with documentation of a daily bath or shower. A $c2$ test for independence indicated a statistically significant increase between the pre- and post-assessments of compliance with a daily bath or shower ($c2[1, N = 80] = 11.736, P = .001$).

CVC daily maintenance compliance was defined as "met" if the audit revealed that 100% of the components that can be measured were documented in EMR. Compliance with the CVC daily maintenance care bundle was 28.8% pre-intervention. Post-intervention compliance with the CVC daily maintenance care bundle was significantly higher at 71.2% ($c2[1, N = 80] = 13.410, P =.000$).

In 2013, there were a total of 10 CLABSI. In the 6-month period prior to the re-implementation of the CVC daily care bundle from January 2013 to June 2013, there were eight CLABSI reported. During the 6-month period of the re-implementation of the CVC daily maintenance care bundle (July 2013 to December 2013), there were two CLABSI reported. The Mann-Whitney U test comparing rates demonstrated a trend toward significance ($U = 8.00, z = -1.66, P = .096$) with the infection rate showing a decrease from pre (Mdn = 1.63, Mrank = 8.17) to post (Mdn = 0, Mrank = 4.83; **FIGURE 1**).

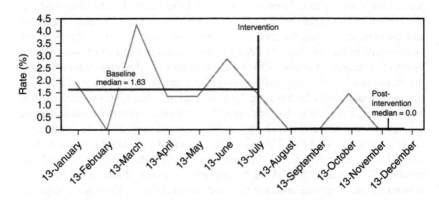

FIGURE 1 Comparison of median infection rates, baseline and intervention.

Discussion

The rate of CLABSI was higher during pre-intervention (January 2013 to June 2013) than post-intervention (July 2013 to December 2013). During the intervention there was a stretch of 89 days without a CLABSI. Four of the six months during the intervention period had a CLABSI rate of zero. Although not statistically significant, the small decrease in CLABSI is clinically significant with a potential decrease in the healthcare costs and avoidance of negative patient outcomes (Rinke et al., 2013).

Beginning in May 2013, there was a practice change for nursing staff to use a stopcock system to draw patient labs which decreased the number of times the CVC was accessed. Only nursing staff accessed the CVC, which decreased variance in practice. The practice change was consistent with the CVC daily maintenance care bundle recommendation for batched tasks and limited the number of time that the line was accessed (Choi et al., 2012).

Re-implementation of a CVC daily maintenance care bundle on the inpatient pediatric oncology unit was associated with a statistically significant increase in staff nurses' compliance with the completion of a daily patient bath or shower. Consistent with any documentation audit, tasks that were not recorded were assumed to be not completed. Therefore, if a daily bath or shower was not documented in the EMR, it was considered not performed. Recognizing the importance of compliance to this part of the CVC daily maintenance care bundle, the pre-implementation data were shared with nursing staff during the implementation phase in an effort to increase compliance (McMullen et al., 2013).

Data results revealed that adolescent patients had a higher rate of CLABSI. Five of the ten cases of CLABSI were attributed to adolescent males and one to an adolescent female; the organisms associated with the infections were consistent with skin or gastrointestinal organisms. Further analysis determined that these adolescent patients did not consistently have a daily bath or shower. In addition, one adolescent male patient acquired three of the five infections attributed to adolescent males. The other five cases of CLABSI did not demonstrate any common patient demographics.

Limitations

There are several limitations to this quality improvement project. First, the EMR chart audit did not measure compliance with all components of the daily maintenance care bundle. Critical infection control interventions such as hand washing, the amount of time spent rubbing the cap with alcohol prior to needle insertion, and the number of times the CVC was accessed were not documented and cannot be measured in this pre-/post-test design using a random EMR chart audit. Observation of nursing practice is needed to accurately measure this intervention. Second, the change from phlebotomy staff drawing all patient labs to nursing staff assuming complete responsibility for batching the amount of times the CVC was accessed was not measured. In addition, the decrease in the number of times the line was accessed through the use of the stopcock system for lab draws may also have contributed to the decrease in CLABSI. Third, compliance with CHG bathing was not measured through this project. Fourth, the timeframe for data collection was only six months. When measuring CLABSI rates, a longer duration of time is advantageous to demonstrate trends in infection rate and sustainability of the quality improvement project. There are positive indications that the intervention has been sustained extending the outcome period is suggested.

Conclusions and Recommendations

The results from the re-implementation of the CVC daily maintenance care bundle are consistent with the findings from the multidisciplinary quality improvement project that ended in 2011. This project confirms that the use of a CVC daily maintenance care bundle decreases CLABSI and demonstrates the pivotal role the pediatric oncology nurse plays in prevention. The first implementation did not take into account the impact of nursing champions at the staff level and their direct positive impact on adherence. There is consensus in the literature that evidence-based nursing practice is the gatekeeper for CLABSI prevention through CVC daily maintenance care; the goal is to sustain this best nursing practice. The integration of nursing champions that understand the importance of standardizing practice based on evidence is vital in current and future CLABSI prevention strategies.

Acknowledgments

A special thank you to all of the dedicated nursing staff, nursing leadership, and physician staff for their support and participation in this project. In addition, thank you to the infection control practitioner for her expertise and leadership throughout the quality improvement process.

Declaration of Conflicting Interests

The author(s) declared no potential conflicts of interest with respect to the research, authorship, and/or publication of this article.

Funding

The author(s) received no financial support for the research, authorship, and/or publication of this article.

References

Brungs, S. M., & Render, M. L. (2006). Using evidence-based practice to reduce central line infections. *Clinical Journal of Oncology Nursing, 10*, 723–725.

Centers for Disease Control and Prevention (CDC). (2010). *Healthcare-associated infections.* Retrieved from http://www.cdc.gov/ncidod/dhqp/gl_intravascular.html

Choi, S. W., Chang, L., Hanauer, D., Shaffer-Hartman, J., Teitelbaum, D., Lewis, I., . . . Niedner, M. F. (2012). Rapid reduction of central line infections in hospitalized pediatric oncology patients through simple quality improvement methods. *Pediatric Blood Cancer, 10*(1002), 1–8.

Jeffries, H. E., Mason, W. B., Brewer, M., Oakes, K. L., Munoz, E. I., Gornick, W., . . . Jarvis, W. R. (2009). Prevention of central venous catheter-associated bloodstream infections in pediatric intensive care units: A performance improvement collaborative. *Infection Control and Hospital Epidemiology, 30*, 645–651.

McMullen, C., Propper, G., Schuhmacher, C., Sokoloff, L., Harris, D., Murphy, P., & Greene, H. (2013). A multidisciplinary approach to reduce central line-associated bloodstream infections. *Joint Commission on Quality and Patient Safety, 39*(2), 61–71.

Miller, M. R., Griswold, M., Harris, J. S., Yenokyan, G., Moss, M., Rice, T. B., . . . Brilli, R. J. (2010). Deceasing PICU catheter-associated bloodstream infections: NACHRI's quality transformation efforts. *Pediatrics, 125*(2), 206–213.

National Association of Children's Hospitals and Related Institutions (NACHRI). (2008). Retrieved from http://www.childrenshospitalsnet/AM/Template.cfm/Section=Blood_Stream_Infections_Project&Template=/TaggedPage/TaggedPageDisplay.cfm&TPLID=123&Content ID=21390

Pronovost, P., Marsteller, J., & Goeschel, C. (2011). Preventing bloodstream infections: A measurable national success story in quality improvement. *Health Affairs (Millwood), 30*(4), 628–634.

Rinke, M. L., Bundy, D. C., Chen, A. R., Milstone, A. M., Colantuoni, E., Peher, M., . . . Miller, M. R. (2013). Central line maintenance bundles and CLABSIs in ambulatory oncology patients. *Pediatrics, 132*(5), e1403–e1412.

Secola, R. N., Lewis, M. A., Pike, N., Needleman, J., & Doering, L. (2012). "Targeting to Zero" in pediatric oncology: A review of central venous catheter-related blood-stream infections. *Journal of Pediatric Oncology Nursing, 29*(1), 14–27.

White, K. M., & Dudley-Brown, S. (2012). *Translation of evidence into nursing and health care practice.* New York, NY: Springer.

Author Biographies

Elizabeth A. Duffy, DNP, RN, CPNP, is clinical faculty at The University of Michigan School of Nursing and practices as a pediatric nurse practitioner.

Cheryl C. Rodgers, PhD, RN, CPNP, CPON, is an Assistant Professor at the Duke University School of Nursing.

Leah L. Shever, PhD, RN, is currently the Director of Nursing Research, Quality, and Innovation at the University of Michigan Health System.

Marilyn J. Hockenberry, PhD, RN, PNP-BC, FAAN, is the Bessie Baker Professor of Nursing and Professor of Pediatrics at Duke University School of Nursing and also serves as one of the 11 chairs of the Duke Institutional Review Board.

CHAPTER 16

The Rest of the Story— Evaluating the Doctor of Nursing Practice

Dianne Conrad and David G. Campbell-O'Dell

CHAPTER OVERVIEW

Throughout this text, the doctor of nursing practice (DNP) project has been highlighted as an important product of DNP education that reflects the attainment of the skill set that launches the DNP graduate into scholarly practice. However, it is also important to recognize that the practice doctorate degree for nursing will need to be evaluated for effectiveness in accomplishing the goals of improving the nursing profession, health care, and society. In an attempt to begin this process, a model of evaluation of the practice doctorate is proposed using the Actualized DNP Model that focuses on structure, process, and outcome measures (Burson, Moran, & Conrad, 2016). Current trends reflected in DNP practice as well as DNP exemplars applying the model are explored. Finally, an exemplar by Dr. Lisa Chism illustrates how the *Essentials* of DNP education are reflected in her DNP practice and scholarship.

CHAPTER OBJECTIVES

After completing this chapter, the learner will be able to:

1. Discuss the impact of the practice doctorate on the nursing profession, health care, and society.
2. Explain the evaluation of the impact of the DNP in terms of the structure of DNP education, the process of advanced nursing practice, and the various types of outcomes expected as illustrated in the Actualized DNP Model.

(continues)

CHAPTER OBJECTIVES   *(continued)*

3. Review how contributions to the literature and practice are made by DNP-prepared nurses, beginning with the DNP project as a launching pad to practice scholarship.

The DNP degree is reflective of the rigorous education that students receive to be high quality clinicians, leaders in interprofessional health care team delivery, and contributors to the redesign and improvement of health care delivery models. (National Organization of Nurse Practitioner Faculties, 2015, para. 4)

As discussed in Chapter 2, Defining the Doctor of Nursing Practice: Current Trends, the DNP educational program is the foundation for the practice doctorate and is built on the American Association of Colleges of Nursing (AACN) *Essentials of Doctoral Education for Advanced Nursing Practice* (2006). The DNP project reflects the culmination of the attainment of the *Essentials* by the DNP student. However, the ultimate impact of the DNP graduate on nursing as a profession, health care, and society will be "the rest of the story. . ."

Montgomery and Porter-O'Grady (2010) summarize the value of the scholarly project in DNP education by stating that it "provides students with an opportunity for rigorous and scholarly development of a clinical issue, demonstrating the ability to apply knowledge, translate learning and exhibit evidence-driven outcomes in their areas of practice expertise" (p. 45).

> *The DNP project reflects the culmination of the attainment of the DNP Essentials.*

Marie Annette Brown (2011) challenges us to imagine the reality where the DNP project accomplishes multiple goals, such as:

- Building student expertise in practice inquiry
- Contributing to advancing and improving care in institutions, local communities, and all types of healthcare settings by affecting care delivered and assisting agencies to innovate better models of care delivery, thus improving outcomes of care
- Contributing to advancing the practice of registered nurses (RNs) and advanced practice registered nurses (APRNs)
- Contributing to the nursing profession and nursing science
- Contributing to practice inquiry, translational science, and comparative effectiveness research

The completion of the DNP project prepares the graduate for the art and science of practice scholarship, as well as to contribute to the body of translational research knowledge and clinical practice knowledge development for the nursing profession. The ultimate value and impact of practice scholarship in advanced nursing practice will be reflected in a variety of healthcare outcomes.

▶ The DNP: Continuous Quality Improvement of the Degree, DNP Graduate Practice, and the Impact on Outcomes

Fontaine and Langston (2011) state that DNP programs are "forging new territory for translational science" and that "outcomes will need to be assessed in a robust manner" (p. 122). As the practice doctorate continues to mature, the present and future of the DNP degree and its impact on health care can be examined in the context of the Actualized DNP Model (see **FIGURE 16-1**; Burson, Moran, & Conrad, 2016). The Actualized DNP Model illustrates the relationship of the critical features of DNP education and practice that produce outcomes to improve health care at multiple levels. The attainment of the DNP *Essentials* (AACN, 2006) competencies produces a nursing practice doctorate with critical skills in advanced nursing practice, leadership, policy, and informatics who can apply evidence-based practice in the clinical arena. Through the use of leadership skills in traditional and innovative roles, implementation science, and interprofessional collaboration, the practice doctorate uses an *evidence-based practice* application component to generate new knowledge in practice, developing *practice-based evidence*. This is the added value that the DNP-prepared nurse brings to health care to impact outcomes in patient care, population health, systems, and policy. Generating practice-based knowledge

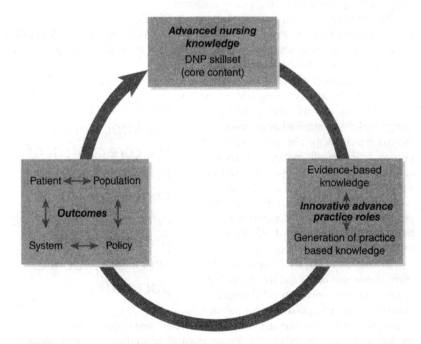

FIGURE 16-1 The Actualized DNP Model.

Reproduced from Rosanne Burson, D. N. P., & Dianne Conrad, D. N. P. (2016). Why Hire a Doctor of Nursing Practice-Prepared Nurse? The Value Added Impact of the Practice Doctorate. *Journal of Doctoral Nursing Practice, 9*(1), 152.

then informs the core skill set needed for the practice doctorate, hence completing and continuing the circular process (Burson, Moran, & Conrad, 2016).

This threefold approach to assessing the value and impact of the practice doctorate acknowledges the linkage between all the components: Good structure leads to good process, which in turn increases the likelihood of good outcomes, as demonstrated by Donabedian (1988) in his classic approach to quality improvement. In assessing the impact of the DNP degree now and in the future, the *structure* of how DNP students are prepared and educated, the *process* of how care is delivered by the DNP-prepared nurse, as well as the *outcomes* of that care and how it impacts patients and society can be explored using the Actualized DNP Model.

▶ Advanced Nursing Knowledge— DNP Education

As the nursing profession grows, matures, and stretches to meet the needs of patients in an evolving healthcare delivery system, the terminal practice degree in nursing is also evolving. Though the intentions of improving healthcare outcomes are understood, the question is: How well are DNP graduates succeeding in this challenge? How has nursing education evolved to meet the growing demands of educating practice doctorates? The Actualized DNP Model begins with the importance of the core content of advanced nursing knowledge in DNP education to develop the unique skill set of the practice doctorate.

The foundation of the practice doctorate is *The Essentials of Doctoral Education for Advanced Nursing Practice (DNP Essentials)* (AACN, 2006) (see **FIGURE 16-2**). Regardless of the role in advanced nursing practice that the graduate undertakes, the core competencies attained are in the areas of leadership, advanced practice based on an evidence-based science, working in interprofessional teams, and influencing policy. All competencies are enhanced by the use of information technology. The roles of advanced nursing practice will continue to develop, and DNP education will evolve to meet the demands of these roles. The DNP project is the first venture of the DNP student into practice scholarship and demonstrates that the student has met the DNP *Essentials* (AACN, 2006) *outcome expectations.*

Evaluation of the DNP degree will involve assessment of the quality of DNP education. As more university DNP programs attain accreditation, quality and consistency across programs will continue to improve. There are two major accreditation bodies that are recognized by the U.S. Department of Education: the Commission on Collegiate Nursing Education (CCNE), which began accrediting DNP programs in 2008 and 2009, and more recently, the Accreditation Commission for Education in Nursing (ACEN).

> *The Actualized DNP Model begins with the importance of the core content of advanced nursing knowledge in DNP education to develop the unique skill set of the practice doctorate.*

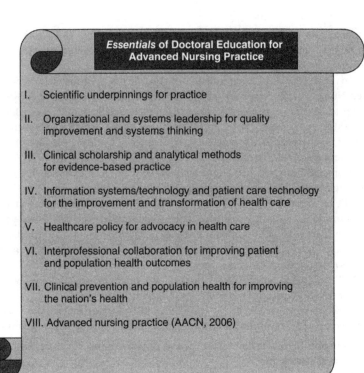

FIGURE 16-2 *Essentials* of Doctoral Education for Advanced Nursing Practice.

Data from American Association of Colleges of Nursing (AACN). (2006). *The essentials of doctoral education for advanced nursing practice.* Retrieved from https://www.aacnnursing.org/Portals/42/Publications/DNPEssentials.pdf

Currently, both organizations accredit only the practice doctorate; research doctorates such as the PhD and Doctor of Nursing Science (DNSc) are not eligible for CCNE or ACEN accreditation (ACEN, 2017; CCNE, 2016). DNP programs presented for CCNE accreditation are required to demonstrate incorporation of the DNP *Essentials* (AACN, 2006). In keeping with the two foci for DNP programs identified in the DNP *Essentials*, CCNE accredits DNP programs with (1) an advanced practice nursing direct care focus, (2) an aggregate/systems/organizational focus, or (3) both foci (CCNE, 2016, para. 2). Programs with ACEN accreditation meet standards and criteria for the clinical doctorate/DNP specialist certificate (ACEN, 2017).

Accreditation has traditionally signified quality in curriculum and university resources to achieve the goal of preparing students for the degrees they seek. Students evaluating DNP programs can investigate the accreditation status of the program, as well as the standards of the certifying body to help choose a quality educational experience. Current accreditation status of DNP programs can be found at the Doctor of Nursing Practice, Inc. website: www.doctorofnursingpracticednp.org /accredited-dnp-programs-by-state/.

Evaluation of the quality of DNP education also involves assessment of the achievement of the *Essentials* (AACN, 2006) of DNP education outcomes by DNP graduates. The Implementation of the DNP Task Force (AACN, 2015) emphasizes that DNP programs must demonstrate that the graduate has attained all of the DNP *Essentials* outcomes. Evaluation tools such as the *Self-Assessment Tool–Competency*

Assessment for Practicum Design found in Chapter 13, The DNP Project Toolbox, can be used for documentation of student progression toward attaining the DNP *Essentials* throughout the curriculum.

In 2016, the AACN commissioned the APRN (Advanced Practice Registered Nurses) Competency-Based Education for Doctoral-Prepared APRNs Work Group to develop a common taxonomy for role-specific competencies for APRN doctoral-level education. Read more about this report, which includes the definitions of competence and competency, in Chapter 2, Defining the Doctor of Nursing Practice: Current Trends. Competency-based evaluation for the DNP-prepared nurse practitioner (NP) that aligns with the AACN DNP *Essentials* has also been addressed by the National Organization of Nurse Practitioner Faculties (NONPF). NONPF has developed a DNP Nurse Practitioner Toolkit for programs that have NP tracks to address specific knowledge, skills, and attitudes students should possess at the culmination of an educational program, including scientific foundation, leadership, quality, practice inquiry, information technology literacy, policy, health delivery system, and ethical and independent practice competencies (NONPF, 2013). NONPF has joined other APRN organizations in endorsing doctoral-level education for advanced practice nursing roles (NONPF, 2018).

A white paper produced by NONPF in 2016 further emphasized that DNP-prepared nurse practitioners are *clinical scholars* and all educational programs should:

- Function in an academic culture and organizational structure that supports clinical scholarship
- Have progressive evidence of the introduction, reinforcement, and mastery of clinical scholarship across the curriculum
- Have criteria to effectively measure the quality of clinical scholarship being produced

Another process for tracking the growth and development of DNP education and outcomes was created by an organization dedicated to enhancing the caliber of the DNP graduate. Doctors of Nursing Practice, Inc. was founded in 2006 by a group of DNP students at the University of Tennessee Health Science Center College of Nursing in Memphis, Tennessee. An online discussion about the growth and needs of the DNP-prepared professional began in 2005 during an assignment for one of the first courses in the program. Issues of sharing and growing as a group were discussed. There were fewer than 10 universities offering the DNP degree at the time, and the classmates recognized that, as a cohort, there were few colleagues nationally to connect to and share insights and challenges associated with this degree. In the fall of 2006, during an Advanced Leadership class, classmates agreed to develop a business plan with the mission of enhancing the DNP degree. This plan led to the development and implementation of DNP, Inc.

The mission of DNP, Inc. is to improve healthcare outcomes by promoting and enhancing the doctoral-prepared nursing professional. The organization is dedicated to:

- Providing accurate and timely information
- Supporting, developing, and disseminating professional practice innovation
- Collaborating in a professional manner that demonstrates universal respect for others, honesty, and integrity in communications
- Responding with open discussions and dialogues that promote the evolution of advanced nursing practice and the growth of the DNP degree

In 2010, DNP, Inc. began collecting data regarding DNP outcomes and education via the first national DNP outcomes survey. Successive and evolving studies have taken place in 2011, 2012, 2013, 2015, and 2017, allowing for comparison and trending of collected data from DNP graduates.

Characteristics of survey respondents were compared over the years. The total number of respondents to the survey has increased from approximately 350 in 2011 to over 700 in 2017. Overall, respondents to the survey reflect the predominantly female gender of the nursing profession. In 2017, Auerbach, Buerhaus, Skinner, and Staiger found that the male full-time equivalent RN in the workforce has remained steady at 11% for the past 5 years, similar to the male graduates of DNP programs that represent between 10% and 14.6% of the nurses that responded to the DNP surveys (See **FIGURE 16-3**).

DNP Practice Outcomes Survey graduate respondents have also clearly indicated a vital educational program outcome: the incorporation of the eight DNP *Essentials* (AACN, 2006) into their practice. In the 2011, 2012, and 2013 surveys, a simple yes/no response indicated that between 95.6% and 98% of respondents believed that the eight *Essentials* were met in their programs. In following surveys that took place in 2015 and 2017, this question was expanded to ask respondents to respond to a Likert scale of strongly disagree, disagree, agree, and strongly agree. Clearly, the majority of respondents reflected perceptions that they felt that each of the eight *Essentials* were integrated into their practice by agreeing or strongly agreeing (See **FIGURE 16-4**).

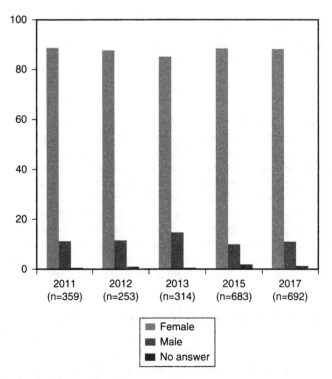

FIGURE 16-3 Gender of respondents (percentages).

Data from Doctors of Nursing Practice, Inc. (2017). *2017 DNP practice outcomes survey.*

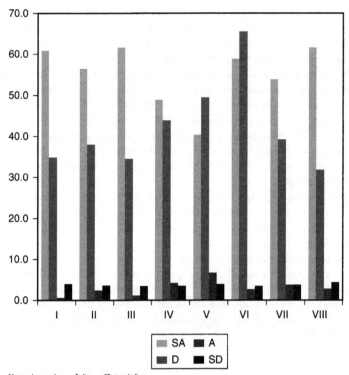

SA: strongly agree; A: agree; D: disagree; SD: strongly disagree

FIGURE 16-4 DNP Practice Outcomes Survey 2015–2017: Percentage of DNP graduate integration/application of the DNP *Essentials* (*n* = 697).

Average of 2015 and 2017 survey question: Indicate your level of agreement that each *Essential* is integrated into practice.

Data from Doctors of Nursing Practice, Inc. (2017). *2017 DNP practice outcomes survey.*

The results of the survey indicate that the DNP-prepared nurse can clearly articulate the core elements of DNP education as they relate to postgraduate practice. Incorporation of the skills and knowledge related to the *Essentials* are critical for the DNP graduate to develop and evaluate models of care delivery that can be sustained at multiple organizational levels in the healthcare system (AACN, 2015).

Attainment of the *Essentials* of DNP education by DNP students is one of the first steps in evaluating the effectiveness of the degree to prepare nurses for advanced nursing practice roles. Further, by evaluating the DNP degree through various mechanisms, adherence of DNP educational programs to prepare the practice doctorate is assured by accreditation status, program self-evaluation, and commitment to continuous quality improvement of the educational process.

Preparation for Advanced Nursing Practice Roles

Though the majority of DNP programs have tracks to prepare students for established roles such as nurse practitioner, clinical nurse specialist, nurse midwife, and nurse anesthetist, other advanced nursing practice roles are now needed for the practice doctorate to assist in the transformation of health care. Alternative

DNP educational tracks are evolving to prepare graduates with specialty knowledge beyond the traditional APRN roles. The AACN conducts a survey of DNP programs periodically to assess the various major areas of study offered across the country (see **TABLE 16-1**). The data from 2017–2018 AACN (2018) survey illustrate the numbers of programs, students, and graduates from the APRN majors of study in both post-baccalaureate and post-MSN DNP programs. In both BSN-DNP and post-master's programs, APRN tracks make up the largest percentage of students and graduates. Interestingly, the students in the post-MSN DNP programs chose tracks in administration/management and leadership more often than BSN-DNP students. In addition to preparation for APRN roles, the surveyed DNP schools offer additional programs of study in administration/management, health management and policy, informatics, community/public health, leadership, advanced practice, and other majors. With in-depth preparation for innovative practice roles, the DNP graduate has the skill set to respond to the challenges of leading change in healthcare organizations.

The DNP Project

The DNP project is also evolving to meet the changing needs of the nursing profession, practice, and society. The DNP project is the entry into practice scholarship by the nurse with the DNP degree. With the rapid growth of DNP programs since 2004, a wide variation in requirements for the DNP projects was noted across the nation. As a result, the AACN Implementation of the DNP Task Force (2015) was charged with clarifying the purpose of the DNP final project and the clinical learning expectations for DNP programs to require of their graduates. See Chapter 2 for a summary of the Implementation of the DNP Task Force recommendations regarding the DNP project. The task force outlined critical recommendations for standardizing the name of the final product as "The DNP Project" and clarified the expectations for the foci, content, and dissemination of DNP projects. The leadership of the AACN took action to standardize expectations for the DNP project with this report. This is a crucial outcome in the evolution of the DNP degree to ensure quality and rigor for the final product of DNP education.

Efforts have continued to evaluate the content and rigor of DNP projects. Terhaar and Sylvia (2015) used the UPC (Uncertainty, Pace, and Complexity) model adapted from industry to evaluate DNP projects. Roush and Tesoro (2018) assessed the value and rigor of 80 DNP projects using the DNP-ACAT tool based on the DNP *Essentials* and SQUIRE guidelines for quality improvement. Using this tool, 65 projects from 2013 to 2016 were analyzed with the conclusion that there is still wide variability in DNP projects, with many of the projects reviewed lacking critical evaluation of implementation and outcomes, including invalid data analysis. At the University of Colorado, Nelson, Cook, and Raterink (2013) have also incorporated the SQUIRE guidelines along with the DNP *Essentials* in rubrics for evaluating quality improvement projects. Outcomes using this methodology have resulted in 113 student projects published or presented at national conferences.

Continued evaluation of the final deliverable by the DNP student, the DNP project, will be important in the overall evaluation of DNP education. Attaining the core skill set of DNP competencies as outlined in the DNP *Essentials* is critical to contribute to the formation of transformational leaders in the areas of informatics,

Major Area of Study[1]	Number of Schools Offering Major	Post-Baccalaureate DNP Enrollment						Graduations	
		Full-Time		Part-Time		Total			
		Number	%	Number	%	Number	%	Number	%
Nurse-Midwifery	17	100	1.0	72	1.2	172	1.1	31	1.2
Nurse Anesthesia	43	2,077	20.3	182	3.1	2,259	14.0	386	14.6
Clinical Nurse Specialist (CNS)	32	71	0.7	71	1.2	142	0.9	23	0.9
Nurse Practitioner (NP)[2]	187	7,798	76.1	5,052	86.0	12,850	79.7	2,101	79.4
Administration/Management	30	38	0.4	265	4.5	303	1.9	16	0.6
Informatics	11	24	0.2	10	0.2	34	0.2	7	0.3
Community Health/Public Health	17	21	0.2	51	0.9	72	0.4	21	0.8
Leadership	59	79	0.8	109	1.9	188	1.2	25	0.9
Education	2	0		1	0.0	1	0.0	0	
Advanced Practice	12	12	0.1	10	0.2	22	0.1	4	0.2
Other Majors	13	26	0.3	10	0.2	36	0.2	11	0.4
Major Area Not Specified	15	5	0.0	39	0.7	44	0.3	21	0.8
TOTAL		10,251		5,872		16,123		2,646	

	Post-Master's DNP								
		Enrollment						Graduations	
		Full-Time		Part-Time		Total			
		Number	%	Number	%	Number	%	Number	%
Nurse-Midwifery	16	17	0.3	4	0.1	21	0.2	4	0.1
Nurse Anesthesia	37	88	1.7	70	0.9	158	1.2	56	1.6
Clinical Nurse Specialist (CNS)	30	16	0.3	60	0.8	76	0.6	27	0.8
Nurse Practitioner (NP)[2]	158	986	19.2	2,007	25.6	2,993	23.1	859	24.9
Administration/Management	53	301	5.9	980	12.5	1,281	9.9	289	8.4
Health Management & Policy	4	12	0.2	17	0.2	29	0.2	7	0.2
Informatics	13	6	0.1	29	0.4	35	0.3	1	0.0
Community Health/Public Health	19	17	0.3	99	1.26	116	0.9	37	1.07
Leadership	121	1,596	31.1	1,882	24.0	3,478	26.8	981	28.5
Education	3	92	1.8	256	3.3	348	2.7	83	2.4
Advanced Practice	33	183	3.6	588	7.5	771	5.9	208	6.0
Other Majors	20	27	0.5	266	3.4	293	2.3	74	2.1
Major Area Not Specified	49	1,787	34.8	1,584	20.2	3,371	26.0	818	23.8
TOTAL		5,128		7,842		12,970		3,444	

[1]Functional or professional role.

[2]Information in this report pertaining to nurse practitioners is the result of a collaborative effort between the *American Association of Colleges of Nursing* and the *National Organization of Nurse Practitioner Faculties*.

Note: Percents may not total to 100.0 due to rounding.

Reproduced from the American Association of Colleges of Nursing (AACN). (2018a). *2017–2018 Enrollment and Graduations in Baccalaureate and Graduate Programs in Nursing.* Washington, DC: Author.

policy, and advocacy to impact legislation and the development of new, innovative roles and entrepreneurship in advanced nursing practice (Prithham & White, 2016).

The DNP Actualized Model has been used as a framework to improve the efficiency and efficacy of DNP projects. See the exemplar by Dr. Marie Vanderkooi, Dr. Sandra Spoelstra, and Dr. Dianne Conrad (**EXEMPLAR 16-1**).

EXEMPLAR 16-1   Enhanced Actualized DNP Model for DNP Projects

Marie Vanderkooi, DNP, RN; Sandra L. Spoelstra, PhD, RN, FAAN; and Dianne Conrad, DNP, FNP-BC, FNAP

A DNP project is a "scholarly" summative evaluation, demonstrating application of the DNP *Essentials* (AACN, 2006). However, there is a paucity of literature on how to operationalize the DNP project. As a faculty team (PhD-DNP prepared), we felt challenged by the AACN Task Force recommendation to explore new models for DNP project enactment. We envisioned use of our unique knowledge and skills, the PhD-prepared faculty member with design, methods, analytical, and dissemination experience and the DNP-prepared faculty member with DNP *Essentials* skills, to guide students conducting DNP projects. Our PhD-DNP vision was deployment of the DNP *Essentials* via DNP projects that were data driven, addressed "wicked" clinical problems, were meaningful to the site, and sustainable.

Our DNP program had already embraced the Actualized DNP Model for 3 years. To operationalize our vision, we critically examined the Model elements and, using an iterative process; defined structural elements, actionable processes, and measurable outcomes; and met with the Model authors to seek guidance.

We designed a study to test our "Enhanced" Actualized DNP Model (**FIGURE 16-5**). We selected one site. Faculty met with students and mentors at the site and collaboratively identified "wicked" problems that the DNP project could address. We informed the site mentors about the DNP *Essentials*, student assessment of the organization, appraisal of evidence, and implementation of practice improvements, as well as the mentor role and responsibilities.

Students enacted several projects at the site using the "Enhanced" Actualized DNP Model. The mentors provided data to inform the assessment. A folder was set up on an internal electronic drive for data storage for student projects. Each student had several measures and mentors supported data collection or connected students with others in the health system to obtain data. Each of these actions resulted in data-informed organizational assessments, which led to focused, tailored project plans.

Student outcomes were remarkable, with more on-time graduates and a longer period to conduct the DNP project during the curriculum. Students expressed satisfaction with the structure and process elements of the "Enhanced" Actualized DNP Model and PhD-DNP team support, and appreciated the PhD's expertise in methodology, particularly measurement, and the DNP's expertise in DNP *Essential* skills. Mentors and leadership at the site expressed a high level of satisfaction with the PhD-DNP team support and impact projects had on the "wicked" problems. Faculty expressed high satisfaction with format of written papers, which reduced the number of draft papers reviewed. Notably, the number of students conducting projects and employed after graduation at the site tripled the year following the study. Study results were reported at two national conferences and are accepted for publication.

Moving forward, our DNP program embraced lessons learned and revised the DNP Immersion Toolkit, forms, and rubrics. A collegial relationship formed with the site and the number of DNP projects at the sites is growing exponentially. In summary, we found operationalizing the Actualized DNP Model supported achievement of our vision and allowed us to attain improved student, faculty, and site outcomes.

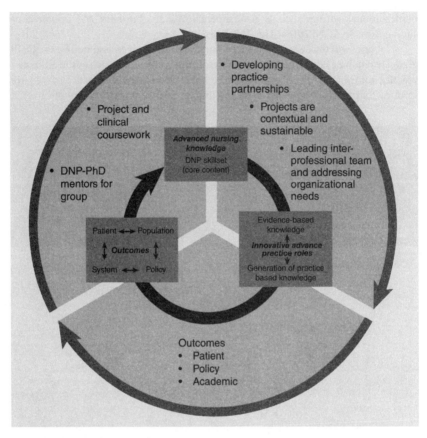

FIGURE 16-5 Enhanced Actualized DNP Model for DNP projects.

Reproduced from Rosanne Burson, D. N. P., & Dianne Conrad, D. N. P. (2016). Why Hire a Doctor of Nursing Practice-Prepared Nurse? The Value Added Impact of the Practice Doctorate. *Journal of Doctoral Nursing Practice*, 9(1), 152.

▶ Healthcare Delivery by the DNP-Prepared Nurse

Innovative Advanced Practice Roles

Evaluation of the effectiveness of the DNP-prepared nurse will include assessment of healthcare delivery by the DNP graduate, the second step in the Actualized DNP Model. Currently, the roles of the nurse in advanced practice are varied, ranging from traditional APRN clinical roles to administrative roles. The DNP graduate is employed in a variety of settings including academic, hospital, and ambulatory clinical positions, as well as

Evaluation of the DNP-prepared nurse will include assessment of healthcare delivery by the DNP graduate, the second step in the Actualized DNP Model.

nontraditional settings such as governmental/military, business, and private consulting firms (AACN, 2018a) (see **TABLE 16-2**).

Not only will the current advanced nursing practice roles assumed by the DNP graduate require evaluation, but the emerging, innovative roles such as the advanced practice informatics nurse and advanced practice policy nurse will also require scrutiny for quality of care delivered and impact on outcomes. Delivery of care, via

TABLE 16-2 Employment Commitments of Doctor of Nursing Practice Graduates

	Graduates	
Employment Commitment	Number	%
Doctoral (Research-Focused)		
Faculty position: School/College of Nursing	348	43.7
Faculty position: Other type of school/college	22	2.8
Post-doctoral fellowship	58	7.3
Hospital nursing service research and/or clinical position	53	6.7
Hospital nursing service administrative or executive position	57	7.2
Ambulatory (non-hospital) research position and/or clinical position	15	1.9
Ambulatory (non-hospital) administrative or executive position	7	0.9
Private consultation or consulting firm	6	0.8
Federal or state governmental agency	6	0.8
Military	4	0.5
Business or industry	2	0.3
No employment commitment	32	4.0
Other	13	1.6
Do not know	173	21.7
TOTAL	796	

Employment Commitment	Graduates	
	Number	%
Doctor of Nursing Practice		
Faculty position: School/College of Nursing	463	7.6
Faculty position: Other type of school/college	48	0.8
Post-doctoral fellowship	6	0.1
Hospital clinical position	1,150	18.9
Hospital administrative or executive position	306	5.0
Ambulatory (non-hospital) clinical position	693	11.4
Ambulatory (non-hospital) administrative or executive position	70	1.1
Private consultation or consulting firm	152	2.5
Federal or state governmental agency	70	1.1
Military	153	2.5
Business or industry	28	0.5
No employment commitment	281	4.6
Other	207	3.4
Do not know	2,463	40.4
TOTAL	6,090	

Note: Percents may not total to 100.0 due to rounding.
Reprinted with permission from the American Association of Colleges of Nursing (AACN). (2018b). *Employment Commitment of Doctoral (Research-Focused) and Doctor of Nursing Practice Graduates.* Washington, DC: Author.

whatever role is assumed by the DNP graduate in new and traditional types of organizations, needs to be assessed for use and generation of evidence-based science as well as effectiveness in improving outcomes.

Dr. Amy Manderscheid, a DNP-prepared faculty member, applied the DNP Actualized Model to an innovative faculty practice role to illustrate the effectiveness each step in the model to guide faculty practice and lead to improved outcomes with an academic practice partner (see **EXEMPLAR 16-2**).

EXEMPLAR 16-2 The Actualized DNP Model: Building a Roadmap for a Doctoral of Nursing Practice Faculty Scholarship

Amy Manderscheid, DNP, RN, CMSRN

Developing a program of scholarship in academia can be challenging for DNP-prepared faculty, considering the emphasis is on research in most colleges of nursing. The increase in DNP-prepared nurses in academic faculty positions and the dynamic roles of practice-based faculty emphasize the need to clarify clinical practice-based criteria for promotion and tenure.

Since the Actualized DNP Model is applicable to the unique role of the practice doctorate, the model concepts provide a solid foundation to guide faculty in their scholarship journey. Rooted in advanced nursing knowledge and expertise, faculty scholarship is uniquely designed through new roles within practice-academic partnerships, impacting both organizational and scholarly outcomes.

The Actualized DNP Model for Faculty Scholarship (**FIGURE 16-6**) provides a framework for practice-based faculty to plan, implement, and document scholarly activities and outcomes contributing to tenure and promotion. The model includes: (1) expanding advanced nursing knowledge through activities related to teaching,

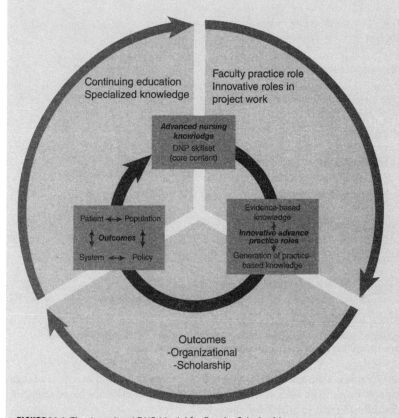

FIGURE 16-6 The Actualized DNP Model for Faculty Scholarship.

Reproduced from Rosanne Burson, D. N. P., & Dianne Conrad, D. N. P. (2016). Why Hire a Doctor of Nursing Practice-Prepared Nurse? The Value Added Impact of the Practice Doctorate. *Journal of Doctoral Nursing Practice, 9*(1), 152.

scholarship, and nursing expertise; (2) developing existing and new roles in practice-academic partnerships; and (3) quantifying the impact of practice-related outcomes as a result of scholarship activities.

Doctoral-prepared nurses embrace lifelong learning and continue to develop, grow, and possibly expand one's expertise. Specialized *knowledge through continuing education* and enhanced skills may influence scholarly activities as a faculty member. Through faculty practice, the DNP-prepared nurse may engage in *innovative roles* fostered by practice-academic partnerships in embedded faculty or consulting roles. These roles may consist of partnering with the interprofessional team to improve quality, care processes, and outcomes to align with national benchmarks. Through these traditional and innovative roles, DNP project work continues in the organization, with application of evidence to produce outcomes. *Outcomes* transcend patient- and system-level impact in the organization and include scholarly outputs such as articles and publications to enhance the wide repository of knowledge in health care. However, organizational impact is not to be minimized and may include decreased length of stay, decreased healthcare complications, and improved quality scores. Proactive quality improvement planning may mitigate risk of clinical complications or unfavorable quality outcomes. The important feature of the model is that faculty scholarship has structural and process components that lead to faculty output and outcomes. Each area of the model may be populated with exemplars of faculty scholarship components that demonstrate the competencies attained in the tenure journey. Activities outlined in each construct in the model are critical to a DNP-prepared faculty member demonstrating the competencies required for the scholarship of practice in the tenure journey.

Engaging in a DNP faculty scholarship plan contributes to outcomes and dissemination of findings across the nursing profession. Dissemination of patient, clinical, team, and organizational outcomes may include joint presentations among faculty and organizational representatives at academia and clinically based forums. Application of the Actualized DNP Model undoubtedly elevates value offered to healthcare organizations and academic environments as outcomes impact the Institute for Healthcare Improvement Triple Aim (quality, cost, and experience) across patients, populations, and systems.

To explore the evolving roles of DNP-prepared nurses, Clark and Allison-Jones (2011) surveyed recent graduates regarding their practice environments and organizational factors that impact their roles. The graduates confirmed that their practices had changed with incorporating DNP competencies of evidence-based practice utilization, clinical leadership, advanced practice clinician, and change agency. Even if the DNP graduates were in faculty roles as educators, they were maintaining a clinical role as well. However, the acceptance of the DNP-prepared nurse in both academic and research environments was identified as a concern as the unique contributions of the DNP-prepared nurse continue to evolve.

Though the recommendations from the Implementation of the DNP Task Force (AACN, 2015) state that DNP programs are not to focus on preparing the nurse educator role, the nurse with a practice doctorate has a critical presence in nursing education. See Table 16-2 for numbers of DNP graduates accepting faculty positions in colleges of nursing (AACN, 2018b). In 2017, the AACN reported that 97 out of 765, or 13%, of chief nursing administrators in nursing education programs held the DNP degree (AACN, 2017). Nursing is a *practice profession* that requires educators with nursing practice expertise to educate and mentor future nurses at all educational levels. All doctoral-prepared nurses, including research doctorates, should have additional training in the pedagogy of teaching as the discipline of education encompasses an entirely separate body of knowledge and competence (AACN, 2015).

Innovative Healthcare Delivery Through Evidence-Based Practice

Changes in practice related to healthcare delivery were assessed in DNP, Inc.'s 2017 Practice Outcomes Survey of over 700 DNP graduates. Over 60% of DNP graduates responded that they are better able to incorporate the following activities in their roles as a practice doctorate more often since obtaining their degree:

- Translate evidence into new practice initiatives.
- Incorporate evidence into their practice.
- Translate practice guidelines.
- Develop, implement and/or evaluate practice initiatives.

These practice initiatives by DNP graduate respondents occurred for most while participating in and/or leading interdisciplinary teams. Other important changes in practice in the 2017 survey included using technology to promote change and increased cultural awareness as a result of DNP education. These are important expectations of the practice doctorate in transforming health care. Recognition of the value of DNP graduates was reflected in the 2017 DNP Practice Outcomes Survey, with over 48% of respondents indicating that they had experienced an increase in salary with the same or different employer. These important changes in areas of practice will need to be addressed in future surveys to assess both post-BSN and post-master's–prepared DNP graduate effectiveness as these practitioners develop healthcare delivery innovations.

However, the reported ability to apply evidence to practice by the respondents in the 2017 DNP Practice Outcomes Survey cannot be minimized. The number of respondents reporting increased skills in evidence-based practice is important and reflective of the continuing potential for improving healthcare outcomes as a result of this skill learned as a DNP student. These changes in practice outcomes by the DNP graduate are also reflective of achievement of the goals of the Institute of Medicine's (2003) call for improved healthcare professional educational competencies to impact and transform care, signaling the nursing profession's ability to prepare qualified practitioners responsive to healthcare challenges now and in the future.

▶ The Impact of the DNP-Prepared Nurse on Patients, Systems, Populations, and Policy

The ultimate goal of the practice doctorate is to improve *outcomes* by introducing evidence and innovation into practice across diverse settings and communities, both nationally and internationally (Terhaar & Sylvia, 2016). The type of outcomes to be evaluated in the third step of the DNP Actualized Model include how DNP-prepared nurses affect patients and their care, how DNP-prepared nurses affect health policy, how DNP-prepared nurses improve care at the systems level to improve outcomes, and how DNP-prepared nurses improve the quality of care delivered to populations to improve health outcomes.

The ultimate goal of the practice doctorate is to improve outcomes, the third step of the Actualized DNP Model.

Examples of DNP graduates with their roles, DNP project titles, and impact on practice outcomes are illustrated in **TABLE 16-3**.

Dissemination of Outcomes

Dissemination of DNP project results is critical to impacting healthcare outcomes. Dissemination of the project outcomes will need to become more systematic to close the gap in evidence-based practice implementation at the point of care. See Chapter 15, Disseminating the Results, for more information on communicating the results of the DNP project.

As more DNP graduates enter the workforce equipped with this skill set and knowledge of practice inquiry, the impact on improving outcomes with evidence-based practice has continued to grow. From 2001 to 2012, DNP authors published over 300 papers in 59 journals (Broome, Riner, & Allum, 2013). The publications included practice- and patient-focused database papers, evaluation of clinical interventions and evidence-based practice guidelines, clinical teaching, and organizational/systems improvement studies. Redman, Pressler, Furspan, and Potempa (2014), in an analysis of publication activity, found over 690 publications from 417 different authors with a DNP credential. The DNP-prepared nurse was a solo or first author on 79.5% of the publications. More than half of the articles dealt with clinical practice and included the areas of research, evidence-based guidelines, program evaluation, reviews, case studies, and opinions.

The Implementation of the DNP Task Force (AACN, 2015) has also recommended that a digital repository for DNP projects be formed to advance nursing practice by archiving and sharing project outcomes. The goal of the repository is to showcase practice outcomes of the DNP-prepared nursing professional in an interactive format. Since 2007, DNP, Inc. has continued to collect and catalog DNP project data via their website (www.doctorsofnursingpractice.org/resources/dnp-scholarly-projects/). Another repository for DNP projects along with PhD dissertations, MSN theses, and exceptional undergraduate student submissions is maintained by the Virginia Henderson Global Nursing e-Repository, a resource of the Honor Society of Nursing, Sigma Theta Tau International. Access this repository at www.nursinglibrary.org/vhl/handle/10755/223051.

However, evaluating the impact of the DNP-prepared nurse on practice should not be determined solely by the amount of publications, as the literature may not reflect the added value of DNP project outcomes and the contributions by DNP graduates at the organizational, public, and societal level.

Through the 2017 DNP Practice Outcomes Survey, data were obtained related to the dissemination practices of DNP graduates (see **TABLE 16-4**). Surprisingly, the highest rate of dissemination modalities is podium and poster presentations followed by publications, then book contributions. These dissemination techniques are important avenues that demonstrate the breadth and depth of the practice doctorate impact on health care.

TABLE 16-3 DNP Exemplars

Name/ Preparation	Role	DNP Project	DNP Practice Impact
Sue Sirianni, Nurse Practitioner	▪ Hospital lead for sepsis quality improvement project and other QI efforts ▪ Resident and nursing education	An Interprofessional Approach to Sepsis Care	▪ Improved application of evidence. ▪ Decreased mortality rate. ▪ Decreased costs. ▪ Increased collaboration. ▪ Saved $1 million – Choose Wisely Campaign.
Denise O'Brien, Clinical Nurse Specialist	▪ Perianesthesia nursing quality care	Intraoperative Risk Factors Associated with Pressure Ulcer Development in Critically Ill Patients	▪ Focused on perioperative outcomes; national and international dissemination. ▪ Collaborated with a PhD-prepared faculty member at the University of Michigan School of Nursing, exploring the development of a clinically useful risk stratification tool to identify patients at risk for development of pressure ulcer intraoperatively and to determine best practices for positioning, padding, and protecting patients from skin injury in the perioperative and perianesthesia setting. ▪ Developed and tested nurse-sensitive outcomes associated with care in the perianesthesia setting.
Lisa Fetters, Clinical Nurse Specialist	▪ Director of Quality and Patient Safety ▪ Emergency Physicians Medical Group: 35 emergency department and 8 urgent care sites	Fall Risk Factors in Emergency Department (ED) Patients	▪ Increased patient satisfaction. ▪ Increased collaboration. ▪ Improved systems that increase safety. ▪ Decreased cost within the ED setting.
Kristel Ray, Nurse Practitioner	▪ Associate Professor	High Fidelity Simulation as a Strategy for Inter-professional Education: A Teaching Innovation Within the Community College	▪ Development of interprofessional education using simulation in combination with other technology.
Judy Paull, Nurse Executive	▪ Chief Nurse Executive	An Examination of Nurse Caring and Hospital Acquired Pressure Ulcers	▪ Used program design best practice; capitalized on opportunities to meet population health needs. ▪ Drove organizational business objectives to achieve regulatory requirements. ▪ Centralized telemetry, which improved efficiency and increased patient safety.

Name/ Preparation	Role	DNP Project	DNP Practice Impact
Ann Sheehan, Nurse Practitioner	■ Assistant Dean for Practice ■ State NP organization, President elect	Growing Grassroots Advocacy: Implementation of a Legislative Tracking Tool	■ Multidimensional role: university faculty-, student-, and nurse-managed clinic responsibilities. ■ Strategic planning has resulted in a 60% increase in patient visits and revenue.
Stephanie Brady, Mental Health Clinical Nurse Specialist	■ Nurse Executive, Vice President of Care Transitions	The Impact of Mindfulness Meditation on a Culture of Safety on an Inpatient Psychiatric Unit	■ Spearheaded 5 CMS demonstration projects. ■ Was awarded $6 million dollars to evaluate 5 care coordination models (community care transitions, high-intensity care model, patient care liaison role, telephonic case management program with 24/7 nurse rescue line, telephonic high-intensity care management to reduce readmissions). ■ Restructured ambulatory rehabilitation services, saving $500,000. ■ Wrote business plan for senior services—resulting in $250,000 additional revenue.
Susan Burke-Bebee, Informatics	■ Senior Health Informatician ■ Office of the Assistant Secretary for Planning and Evaluation at the U.S. Department of Health and Human Services (HHS).	Building Health Information Technology Capacity: They May Come but Will They Use It?	■ Health informatics policy specialist. ■ Part of the original team organizing and facilitating HHS activities promoting the National Health Information Infrastructure (NHII) leading to the creation of Office of the National Coordinator for Health Information Technology (ONC).
Kim Kuebler, Nurse Practitioner	■ Associate Professor ■ Owner, Advanced Disease Concepts LLC ■ Director, Multiple Chronic Conditions Resource Center	Comparing Perceived Knowledge of Chronic Disease Management to Quantitative Knowledge Measurement in a Sample of Baccalaureate Nursing Students: Implications for Palliative Care Nursing Education	■ Principal investigator: Systematic review to evaluate evidence to support chronic disease, symptom, and self-management content in graduate nursing curriculum. ■ Principal investigator: National graduate nursing survey queried 800 U.S. nursing programs on self-knowledge and actual knowledge of chronic disease, symptoms, and self-management. ■ Developed the Multiple Chronic Conditions Resource Center—virtual center with the most current evidence to support the care management of patients with symptomatic chronic conditions and policy specific topics.

Reproduced from Burson, R., Moran, K., & Conrad, D. (2016). Why hire a DNP? The value-added impact of the practice doctorate. *Journal of Doctoral Nursing Practice, 9*(1).

TABLE 16-4   2017 DNP Practice Outcomes Survey: Dissemination Activities of DNP Graduates ($n = 750$)

Answer Options	Response Percentage	Response Count
Published a research article.	34.4 %	258
Published an evidence-based guidelines article.	17.7 %	133
Published a quality improvement article.	21.1 %	158
Published a case study.	11.1 %	83
Presented a poster at a professional a meeting.	72.0 %	540
Provided a podium presentation at a professional meeting.	61.3 %	460
Contributed to a book or professional journal.	31.7 %	238
Peer reviewed or edited a book or journal article.	38.0 %	285
Developed and published a continuing education module for nursing.	24.8 %	186
Developed and published a continuing education module for a discipline other than nursing.	7.9 %	59
Published an article for a nonprofessional journal (not peer reviewed).	14.8 %	111
	Total	750

Data from Doctors of Nursing Practice, Inc. (2017). *2017 DNP practice outcomes survey.*

▶ The Impact of the DNP Graduate in Practice

Graduates of DNP programs are impacting the nursing profession and the people they serve. Montgomery and Porter-O'Grady (2010) find that "in health care delivery systems, many DNP nurse leaders are disrupting traditional practices by evidencing their value; offering a broader, more integrated perspective on practice or system issues; and using innovation to positively impact patient and system outcomes" (p. 45).

The definitive impact of evaluating the effectiveness of the practice doctorate must come from the practice arena. The Rand Corporation Report (Auerbach et al.,

2014) recommended that the next steps in promoting and evaluating the DNP-prepared nurse are to conduct outcome studies to better understand the impact of DNP graduates on patient care, and secondly to provide outreach data to help employers and healthcare organizations understand the comprehensive competencies and capabilities of DNP-educated nurses. The generation of practice-based knowledge by DNP-prepared nurses in innovative roles, resulting in improved outcomes, completes and continues the cycle of value and impact of the practice doctorate in the Actualized DNP Model.

The generation of practice-based knowledge by DNP-prepared nurses in innovative roles, resulting in improved outcomes, completes and continues the cycle of value and impact of the practice doctorate in the Actualized DNP Model.

The DNP graduate must be able to continually articulate, define, and promote their added value to practice leaders to demonstrate in practice the skill set attained with the DNP degree. To maximize their impact on health care, DNP graduates must reach out and partner with healthcare leaders, scientists, clinicians, patients, families, and community members. The practice doctorate also must demonstrate the ability to balance the demands of population data with individualized, patient-centered care, connecting research into care systems with an informed local context. Most importantly, the DNP graduate must courageously demonstrate the DNP *Essentials* to move organizations forward. The impact of the DNP-prepared nurse will need continuous and intentional evaluation by the profession. How the DNP graduate will affect patients, populations, systems, and policy will need systematic evaluation focusing on the impact and outcomes realized in practice. The ultimate impact will be the change in how health care is delivered and how the health of society is improved by innovative DNP-prepared nurses' practice.

Dr. Lisa Chism was one of the first DNP graduates in the United States. She shares her story in **EXEMPLAR 16-3** of how the DNP *Essentials* are reflected in her daily nursing practice.

EXEMPLAR 16-3 A Personal Journey

Lisa Chism, DNP, GNP, BC, NCMP, FAANP

I began researching DNP degree programs in 2005. At the time, there were less than 10 DNP programs in the country. I was the first applicant at Oakland University in Rochester, Michigan, and I began my DNP program in the fall of 2006. It was a pilot program and the first in Michigan. My cohort and I were supported through a wonderful grant provided by the state of Michigan and experienced novel approaches in distance learning. We met for workshops across the state, stayed on campus for a week of concentrated coursework, and participated in web-based "live" meetings and traditional online coursework. It was a wonderful experience. I met my first mentor in

(continues)

my DNP program, Dr. Morris Magnan, and with his guidance and support I graduated from my program 18 months later.

It was about 2 months after graduation when I realized that I wasn't sure how to develop my role as a DNP graduate. I figured that if I had questions about my new role, so did others. This notion sparked the idea for a resource I thought was needed for DNP students and graduates. This was my first opportunity to spread my leadership wings and incorporate *Essential* II: Organizational and Systems Leadership for Quality Improvement and Systems Thinking of the *Essentials of Doctoral Education for Advanced Nursing Practice* (AACN, 2006) into my role as a DNP graduate.

Understanding the importance of interprofessional collaboration (*Essential* VI: Interprofessional Collaboration for Improving Patient and Population Health Outcomes) (AACN, 2006), I consulted with another of my mentors, Dr. Elizabeth Johnston Taylor, regarding the process of writing and publishing a book. Dr. Taylor had published a book on spiritual care and helped me formulate a query letter to send to publishers. This query letter led to a meeting with Jones & Bartlett Learning, and later, a contract. I incorporated *Essential* VI and collaborated with colleagues to contribute chapters and interviews for the project. Through collaboration and leadership, I completed the project and the first edition of *The Doctor of Nursing Practice: A Guidebook for Role Development and Professional Issues* was published in May 2009. The fourth edition of this text was recently published (Chism, 2019). As the first DNP-related text written by DNP graduates for DNP graduates, this project truly exemplified leadership and collaboration.

I continued to develop my scholarship through regular presentations and guest lectures. I also partnered with my mentor, Dr. Morris Magnan, and published my DNP research project, which included the development and testing of a middle-range nursing theory. For myself and other DNP graduates, completing, publishing, and presenting the DNP project is an example of *Essential* III: Clinical Scholarship and Analytical Methods for Evidence-Based Practice (AACN, 2006).

As a DNP graduate practicing as a nurse practitioner in a comprehensive breast center, I credit my DNP degree for expanding my perspective regarding my clinical knowledge. I had an interest in menopause and became certified as a menopause practitioner through the North American Menopause Society (NAMS). Developing scientific knowledge related to my practice is an example of *Essential* I: Scientific Underpinnings for Practice (AACN, 2006). This experience led me to another mentor, Dr. Diane Pace, who is Dean of Faculty Practice at the University of Tennessee Health Science Center and immediate past president of NAMS. Dr. Pace mentored me and invited me to join the Patient Education and Scientific Programming Committees through NAMS. This experience was invaluable and led me to be able to develop *Essential* V: Healthcare Policy for Advocacy in Health Care (AACN, 2006). My work on these committees allowed me to impact policy regarding patient education materials program development and membership in the organization. In October 2015, I was elected to the NAMS Board of Trustees.

My work in menopause also led me to develop a practice dedicated to meeting the needs of women experiencing menopausal symptoms who have cancer or who are at risk for cancer. Through caring for these patients, I recognized the need to care for their sexual health concerns as well. I completed a certificate as a sexual health counselor and educator and in May 2017, I became a certified sexuality counselor through the American Association of Sexuality Counselors, Educators, and Therapists (AASECT). The menopause clinic has transitioned to a menopause and sexual health clinic caring for patients with menopause- or sexual health–related concerns. I credit my DNP degree for helping me recognize the need for a clinic dedicated to meeting the needs of these patients. This is an example of *Essential* VII: Clinical Prevention and Population Health for Improving the Nation's Health (AACN, 2006).

Finally, I credit the skills I developed in leadership *Essential* II: Organizational and Systems Leadership for Quality Improvement and Systems Thinking (AACN, 2006) through the DNP degree to enable me to develop my current position. I practice within a comprehensive breast center in a clinic called the Women's Wellness Clinic (WWC) staffed by three nurse practitioners. We are the only independent nurse-managed clinic within the organization. I sensed a need for leadership within the clinic and developed a proposal for a clinical director position. I approached my nursing leadership with the proposal and received invaluable support. I was fortunate enough to write my own job description and have been in this role for approximately 2 years. I continue to grow within this role and develop additional skills related to the finances and productivity of the WWC clinic.

Ten years after graduating from a DNP program, I realize that my role as a DNP graduate continues to develop. With each year, I gain new perspectives about patient care and solutions to complex, challenging healthcare problems. I offer this advice to graduating DNP students: Take the time to allow yourself to grow and develop. You will need time to actualize your roles as DNP graduates. Be ready to change your perspective and widen your views. You will view health care through a different lens and be challenged in new ways to find new solutions. It is a journey, one most definitively worth taking.

▶ Summary

The practice doctorate in nursing is evolving to meet the needs of the society it serves. Evaluation of this new preparation for nurses at the practice doctorate level requires scrutiny and systematic evaluation to assess its value. The Actualized DNP Model is a framework to assess the impact of the DNP education, projects, and innovative practice roles to produce outcomes. Assessment of the DNP degree is needed to determine the quality of education delivered and to produce practitioners who are prepared to deliver high-quality, innovative, evidence-based care. Assessment of the impact of outcomes achieved with patients, populations, systems, and policy is also needed to evaluate the DNP-prepared nurse at multiple levels. This will be an ongoing process that will improve the quality of education and care delivered, as well as impact outcomes for society. It is an exciting time for nursing to take an active part in transforming health care. Donabedian (1988) acknowledges the journey with the statement, "I hope it is clear that there is a way, a path worn rather smooth by many who have gone before us. I trust it is equally clear that we have, as yet, much more to learn" (p. 1748).

Key Messages

- The DNP project reflects the culmination of the attainment of the DNP *Essentials*.
- Evaluation of the impact of the DNP-prepared nurse can be assessed using The Actualized DNP Model.

- DNP education provides the structure for developing an advanced nursing practice role as well as developing scholarly practice through the completion of the DNP project.
- Innovative healthcare delivery in advanced nursing practice roles is the process through which the DNP-prepared nurse will impact evidence-based practice.
- The impact of DNP practice will be realized in improved policy outcomes, improved patient outcomes, improved population outcomes, and improved system outcomes.

Action Plan—Next Steps

1. Successfully complete your DNP project.
2. Disseminate the results of the project.
3. Use the competencies gained in attaining the *Essentials* of DNP education in an advanced nursing practice role to impact healthcare outcomes.
4. Continually articulate, define, and promote the value-added impact of the DNP-prepared nurse to practice leaders, colleagues, and society.
5. Transform health care!

References

Accreditation Commission for Education in Nursing (ACEN). (2017). *ACEN 2017 standards and criteria clinical doctorate/DNP specialist*. Retrieved from http://www.acenursing.net/manuals/sc2017_C.pdf

American Association of Colleges of Nursing (AACN). (2006). *The essentials of doctoral education for advanced nursing practice*. Retrieved from https://www.aacnnursing.org/Portals/42/Publications/DNPEssentials.pdf

American Association of Colleges of Nursing (AACN). (2015). *The doctor of nursing practice: Current issues and clarifying recommendations*. Retrieved from https://www.aacnnursing.org/Portals/42/DNP/DNP-Implementation.pdf

American Association of Colleges of Nursing (AACN). (2017). *Number of chief nursing administrators by degree, Fall 2017*. Washington, DC: Author.

American Association of Colleges of Nursing (AACN). (2018a). *2017–2018 enrollment and graduations in baccalaureate and graduate programs in nursing*. Washington, DC: Author.

American Association of Colleges of Nursing (AACN). (2018b). *Employment commitment of doctoral (research-focused) and doctor of nursing practice graduates*. Washington, DC: Author.

Auerbach, D., Buerhaus, P., Skinner, L., & Staiger, D. (2017). *2017 data brief update: Current trends of men in nursing*. Bozeman, MT: Montana State University. Retrieved from http://healthworkforcestudies.com/publications-data/data_brief_update_current_trends_of_men_in_nursing.html

Auerbach, D., Martsolf, G., Pearson, M., Taylor, E., Zaydman, M., Muchow, A., . . . Dower, C. (2014). The *DNP by 2015: A study of the institutional, political, and professional issues that facilitate or impede establishing a post-baccalaureate doctor of nursing practice program*. Boston, MA: RAND Corporation. Retrieved from https://www.rand.org/pubs/research_reports/RR730.html

Broome, M. E., Riner, M. E., & Allam, E. S. (2013). Scholarly publication practices of doctor of nursing practice-prepared nurses. *Journal of Nursing Education, 52*(8), 429–434.

Brown, M. A. (2011, January). *Advancing practice through the DNP capstone*. Paper presented at American Association of Colleges of Nursing Doctoral Conference, San Diego, CA.

Burson, R., Moran, K., & Conrad, D. (2016). Why hire a DNP? The value added impact of the practice doctorate. *Journal of Doctoral Nursing Practice, 9*(1).

Chism, L. A. (2019). *The doctor of nursing practice: A guidebook for role development and professional issues (4th ed.)*. Burlington, MA: Jones & Bartlett Learning.

Clark, R. C., & Allison-Jones, L. (2011). The doctor of nursing practice graduate in practice. *Clinical Scholars Review, 4*(2), 71–77.

Commission on Collegiate Nursing Education (CCNE). (2016). *Frequently asked questions on DNP programs and DNP accreditation.* Retrieved from http://www.aacnnursing.org/CCNE -Accreditation/FAQs/DNP

Doctors of Nursing Practice, Inc. (2017). *2017 DNP practice outcomes survey.*

Donabedian, A. (1988). The quality of care: How can it be assessed? *Journal of the American Medical Association, 260,* 1743–1748.

Fontaine, D. K., & Langston, N. F. (2011). The master's is not broken: Commentary on "The doctor of nursing practice: A national workforce perspective." *Nursing Outlook, 59,* 121–122. doi: 10.1016/j.outlook.2011.03.003

Institute of Medicine (IOM). (2003). *Health professions education: A bridge to quality.* Retrieved from http://www.nap.edu/openbook.php?record_id=10681&page=45

Montgomery, K. L., & Porter-O'Grady, T. (2010). Innovation and learning: Creating the DNP nurse leader. *Nurse Leader, 8,* 44–47. doi: 10.1016?j.mn/2010.05.001

National Organization of Nurse Practitioner Faculties (NONPF). (2013). *DNP NP toolkit: Process and approach to DNP competency based evaluation.* Retrieved from https://www.nonpf.org /general/custom.asp?page=27

National Organization of Nurse Practitioner Faculties (NONPF). (2015). *Sample curriculum templates for practice doctorate education.* Retrieved from https://www.nonpf.org/resource /resmgr/DNP/NONPFDNPStatementSept2015.pdf

National Organization of Nurse Practitioner Faculties (NONPF). (2016). White paper: *The doctor of nursing practice nurse practitioner clinical scholar.* Retrieved from https://www.nonpf.org /resource/resmgr/docs/ClinicalScholarFINAL2016.pdf

National Organization of Nurse Practitioner Faculties (NONPF). (2018). *The doctor of nursing practice degree: Entry to nurse practitioner practice by 2025.* Retrieved from https://www.nonpf .org/resource/resmgr/dnp/v3_05.2018_NONPF_DNP_Stateme.pdf

Nelson, J. M., Cook, P. F., & Raterink, G. (2013). Nursing practice capstone process: Programmatic revisions to improve the quality of student projects. *Journal of Professional Nursing, 29*(6), 370–380, doi: 10.1016/j.profnurs.2012.05.018

Pritham, U. A., & White, P. (2016). Assessing DNP impact: Using program evaluations to capture healthcare system change. *The Nurse Practitioner, 41*(4), 44–53.

Redman, R. W., Pressler, S. J., Furspan, P., & Potempa, K. (2014). Nurses in the United States with a practice doctorate: Implications for leading in the current context of health care. *Nursing Outlook, 63*(2), 124–129.

Roush, K., & Tesoro, M. (2018, March). An examination of the rigor and value of final scholarly projects completed by DNP nursing students. *Journal of Professional Nursing.* doi: 10.1016/j .profnurs.2018.03.003

Terhaar, M. F., & Sylvia, M. (2015). Scholarly work products of the doctor of nursing practice: One approach to evaluating scholarship, rigour, impact and quality. *Journal of Clinical Nursing, 25,* 163–174, doi: 10.1111/jocn.13113

Index

Note: Page numbers followed by *b*, *f*, or *t* indicate material in boxes, figures, and tables, respectively.

E

F